Health and Social Care Policy

Health and Social Care Policy

Editors
Sofia Koukouli
Areti Stavropoulou

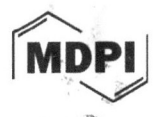

Basel • Beijing • Wuhan • Barcelona • Belgrade • Novi Sad • Cluj • Manchester

Editors

Sofia Koukouli
Department of Social Work
Hellenic Mediterranean University
Heraklion
Greece

Areti Stavropoulou
Department of Nursing
University of West Attica
Egaleo
Greece

Editorial Office
MDPI
St. Alban-Anlage 66
4052 Basel, Switzerland

This is a reprint of articles from the Special Issue published online in the open access journal *Healthcare* (ISSN 2227-9032) (available at: www.mdpi.com/journal/healthcare/special_issues/health_care_policy).

For citation purposes, cite each article independently as indicated on the article page online and as indicated below:

Lastname, A.A.; Lastname, B.B. Article Title. *Journal Name* **Year**, *Volume Number*, Page Range.

ISBN 978-3-7258-0970-7 (Hbk)
ISBN 978-3-7258-0969-1 (PDF)
doi.org/10.3390/books978-3-7258-0969-1

© 2024 by the authors. Articles in this book are Open Access and distributed under the Creative Commons Attribution (CC BY) license. The book as a whole is distributed by MDPI under the terms and conditions of the Creative Commons Attribution-NonCommercial-NoDerivs (CC BY-NC-ND) license.

Contents

About the Editors ix

Preface xi

Maria Moudatsou, Areti Stavropoulou, Michael Rovithis and Sofia Koukouli
Evaluation of Online Counseling through the Working Experiences of Mental Health Therapists Amidst the COVID-19 Pandemic
Reprinted from: *Healthcare* **2024**, *12*, 495, doi:10.3390/healthcare12040495 1

Eugenia Halki, Maria Kapiri, Sotirios Plakas, Chrysoula Tsiou, Ourania Govina and Petros Galanis et al.
Fatigue among Greek Parents of Children with Autistic Spectrum Disorder: The Roles of Spirituality and Social Support
Reprinted from: *Healthcare* **2024**, *12*, 455, doi:10.3390/healthcare12040455 16

Petros Galanis, Ioannis Moisoglou, Ioanna V. Papathanasiou, Maria Malliarou, Aglaia Katsiroumpa and Irene Vraka et al.
Association between Organizational Support and Turnover Intention in Nurses: A Systematic Review and Meta-Analysis
Reprinted from: *Healthcare* **2024**, *12*, 291, doi:10.3390/healthcare12030291 27

Younyoung Choi, Mirim Kim and Jeongsoo Park
Mental Healthcare through Cognitive Emotional Regulation Strategies among Prisoners
Reprinted from: *Healthcare* **2023**, *12*, 6, doi:10.3390/healthcare12010006 40

Dieudonne Bwirire, Inez Roosen, Nanne de Vries, Rianne Letschert, Edmond Ntabe Namegabe and Rik Crutzen
Maternal Health Care Service Utilization in the Post-Conflict Democratic Republic of Congo: An Analysis of Health Inequalities over Time
Reprinted from: *Healthcare* **2023**, *11*, 2871, doi:10.3390/healthcare11212871 52

Ho-Jui Tung and Ming-Chin Yeh
Use of Advance Directives in US Veterans and Non-Veterans: Findings from the Decedents of the Health and Retirement Study 1992–2014
Reprinted from: *Healthcare* **2023**, *11*, 1824, doi:10.3390/healthcare11131824 77

Pelagia Soultatou, Stamatis Vardaros and Pantelis G. Bagos
School Health Services and Health Education Curricula in Greece: Scoping Review and Policy Plan
Reprinted from: *Healthcare* **2023**, *11*, 1678, doi:10.3390/healthcare11121678 86

Jacqueline A. Krysa, Mikayla Buell, Kiran Pohar Manhas, Katharina Kovacs Burns, Maria J. Santana and Sidney Horlick et al.
Understanding the Experience of Long COVID Symptoms in Hospitalized and Non-Hospitalized Individuals: A Random, Cross-Sectional Survey Study
Reprinted from: *Healthcare* **2023**, *11*, 1309, doi:10.3390/healthcare11091309 95

Elli D. O. Kyriakaki, Efstathios T. Detorakis, Antonios K. Bertsias, Nikolaos G. Tsakalis, Ioannis Karageorgiou and Gregory Chlouverakis et al.
Clinical and Social Features of Patients with Eye Injuries Admitted to a Tertiary Hospital: A Five-Year Retrospective Study from Crete, Greece
Reprinted from: *Healthcare* **2023**, *11*, 885, doi:10.3390/healthcare11060885 109

Areti Efthymiou, Argyroula Kalaitzaki and Michael Rovithis
Cultural Adaptation of a Health Literacy Toolkit for Healthcare Professionals Working in the Primary Care Setting with Older Adults
Reprinted from: *Healthcare* 2023, 11, 776, doi:10.3390/healthcare11050776 121

Emma Altobelli, Paolo Matteo Angeletti, Giovanni Farello and Reimondo Petrocelli
The Effects of the Ukrainian Conflict on Oncological Care: The Latest State of the Art
Reprinted from: *Healthcare* 2023, 11, 283, doi:10.3390/healthcare11030283 134

Stelios Parissopoulos, Fiona Timmins, Meropi Mpouzika, Marianna Mantzorou, Theodore Kapadochos and Eleni Papagaroufali
Intensive Care Nurses' Experience of Caring in Greece; A Qualitative Study
Reprinted from: *Healthcare* 2023, 11, 164, doi:10.3390/healthcare11020164 142

Firat K. Sayin, Margaret Denton, Catherine Brookman, Sharon Davies and Isik U. Zeytinoglu
Violence, Harassment, and Turnover Intention in Home and Community Care: The Role of Training
Reprinted from: *Healthcare* 2022, 11, 103, doi:10.3390/healthcare11010103 163

Satoko Nagai, Yasuko Ogata, Takeshi Yamamoto, Mark Fedyk and Janice F. Bell
A Longitudinal Study of the Impact of Personal and Professional Resources on Nurses' Work Engagement: A Comparison of Early-Career and Mid-Later-Career Nurses
Reprinted from: *Healthcare* 2022, 11, 76, doi:10.3390/healthcare11010076 175

Yoshiaki Nakagawa, Kaoru Irisa, Yoshinobu Nakagawa and Yasuhiro Kanatani
Hospital Management and Public Health Role of National Hospitals after Transformation into Independent Administrative Agencies
Reprinted from: *Healthcare* 2022, 10, 2084, doi:10.3390/healthcare10102084 189

Despoina Pappa, Ioannis Koutelekos, Eleni Evangelou, Evangelos Dousis, Georgia Gerogianni and Evdokia Misouridou et al.
Investigation of Mental and Physical Health of Nurses Associated with Errors in Clinical Practice
Reprinted from: *Healthcare* 2022, 10, 1803, doi:10.3390/healthcare10091803 211

Maria Sidiropoulou, Georgia Gerogianni, Freideriki Eleni Kourti, Despoina Pappa, Afroditi Zartaloudi and Ioannis Koutelekos et al.
Perceptions, Knowledge and Attitudes among Young Adults about Prevention of HPV Infection and Immunization
Reprinted from: *Healthcare* 2022, 10, 1721, doi:10.3390/healthcare10091721 221

Ioanna Alexandropoulou, Dimitrios G. Goulis, Theodora Merou, Tonia Vassilakou, Dimitrios P. Bogdanos and Maria G. Grammatikopoulou
Basics of Sustainable Diets and Tools for Assessing Dietary Sustainability: A Primer for Researchers and Policy Actors
Reprinted from: *Healthcare* 2022, 10, 1668, doi:10.3390/healthcare10091668 235

Yun-Ru Zhou and Xiao Zhang
The Experience and Enlightenment of the Community-Based Long-Term Care in Japan
Reprinted from: *Healthcare* 2022, 10, 1599, doi:10.3390/healthcare10091599 255

Areti Stavropoulou, Michael Rovithis, Evangelia Sigala, Maria Moudatsou, Georgia Fasoi and Dimitris Papageorgiou et al.
Exploring Nurses' Working Experiences during the First Wave of COVID-19 Outbreak
Reprinted from: *Healthcare* 2022, 10, 1406, doi:10.3390/healthcare10081406 264

Marianna Drakopoulou, Panagiota Begni, Alexandra Mantoudi, Marianna Mantzorou, Georgia Gerogianni and Theodoula Adamakidou et al.
Care and Safety of Schoolchildren with Type 1 Diabetes Mellitus: Parental Perceptions of the School Nurse Role
Reprinted from: *Healthcare* **2022**, *10*, 1228, doi:10.3390/healthcare10071228 . . . . **277**

About the Editors

Sofia Koukouli

Sofia Koukouli is currently an Associate Professor in Health and Social Care Policy at the Department of Social Work of the Hellenic Mediterranean University (HMU) and a member of the Quality of Life Research Lab. She pursued undergraduate studies in Sociology and Political Science at the University of Paris X-Nanterre (France), continued her postgraduate studies in Political Science at New York University (USA) and completed her PhD thesis at the Medical School of the University of Crete. She teaches social policy at the undergraduate and postgraduate levels. She has participated in various research programs linked to her area of expertise, either as a principal investigator or as a member of the research team. Her research interests focus on social policy for vulnerable groups with an emphasis on assessing needs for health and social care services, the quality of these services, as well as family policy issues. She has co-authored many publications in international and national academic journals and has presented her work at numerous academic conferences. In addition, she served as Head of the Department of Social Work for several years and is currently the Dean of the Faculty of Health Sciences.

Areti Stavropoulou

Areti Stavropoulou is an Assistant Professor in Nursing Management and Education at the Department of Nursing of the University of West Attica. She also holds an Honorary Senior Lecturer post in the Faculty of Health, Science, Social Care, and Education of Kingston University, London, UK. She completed her M.Sc. and Ph.D. at Cardiff University, UK. Her main fields of expertise include nursing education, quality assurance, program planning and evaluation, healthcare innovation, and new technologies. Her academic experience involves research and teaching at undergraduate and postgraduate university programs. She has experience as a project leader and has served as a member of multidisciplinary consortia in several funded research programs (European Union/EPAnEK) directed by Higher Educational Institutes and Research Organisations. She has also edited and published books and papers in international and national academic journals that mainly cover the fields of nursing management, education, and quality assurance.

Preface

The development of health and social care policy is crucial for ensuring the welfare of individuals and communities. It involves a complex interplay of political, economic, social, and ethical factors. It addresses the social determinants that impact health outcomes and seeks to promote equity in healthcare delivery. Health and social care policy aims to address inequalities and improve access to quality care for all individuals. It also focuses on integrating health and social care services to provide holistic support for individuals with complex needs, aiming to improve coordination and communication between healthcare providers and social care professionals to ensure comprehensive and tailored support for individuals. Therefore, it requires careful consideration and collaboration among various stakeholders. Policymakers must take into account the diverse needs of the population and prioritize the allocation of resources effectively. This requires a thorough understanding of epidemiological data and tendencies. It also necessitates collaboration with healthcare professionals and stakeholders to ensure that policies are rooted in best practices, meet the needs of the population, are responsive to emerging health challenges, and adapt to policies accordingly.

In this open access reprint, we seek to explore the complex interplay between health and social care policy, shedding light on the current issues and potential solutions. The papers featured in it encompass a diverse array of subjects, from the impact of healthcare reform to the role of social determinants of health in shaping policy decisions. Topics include the intersection of public health, health and social care, the economic implications of policy decisions, the integration of mental health services, and the impact of technology on healthcare delivery. The diverse range of topics covered in this issue will provide readers with a multifaceted understanding of the complex landscape of health and social care policy.

We believe that the papers featured in this reprint will yield significant effects on the field of health and social care policy, shaping the discourse and inspiring new research and approaches. The insights provided by the contributors offer valuable perspectives that will inform policy decisions and drive positive change within the healthcare system. We are confident that this Special Issue will spark meaningful conversations and drive impactful change in the field of health and social care policy.

We express our gratitude to all the authors who contributed to this endeavor.

Sofia Koukouli and Areti Stavropoulou
Editors

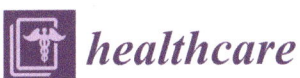

Article

Evaluation of Online Counseling through the Working Experiences of Mental Health Therapists Amidst the COVID-19 Pandemic

Maria Moudatsou [1,2,*], Areti Stavropoulou [2,3,4], Michael Rovithis [2,5] and Sofia Koukouli [1,2]

1. Department of Social Work, Faculty of Health Sciences, Hellenic Mediterranean University, 71410 Heraklion, Greece; koukouli@hmu.gr
2. Laboratory of Interdisciplinary Approaches for the Enhancement of Quality of Life (QoLab), 71410 Heraklion, Greece; astavropoulou@uniwa.gr (A.S.)
3. Department of Nursing, Faculty of Health and Care Sciences, University of West Attica, 12243 Athens, Greece
4. Faculty of Health, Science, Social Care and Education, Kingston University, London KT2 7LB, UK
5. Department of Business Administration and Tourism, School of Management and Economics Sciences, Hellenic Mediterranean University, 71410 Heraklion, Greece
* Correspondence: moudatsoum@hmu.gr

Abstract: This study aimed to reflect on mental health professionals' experiences with online counseling during the COVID-19 pandemic, as well as their perceptions and recommendations for the future. The method of qualitative research with semi-structured interviews was used. The sample consisted of 17 mental health professionals working in the public or private sectors. A framework analysis revealed four main themes, namely (a) the evaluation of online counseling; (b) comparing in-person and online counseling; (c) factors influencing the effectiveness of online counseling; and (d) suggestions for the future use of online counseling. Most therapists reported that their overall experience with online counseling was positive. The main advantages cited were the accessibility for everyone and the reductions in time, money, and distance. Its primary drawbacks included less nonverbal communication, the inability to employ certain therapeutic tools, problems with confidentiality, lack of experience, and technical difficulties during online sessions. Its effectiveness depends on contextual factors and factors related to the therapeutic process itself. Organizational planning, training, and a solid implementation strategy may help ensure that this communication medium is used to its fullest potential. In addition, the possible utilization of remote counseling combined with in-person psychotherapeutic intervention methods will provide solutions for the future, especially in crisis situations.

Keywords: online counseling; mental health professionals; COVID-19 pandemic; internet psychotherapy; qualitative study; Greece

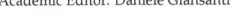

1. Introduction

Prior to the COVID-19 pandemic, counseling and psychotherapy were primarily conducted in-person. Even though remote counseling has been used in the past, there have been few reasons to justify its integration into everyday practice, and mental health professionals were particularly cautious [1,2].

The pandemic of COVID-19 caused great tension and anxiety to people worldwide, influencing their mental health [3]. Even after the end of the first wave, stress remained due to the pandemic's multiple ramifications (such as isolation, social distancing, job loss, and fear of contracting the disease), leading to a secondary epidemic related to negative effects on mental health [4,5]. Remote intervention became necessary because of the pandemic in order to continue the treatments of those who needed them, while also reducing the spread of the virus [6].

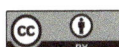

Online counseling was first introduced in the 1960s in order to meet the needs of clients who were isolated in mountainous or remote areas and had to travel a long distance to treatment centers, or to save time and money [7]. However, before the COVID-19 pandemic, counseling and psychotherapy were generally provided in-person. Therefore, most therapists did not have prior knowledge of or experience with online counseling and were quite hesitant to use it, considering that person-to-person intervention is more effective [8]. Nevertheless, due to the challenging circumstances of COVID-19, they were required to initiate or continue their treatments primarily online, without any previous preparation or a well-defined treatment protocol [9].

The rapid changes in health and society have indorsed the use of emerging technologies in many areas of healthcare. More specifically, in the field of counseling, with issues related to immediate accessibility, privacy, and effectiveness, and where the maintenance of communication between therapists and clients in a period in which social distancing was necessary, the use of online practices proved to be a substantial action for the continuation of the therapeutic process [7,8,10,11]. The effectiveness of these practices, however, lies in understanding and being able to manage both the advantages and disadvantages of these technologies, such as security, confidentiality, and the lack of a code of ethics [7,8]. Furthermore, issues of accessibility due to economic, social, and contextual factors should be identified for creating effective platforms for both therapists and clients [9].

In the past, several therapists have successfully utilized online counseling, arguing that it does not differ from in-person therapy [10]. However, in many countries, such as France and Belgium, online counseling was used at least in the first lockdown, without previous experience or training of the therapists, raising concerns about its effectiveness and, more importantly, compliance with counseling ethics [11]. Some therapists still have reservations about ethical and privacy issues, as they believe that ethics are not sufficiently respected [7,8].

Online counseling offers a number of benefits. It can provide opportunities and perspectives like easy access to therapy in case of geographically remote places, or in circumstances of illness or relocation to another area, and resolve issues like reducing distance, saving money, and, in general, making treatment more flexible [9,12].

Despite the advantages of online counseling, there is difficulty for therapists and clients to develop a therapeutic relationship as they cannot sufficiently connect and empathize [13]. Some have mentioned difficulties with the technology and internet connectivity. Others continue to be wary about ethical and privacy issues, considering that ethics are not sufficiently observed [7,8].

The therapist's knowledge, training, practice, work experience, and expertise are central to ensuring appropriate professional ethics [14]. The effectiveness of internet counseling might also be influenced by the therapist's psychotherapeutic approach. It has been found that cognitive therapists are more familiar with it than psychodynamic therapists [15].

Online counseling does not provide the therapist the possibility of global and comprehensive monitoring of the client. As a result, valuable information is lost from non-verbal communication [16]. Additionally, it is not always appropriate for crisis situations, such as when a client expresses suicidal or self-harming intent, or when therapists feel uncomfortable with it [17,18].

Even though it is considered necessary and beneficial, online counseling training is only occasionally offered, at least in European countries [19,20]. The American Association of Psychotherapists' recommendations for online therapy suggest that therapists should feel confident utilizing the technology themselves and have ensured that their clients are also familiar with its use [11]. Additionally, it is essential to establish a secure framework and a comprehensive work protocol that will define the guidelines of online counseling. It is required to be implemented in the context of a contract regulating detailed issues of ethics, methodology, and terminology [11].

As already mentioned, training is necessary for therapists and everyone involved in therapy. The training and specialization should be accompanied by their formal certification following all the rules of ethics and ethics of counseling, while also respecting the client's needs and confidentiality [19,21]. Support from the relevant health agencies is needed in addition to the political, economic, and scientific input from everyone involved in the development of health policies [22].

Remote counseling exhibited several advantages, including the following: (1) it supported people being treated for both their pre-existing and pandemic-related mental health issues, and (2) it helped reduce the transmission of COVID-19. However, it is a topic that has not been thoroughly investigated, especially during the COVID-19 pandemic. Moreover, the endorsement of online counseling in Greece has not been explored adequately, and there is a need to fill in this knowledge gap by providing reliable research evidence. It is important to note that, especially in the public sector, online counseling was endorsed with a considerable delay, as the system was not ready for this abrupt change. In contrast, online procedures were applied faster in the private sector. Not many studies have been conducted to investigate the views and experiences of health professionals on using online counseling under these circumstances. As such, producing qualitative research evidence in this area was considered essential for answering the topic under investigation in depth. This research approach aims to better understand the circumstances surrounding online counseling as a selection of therapy, to evaluate the concerns of experts, the problems identified, and any potential benefits. The present study aimed to investigate the aforementioned issues.

2. Methods

2.1. Aim

This study examined the work contexts, perspectives, and beliefs of mental health practitioners about remote therapy. In particular, their overall experience with online therapy (phone, internet, skype, viber, messenger, etc.) was investigated, as well as the benefits and main obstacles that remote therapy presented to the practitioners, clients, and families. Additionally, recommendations for the usage of online therapy in the future were explored, along with ethical issues.

2.2. Study Design

A qualitative study approach was favored to elucidate the essence of lived experience and develop composite descriptions. Qualitative research investigates the perceptions, feelings, and experiences of the subjects under study in depth through a holistic approach [23,24] As the main goal of this research was to thoroughly examine the subjective experiences of health professionals regarding online counseling, the implementation of a qualitative research design was considered the most appropriate one.

2.3. Population and Study Sample

Mental health professionals, mainly psychologists, and social workers, working either in the public or private sectors constituted the study population. The participants of the sample were selected using a purposeful sampling technique. This non-random sampling technique is also known as judgmental sampling, as the researcher depends on their own judgement for selecting those individuals who are more eligible to participate in a study. According to this technique, the researcher identifies, from the population under investigation, those members who meet the study criteria and can adequately and deeply address the research questions. This means that the selected study participants are extremely knowledgeable about the topic under investigation and can provide a wealth of information about it [24,25]. The inclusion criteria for participating in the study was to practice counseling for at least 2 years and have experience with practicing online counseling during the pandemic period. This experience was considered essential for discussing their experience on online counseling in depth. Specialization in a psychotherapy approach was also considered desirable. The mental health professionals selected were practicing remote counseling either in public agencies or in the private sector. Most of the participants were practicing in the private sector, as the online counseling services in the public sector were not implemented immediately. Our study was advertised through social media (FB and Instagram). Professionals who were therapists were contacted by one member of our authoring team to explore their interest in participating in our study. Access to our sample was also achieved by contacting these professionals directly at their workplaces, or through their professional associations. To obtain the participants' consent, detailed information regarding the nature and the goals of the study as well as the inclusion criteria were initially provided by phone and then via email. The voluntary nature of participation in the survey and the confidentiality of their responses were also assured. The recruitment process lasted approximately 2 months. Twenty-five (25) mental health professionals from four (4) metropolitan cities in northern, central (Attica region), and southern (Grete region) Greece, agreed initially to participate in our study. Eight (8) of them were not finally involved in the study due to time restrictions and lack of availability. Sample size was determined through a data saturation process. Data saturation occurred after completing the 17th interview. At this point, the new data that emerged did not offer new information to allow for further coding and categorization or to seek for additional participants.

2.4. Sample's Socio-Demographic Profile

Seventeen (17) mental health practitioners constituted the final sample, specifically two (2) mental health counselors, five (5) social workers, and ten (10) psychologists. All participants were women and married with children, and most of them were over 50 (50–65 years old). Also, five mental health professionals were university graduates, eleven had a postgraduate degree, and one was a PhD holder. Most of the therapists said that they treat more than thirty clients every week, the majority of whom are adults. Regarding their psychotherapeutic approach, twelve implement a systemic approach, two use a psychodynamic approach, and one did not specify, while two had no specialization. Additionally, seven of them had between twenty and thirty years of experience as psychotherapists, six were public employees, and eleven had a private practice (see Table S1, Supplementary Material).

2.5. Data Collection

For the data collection, semi-structured interviews were used. Semi-structured interviews were used to explore the in-depth personal experiences, perceptions, and thoughts of the participants for the topic under investigation [26].

The interview scheme focused on two main axes: the subjective experience with online counseling and their online counselling challenges as these were confronted by the professionals involved. More specifically, the semi-structured interview guide comprised one introductory open-ended question asking the participants to describe their experience with online counseling. Furthermore, the interview guide focused on the positive and negative aspects of online and recommendations for future use. The relevant literature on online counseling during the period of COVID-19 was the main source of information used for the development of the main axes and the open-ended questions used in the interview guide.

The first author (M.M.), who is experienced in qualitative research approaches, methodically conducted online interviews with all respondents within a designated timeframe (May–June 2022). None of the selected participants withdrew from the study. The average length of an interview was 30 to 40 min.

2.6. Data Analysis

The interviews were first recorded and then transcribed by the first author. To analyze the data, the framework analysis was used [27,28]. This method is popular for managing and analyzing large amounts of qualitative data deriving usually from semi-structured interviews. It is used by multidisciplinary research teams to obtain a clearly descriptive and comprehensive outline of the research data. It leads to structured outcomes and supports the researchers in identifying themes and connotations that might emerge from the data. Framework analysis is valued for following a systematic management and data analysis approach, thus providing a clear audit trail throughout the research process that guarantees the production of reliable findings [24,28,29]. The utilization of framework analysis was considered as most appropriate for our study, as our team consisted of researchers from different scientific backgrounds, and the large amounts of data derived from the semi-structured interviews had to be managed in a highly structured manner.

The framework analysis includes the following stages: (a) familiarization with the data by the researchers as all the results were thoroughly studied; (b) the coding of the data; (c) the identification of the themes and categories that emerged; (d) recording the results based on the existing themes; and (e) writing the results [29].

The trustworthiness of the study was ensured by using mainly two techniques: investigator triangulation and reflexivity. The first technique involved two members of the research team who examined, coded, interpreted, and analyzed the survey data, while the second technique focused on examining how the researchers' preconceptions and values might have influenced the decisions taken throughout the study process. Furthermore, member checking was used to ensure that the findings were representative of the participants' experiences and that no important issues were missed. To accurately present the research data, a backward translation technique was used [23–25].

To report the study results, the COREQ guidelines were used. COREQ is a checklist with 32 items grouped into three domains addressing the (a) research team and reflexivity, (b) study design, and (c) data analysis and reporting. This checklist may assist qualitative researchers to report all the important dimensions of their research design and implementation as well as their findings in a robust and comprehensive manner [30]. In the present study, issues regarding the study design (e.g., sampling strategy and recruitment, sample characteristics, interview guide, and data saturation), the analysis and findings (e.g., theme generation, participants' quotations), and the researchers' profiles and involvement were presented following the COREQ guidelines to the extent possible.

The research team consisted of academics with a wide range of backgrounds in health and social care services (social work, social policy, and nursing), as well as expertise in qualitative research. All of them contributed equally to the design of the research and provided support at all stages of the study process.

2.7. Ethical Issues

Written permission was granted by the university's Research Ethics Committee (A.A. 99, A.P. 65/18-11-2021, accessed on 18 November 2021). The managers of the private practices or the heads of the public agencies where the interviewees worked also granted their approval. Each participant provided her consent after being notified through email or social media (messaging) of the study's purpose, its voluntary nature, and the confidentiality of the information collected.

3. Results

Four main themes were derived from the data analysis, describing the subjective working experience of the participants with online counseling. The four themes revealed are as follows: (1) the evaluation of online counseling (working experience with online counseling, overall assessment, and advantages/disadvantages); (2) comparing in-person with online therapy (similarities, differences); (3) factors influencing the effectiveness of online counseling (contextual factors and the therapeutic process); and (4) suggestions for its future use (a supplementary tool used with caution, create the appropriate conditions) (See Table S2, Supplementary Material).

3.1. Evaluation of Online Counseling

3.1.1. Working Experience with Online Counseling

Some therapists have already been using online counseling services prior to the COVID-19 period due to the specific conditions of their clients (living far away, work conditions, studies, etc.). However, almost all respondents began using online therapy more systematically during the COVID-19 period, albeit with hesitation.

"I started, experimentally a few years before COVID-19 when some of my clients decided to relocate to another city for various reasons". (P11).

"Before COVID it (the online counseling) was possible to serve some cases outside of the county. Then, it was used solely throughout the pandemic and now things are somewhat back to normal". (P8).

"I began using it during the first quarantine. Before, there was no need and I was very reluctant for various reasons...I had to evaluate how the basic principles of our work will be safeguarded..." (P5).

Some, even throughout the COVID-19 period, did not prefer to use it. They did so only in case of illness of themselves or their clients.

"During the COVID period I did face-to-face sessions. My clients didn't want it. Only in situations where a person had received a personal or family diagnosis of COVID we used online therapy". (P4).

3.1.2. Overall Assessment

In the end, for the majority, the overall assessment was favorable. They evaluated online psychotherapy positively, despite the lack of prior experience and the cautiousness of the first transitional phase. They agreed that it was essentially an issue of familiarity of the parties involved, as well as of the therapist's knowledge, experience, ability to adapt, and willingness to learn new things.

"(My experience was...) excellent. Online didn't hinder me in any way. I put new members in groups, graduations took place online. ... (all these were...) concrete signs that everything went well. It matters how one feels comfortable". (P1).

"Now, I prefer it. I sense the closeness. As though we are face to face. There are many benefits and making modifications is simple and easy. I tried myself on something new. Change is never easy, but I was able to adapt". (P10).

"At first, I took each step very cautiously. I believed in face-to-face counseling. Now, however, I am certain. My interventions were successful. It worked well in restrained circumstances. My clients are very satisfied". (P13).

"Although I was afraid that it would be difficult to build a therapeutic relationship between me and the client, eventually it was effective. My experience is very positive". (P11).

3.1.3. Advantages and Disadvantages of Online Counseling

The main advantage mentioned was rendering counseling services more flexible to the therapist and the client. The majority stressed that it reduces travel distance and time and ensures the accessibility of socially excluded people or those who would not attend if the sessions were face-to-face.

"You can work online from any location. The primary benefit is this. The treatment can be continued from anywhere at any time...For people with disabilities and mobility problems, it is very helpful. Also, some of our young clients are worried that their fellow classmates might see them, and, for that reason, they feel more exposed. In that case, video conferences were helpful". (P5).

"It is a valuable supplementary tool. It reduces the physical distance that would make a live session prohibitive. It also helped the clients in teamwork". (P3).

"It gave an opportunity to elderly family members who are not accustomed to technology or therapy to become acquainted with both. Furthermore, after one family member began using it, the others got to know it as well. For instance, a mother we had to call to participate might show up for online sessions, but not for live ones. Through the online program, participants could observe, either directly or indirectly, how the therapist interacts with clients". (P10).

Nevertheless, they enumerated many drawbacks. A primary disadvantage is the difficulty of assessing and using nonverbal communication and the risk of poorer quality of interaction due to contextual factors.

"The internet gives the opportunity to focus on the gaze, but the rest of the body is vanished. The transference and countertransference required, such small qualities are lost.... In face-to-face communication feelings and unconscious experiences are shared differently...". (P8).

"It's less interaction. It is not comprehensive......you don't have the overall image of the person in front of you...there are other distractions during sessions (the phone etc) In other words, there are other stimuli besides counseling and psychotherapy". (P15).

Certain participants mentioned that, in online counseling, they do not have the possibility to use all the therapeutic tools.

"You can't utilize all of your tools, like music or painting. Nonverbal cues are invisible to you; you see them, but not very much". (P7).

Additionally, some raised ethical issues, while for others, there was no question of violating ethics in either context.

"... the professionals suspect that someone is recording them or someone else is in the room. The client is similarly concerned about this...". (P5).

"Also, a difficulty reported by clients was maintaining privacy from their own space. They said that they do not feel safe when people in the next room or apartment are known and can hear. When the client does not feel safe, this limits the session and its benefits". (P9).

A number of professionals view distance as a barrier to establishing a therapeutic relationship. Conversely, others think that developing a therapeutic relationship is unaffected by distance. The client and the therapist jointly determine the extent to which the client wants to engage in therapy.

"I find it facilitates superficiality. There is no particular connection. A more superficial therapeutic relationship". (P17).

"Maybe it takes more time to build a good therapeutic relationship. The information you lose in online you gain along the way. More sessions might be required". (P5).

"In my experience, establishing a therapeutic relationship is not a problem. A person will work on his/her problems if he/she wants to. Additionally, the therapist will grow and acquire new abilities. If it is his desire... For both the therapist and the person treated, it is an issue of free will and decision". (P2).

Certain advantages, such as staying in your own place, may also become drawbacks affecting the quality of the meetings. This is also connected to the lack of a treatment protocol.

"While we can wear comfortable clothing in sessions, previous circumstances taught us the importance of self-care and professional dressing. Personally, I think this is rather negative". (P1).

"In my opinion, both the professional and the person being treated ought to establish clearer boundaries.". (P9).

"People still lack the education necessary for distant learning; they attend online meetings in robes, in the car, at their parents' house, and are not in the controlled setting of a therapist's office where everything is turned off and therapy is the main focus". (P4).

It was also emphasized that online counseling was ineffective for patients with certain conditions.

"Behavioral activation in those suffering from anxiety, social anxiety, or depression is not improved by it. It is not possible to implement therapies for children with behavioral issues, ADHD, or Asperger's syndrome. Some child-centered interventions, such as play therapy, cannot be conducted remotely, unless a protocol is established. I believe these obstacles are difficult to overcome". (P13).

One of the main issues raised was clients' and therapists' unfamiliarity with technology, which tends to immediately exclude those who are less knowledgeable. Concerns were also expressed about whether it is financially feasible for vulnerable social groups to acquire the necessary equipment.

"Not everyone is tech savvy. Age is significant, in my view. The challenges for 60 years old are different from 15 years old. Even for electronic payments". (P14).

"A student eventually stopped coming to class, and I found out that she didn't have a strong signal at home". (P5).

3.2. Comparing In-Person and Online Counseling

3.2.1. Similarities

Regarding the similarities, most respondents focused on the establishment of a therapeutic relationship, its goals and ethical principles, the interview and the verbal and—to a certain extent—the non-verbal communication.

"The goals and fundamental ethical principles, or the interview procedure, for instance, were the same. The interview's format remained unchanged. It took the same amount of time. Case management and referrals were interchangeable". (P5).

"Online privacy is equivalent to that of an office setting. Issues of ethics are similar". (P4).

"I'm still attempting to establish a relationship with my client. Moreover, the therapeutic alliance endures". (P7).

"In both situations, a relationship with certain qualities develops. There's the non-verbal (limited to the face) and the verbal communication. As long as there is a contract, there is a result". (P8).

3.2.2. Differences

The context in which counseling is provided, the non-verbal communication, the whole procedure, and confidentiality issues are the primary areas of distinction.

"There is a screen in online counseling. The therapist does not see the client in its entirety. Inevitably, a loss of information occurs". (P12).

"Live communication requires the person to leave their home and go to the therapist's office, which is a neutral setting. This transition also functions similarly to a commitment process". (P8).

"In live communication you are more focused; when you're online, distractions like the phone and door ringing can happen. When we speak face-to-face and the room is empty, I feel more secure.…..Confidentiality and privacy are important to me". (P7).

3.3. Factors Influencing the Effectiveness of Online Counseling

3.3.1. Contextual Factors

A number of therapists who work in the public sector, in particular, stated that the organization's role is pivotal. Furthermore, it is essential to establish a contract and adhere to procedure.

"The agency's organizational structure is crucial. A communication framework should be established, indicating the platform to be utilized as well. The client must have an informal contract". (P5).

"I believe that therapists need to be trained and that platforms should provide protocols so that they know what cases to take on. For example, if we are communicating remotely with a woman who is experiencing domestic abuse, we need to make sure that she is protected. The same goes for suicidal clients; platforms should provide protocols that are followed. It is vital to preserve quality". (P13).

"An initial framework is necessary…establish guidelines for cooperation. The rules that should be followed…should be outlined in a contract that is agreed at the outset". (P4).

Participants also denoted technical concerns like expertise and network performance.

"I've experienced how having a poor network can make our work more challenging". (P12).

"The network's quality, available technology, tablets, laptops, and cell phones. This could lead to issues. There might be no signal on the cell phone. That creates a problem". (P4).

3.3.2. The Therapeutic Process

For internet counseling to be successful, the therapist's own role is crucial, as well as their expertise, abilities, and background.

"The therapist is important. His/her expertise, experience, disposition, and engagement in the role. The conviction that it's also possible to do it that way. We learn when we are motivated to achieve something. Zoom was a new experience for me. I discovered it". (P1).

A number of participants considered that the therapeutic approach has an impact on the effectiveness of online counseling.

"Systemic therapy adherents are more flexible. Thus, the last group to deal with internet was psychoanalysts. It's not the same for us systemics. We consider distance a useful tool. We are more detached". (P1).

"I'm not sure if it would be effective when applied to psychoanalysis's traditional dimension. Or for those who are body-centered and find it difficult to intervene. As a systemic, I don't find it problematic. In the end, I believe the therapist's method matters". (P7).

However, other participants gave more priority to the therapeutic needs of the person treated.

"I think it has more to do with the therapist and the person's needs rather than the approach used.... if the online process helps you achieve your goal. I work with people who have difficulties in socializing and interacting with others. You realize that in this case it is not in their favor to communicate online.....they didn't improve". (P9).

Almost all respondents agreed that the experiences of the clients positively or negatively influence the course of online counseling. Some had a positive experience, while for others, the experience was negative.

"They found it interesting. It didn't seem difficult for them. I received positive reviews. Perhaps the assessments would differ if the two (online vs. in-person communication) were compared during a typical period (without COVID). They formed a social link, felt very supported, and experienced a sense of belonging to a team..." (P8).

"Many regular clients ceased coming during COVID-19. They did not feel comfortable. Maybe other persons were present in the room during sessions or lacked the resources". (P5).

3.4. Suggestions for the Future Use of Online Counseling
3.4.1. A Supplementary Tool Used with Caution

There are benefits to online counseling, and it can be used in the future where appropriate with some restrictions and by implementing a specific protocol respected by the client. However, almost all respondents agreed that one should use it to supplement in-person counseling rather than to replace it.

"Getting familiar with online will facilitate but not replace in-person..." (P1).

"We have to be careful about tools and confidentiality. For example, I tell them to wear headphones.... I ask them to confirm that they are alone in the room. They are not allowed to use drugs, alcohol, or cigarettes. When they attend the office and when they are online, the indicators will look different for example when a person communicates suicidal thoughts or thoughts of self-destruction. Additionally, the expert will treat you differently online. We must be prepared". (P12).

"A protocol for the management and implementation of the teleconference ought to exist. Anticipate difficulties. Should Skype malfunction, you have the option to utilize an alternative platform". (P5).

It can be utilized by those who are unable to participate in face-to-face therapy for a variety of reasons, such as health issues.

"It is just one additional tool available to therapists. . . .. for those in hospitals, institutions, or with serious illnesses. . .and with a low cost". (P6).

"Only when the person concerned cannot move, is sick, disabled, or far away". (P17).

3.4.2. Create the Appropriate Conditions

The education and training of therapists in online counseling is essential. Some have suggested holding conferences or other scientific processes to exchange views and practices that may help in successful online counseling.

"Exchange of experiences amongst individuals who work in different groups is necessary... participate in conferences and analyze case studies. . ." (P6).

"Education. It would help me to know the experience of others. . ... Networking around such topics". (P3).

"Education is necessary...I recently discovered that there are tools out there that we are unaware of, like the life map". (P16).

Additionally, several therapists offered solutions to technical and practical issues.

"The networks should be better and with optical fibers there are imperfections. There are some connection problems on certain days and times". (P1).

"Good network that is open to everyone. Good know-how and digital accessibility. Encourage having a face-to-face first meeting. It will help in the therapeutic relationship". (P3).

It has been suggested by a number of respondents that the network supporting online counseling be established within the framework of a local government-organized social policy and/or create specific platforms adapted to counseling.

"A strong network throughout the city would be useful. Consequently, local government could provide help. There are places, for example, where a fast network is not supported. . ." (P11).

"I think it would help to have a platform for such cases. Not skype or viber. To make it easier. It would help us therapists to promote such a platform. I have seen it in many colleagues who are promoting such platforms. . ." (P14).

4. Discussion

Our study's findings demonstrate that some therapists had used online counseling occasionally, either as part of their training, or when a client had to leave the place of their treatment for a variety of reasons, such as employment or studies. However, the great majority of therapists started using online counseling more systematically during COVID-19. Despite their initial hesitation and the challenges they encountered, the majority of them reported that the overall experience was positive. Several therapists also had a positive experience with online counseling before the outbreak of the COVID-19 health crisis [9]. Most therapists both in our study and in others stated that when they started using online counseling during the pandemic, their previous experience or relevant training were very limited or completely absent [11].

The factors that, according to our research, can influence the course of a successful online consultation rely both on the organization itself and how well prepared it is, as well as on knowledge-related issues. Mainly, the therapists working in a public agency highlighted the role of the organization. This can be explained by the fact that private sector therapists operate with greater independence and have the resources, know-how, and training necessary to provide online therapy.

All interviewees put an emphasis on the need of having a distinct and clear contract for online counseling. This will eliminate many potential issues and outline a new treatment framework. Previous research has indicated that the existence of a protocol and client and therapist preparation are essential for the process of online counseling because, while it provides practical support, it also serves to lower stress and enhance the therapeutic process as a whole [9].

Our research suggests that the therapist has a crucial role. Their experience and prior knowledge and familiarity as well as the way in which they manage the issues and context of the treatment affect its quality [12,31]. Other findings also support the pivotal role and importance of the therapist's experience in online counseling [7,31]. A therapist who does not feel comfortable with the internet will not be able to convey a feeling of safety to their clients to accept it [14].

In addition, the therapists' psychotherapeutic approach influences the effectiveness of online counseling. Some professionals consider that there are limitations to some psychotherapeutic approaches including psychodynamics. Compared to their counterparts from other methods, such as psychoanalysts, cognitive approach psychotherapists prefer online counseling [15]. In the present study, systemic approach therapists accounted for the majority of participants who indicated a preference for online counseling. One interpretation of these data could be that the therapists of this approach are flexible enough to adopt techniques from other approaches and are receptive to any "innovation" in the field of psychotherapy.

The mode and mechanisms of change used in therapy may explain why some psychotherapeutic approaches favor online counseling. Both our study and others [9,15] report difficulties in the psychodynamic approach of therapists for online counseling. A possible interpretation is that the limited use of non-verbal communication in this particular technique and the difficulty of implementing the change mechanisms that it uses, such as the method of free association on the couch, do not leave room for its successful use [15].

A first evaluation of online counseling, according to our results, states that among its advantages are the arrangement of practical issues such as the reductions in distance, money, and travel time. In addition, the elimination of social exclusion for vulnerable people is an important contribution of online counseling. Related studies [14,32–34] have produced similar results. Of course, online counseling creates another kind of exclusion for those population groups without access to technology. People who belong to vulnerable groups who usually lag behind in terms of the knowledge and management of social media, or who lack an internet connection or the necessary logistical equipment, are thus excluded.

Our findings suggest that, despite the positives of online counseling, it is not recommended for specific categories of psychological disorders, such as interventions for people with psychosis or mental retardation. There are studies that positively evaluate the intervention of online counseling in specific disorders including anxiety and depression [35]. However, other research data highlight its weaknesses in specific disorders as well as in crisis situations, such as suicide attempts [17,18].

The participants of the present study emphasized repeatedly that online counseling does not allow the utilization of non-verbal communication or the use of certain therapeutic tools. This poses significant challenges for the course of the treatment because no information is gathered that could aid in its advancement and development, such as the therapeutic process or the analysis of the clinical picture, which would have provided the therapist with the necessary information to intervene, particularly in crisis situations [12].

According to some study participants, online counseling does not safeguard ethical issues like privacy. Other research has produced similar findings [14,33,35–37]. Mendes-Santos et al. [14] suggest that one plausible reason for the therapists' inability to feel secure in the internet traps could be their inadequate training and lack of knowledge.

Consistent with other studies, divergent opinions on establishing a therapeutic relationship online were found in our results. Some believe that the development of a therapeutic relationship is hampered or prevented by distance [14,34,36–38]. Nonetheless, other therapists disagree, arguing that internet counseling fosters a positive therapeutic alliance [7].

The views of the participants presented in our study appear to recognize that online counseling is a practice that may spread rapidly in the future. This kind of practice may potentially assume a supplementary role in in-person counseling, in cases, for instance, of the clients' disability or health issues that do not allow for physical attendance. Our findings point to the possibility of a uniform, reliable protocol for online therapy. As a result, a stable framework is established, facilitating communication between the therapist and the client as well as the advancement of the healing process. These perspectives corroborate findings from earlier research [7–9].

Finally, the sample's participants endorse the need for therapists to have knowledge and training about online counseling. Knowledge and previous experience in using the internet increase the likelihood of its correct use in the future [39]. According to the APA guidelines for online counseling, therapists must make sure that they have adequate knowledge of the technology required and that online counseling is beneficial to their clients [11]. This is even more evident in the post-COVID-19 era in that online counseling is expected to have an increased utility for people who face health issues requiring systematic monitoring, for elderly people, and for people who experience all kinds of exclusion due to gender, religion, or spiritual peculiarities [40]. The readiness of the therapist to use online counseling should also be underlined. To effectively use these emerging technologies, the therapist should have appropriate skills and experience in managing sensitive issues such as the difficulties in applying online counseling in cases of domestic violence, couple therapy, or when the whole family should be present in the process [41]. The development of supportive technological environments and appropriate and accessible infrastructures are necessary to confine the reluctances of therapists and clients to use online practices within the context of a contemporary therapeutic process [9,41].

5. Limitations

In our study, a qualitative research method was used that does not allow for the generalization of our results. While our analysis covers therapists across Greece, it mostly focused on those in the greater Attica and Crete regions, with a few outliers. This has the consequence of limiting the viewpoints of therapists from smaller towns or other regions of Greece who may have had different perspectives. Moreover, not all therapist backgrounds are represented in our study sample; psychiatrists, for example, would likely have different perspectives and be able to offer us a broader understanding of the online counseling issue. In addition, the majority of the therapists in our sample employed a systemic psychotherapy approach. It is unknown if using different types of treatment methods would add new data to our research. Furthermore, the present study did not include any male therapists. Our findings thus demonstrate a feminine perspective of the topic under investigation. Although, this targeted perspective of our findings can be viewed as an added value for our study, readers should also consider that the gender of a therapist has an impact on their counseling practice. In addition, psychotherapy often investigates the articulation of emotions and the discourse of emotional matters in a manner that is more in line with the gender traits of the counseling therapist and diverges in terms of their communication style with the patient [42].

Finally, the period within which our survey was conducted inevitably affected our results. The therapists' opinions of online counseling might have changed if it had been conducted at a different time, such as at the start or end of the pandemic. As such, the findings of this study should be viewed under these limitations.

6. Conclusions

To our knowledge, this study is one of the few attempts at reflecting on the working experiences of mental health counselors during the COVID-19 pandemic. It provides an idea about the adaptation of these professionals to the pandemic in Greece through the use of online counseling and may contribute to its appropriate use in the future.

Our findings indicate that online therapy has a number of benefits and can be utilized either exclusively or in conjunction with counseling in crisis situations like COVID-19. But future use of it necessitates preparedness. Therapists need to specialize in internet therapy and receive rigorous training in this area. It is still necessary to develop and enforce a treatment protocol that is consistent for all online counseling providers and adhered to by all parties involved.

According to our results, online counseling has several advantages and can be used in combination with counseling or entirely in crisis situations such as COVID-19. However, its use in the future requires preparation. In particular, the systematic training and specialization of therapists in online counseling is required. There is still a need to formulate and have a specific treatment protocol followed by all involved, which is uniform for all therapists practicing online counseling.

Both in the public and private sectors, there must be synchronization and coordination between those responsible for solving respective issues. The contribution of social policy at local and national levels is imperative. It will address training issues, and also finance the actions that need to be performed.

The present research can be continued in the future with other groups of therapists who practice online counseling, such as psychiatrists. It can be extended to other regions of Greece with different social and geographical conditions or combined with quantitative studies. Finally, it would be important to conduct an additional study that would present the views of the clients and their families regarding their experience with online counseling and providing their own suggestions for the future.

Supplementary Materials: The following are available online at https://www.mdpi.com/article/10.3390/healthcare12040495/s1: Table S1: Participants' socio-demographic characteristics; Table S2: Main themes and sub-themes.

Author Contributions: Conceptualization, M.M. and S.K.; methodology, M.M. and S.K; formal analysis, M.M. and A.S.; investigation, M.M.; data curation, M.M., M.R.; writing—original draft preparation, S.K. and M.M.; writing—review and editing, A.S., S.K. and M.R. All authors have read and agreed to the published version of the manuscript.

Funding: This research received no external funding.

Institutional Review Board Statement: The study was conducted according to the guidelines of the Declaration of Helsinki and approved by the Research Ethics Committee of Hellenic Mediterranean University (A.A. 99, A.P. 65/18-11-2021).

Informed Consent Statement: Informed consent was obtained from all subjects involved in the study.

Data Availability Statement: Data generated during the present study cannot be shared due to issues with the subjects' privacy and confidentiality.

Acknowledgments: We express sincere thanks to all therapists who participated in the present study. Without them, this accomplishment would not be possible.

Conflicts of Interest: The authors declare no conflicts of interest.

References

1. Irvine, A.; Drew, P.; Bower, P.; Brooks, H.; Gellatly, J.; Armitage, C.J.; Barkham, M.; McMillan, D.; Bee, P. Are there interactional differences between telephone and face-to-face psychological therapy? A systematic review of comparative studies. *J. Affect. Disord.* **2020**, *265*, 120–131. [CrossRef]
2. Wind, T.R.; Rijkeboer, M.; Andersson, G.; Riper, H. The COVID-19 pandemic: The 'black swan' for mental health care and a turning point for e-health. *Internet Interv.* **2020**, *20*, 100317. [CrossRef]
3. Bao, Y.; Sun, Y.; Meng, S.; Shi, J.; Lu, L. 2019-nCoV epidemic: Address mental health care to empower society. *Lancet* **2020**, *395*, e37–e38. [CrossRef]
4. Galea, S.; Merchant, R.M.; Lurie, N. The mental health consequences of COVID-19 and physical distancing: The need for prevention and early intervention. *JAMA Intern. Med.* **2020**, *180*, 817–818. [CrossRef]
5. Fiorillo, A.; Gorwood, P. The consequences of the COVID-19 pandemic on mental health and implications for clinical practice. *Eur. Psychiatry* **2020**, *63*, e32. [CrossRef]
6. Humer, E.; Stippl, P.; Pieh, C.; Pryss, R.; Probst, T. Experiences of Psychotherapists with Remote Psychotherapy during the COVID-19 Pandemic: Cross-sectional Web-Based Survey Study. *J. Med. Internet Res.* **2020**, *22*, e20246. [CrossRef] [PubMed]
7. Békés, V.; Aafjes-van Doorn, K.; Zilcha-Mano, S.; Prout, T.; Hoffman, L. Psychotherapists' acceptance of telepsychotherapy during the COVID-19 pandemic: A machine learning approach. *Clin. Psychol. Psychother.* **2021**, *28*, 1403–1415. [CrossRef] [PubMed]
8. Topooco, N.; Riper, H.; Araya, R.; Berking, M.; Brunn, M.; Chevreul, K.; Cieslak, R.; Ebert, D.D.; Etchmendy, E.; Herrero, R.; et al. E-COMPARED consortium. Attitudes towards digital treatment for depression: A European stakeholder survey. *Internet Interv.* **2017**, *8*, 1–9. [CrossRef]

9. Békés, V.; Aafjes-van Doorn, K. Psychotherapists' attitudes toward online therapy during the COVID-19 pandemic. *J. Psychother. Integr.* **2020**, *30*, 238–247. [CrossRef]
10. Simpson, S.G.; Reid, C.L. Therapeutic alliance in videoconferencing psychotherapy: A review. *Aust. J. Rural. Health* **2014**, *22*, 280–299. [CrossRef] [PubMed]
11. Haddouk, L.; Milcent, C. Telepsychology in France since COVID-19. Training as key factor for telepsychology practice and psychologists' satisfaction in online consultations. *HAL Sci. Hum. Soc.* 2021; preprint.
12. Cantone, D.; Guerriera, C.; Architravo, M.; Alfano, Y.M.; Cioffi, V.; Moretto, E.; Mosca, L.L.; Longobardi, T.; Muzii, B.; Maldonato, N.M.; et al. A sample of Italian psychotherapists express their perception and opinions of online psychotherapy during the COVID-19 pandemic. *Riv. Psichiatr.* **2021**, *56*, 198–204. [PubMed]
13. Roesler, C. Tele-analysis: The use of media technology in psychotherapy and its impact on the therapeutic relationship. *J. Anal. Psychol.* **2017**, *62*, 372–394. [CrossRef] [PubMed]
14. Mendes-Santos, C.; Weiderpass, E.; Santana, R.; Andersson, G. Portuguese Psychologists' attitudes towards internet interventions: An exploratory cross-sectional study. *JMIR Ment. Health* **2020**, *7*, e16817. [CrossRef] [PubMed]
15. Perle, J.G.; Langsam, L.C.; Randel, A.; Lutchman, S.; Levine, A.B.; Odland, A.P.; Nierenberg, B.; Marker, C.D. Attitudes toward psychological telehealth: Current and future clinical psychologists' opinions of internet-based interventions. *J. Clin. Psychol.* **2013**, *69*, 100–113. [CrossRef] [PubMed]
16. Stoll, J.; Müller, J.A.; Trachsel, M. Ethical issues in online psychotherapy: A narrative review. *Front. Psychiatry* **2020**, *10*, 993. [CrossRef] [PubMed]
17. Sperandeo, R.; Esposito, A.; Maldonato, N.M.; Dell'Orco, S. Analyzing correlations between personality disorders and frontal functions: A pilot study. In *International Workshop on Neural Networks*; Springer: Cham, Switzerland, 2015.
18. Coco, M.; Buscemi, A.; Guerrera, C.S.; Licitra, C.; Pennisi, E.; Vettor, V.; Rizzi, L.; Bovo, P.; Fecarotta, P.; Dell'Orco, S.; et al. Touch and communication in the institutionalized elderly. In Proceedings of the 10th IEEE International Conference on Cognitive Infocomunications (CogInfoCom), Naples, Italy, 23–25 October 2019; pp. 451–458.
19. De Witte, N.A.J.; Carlbring, P.; Etzelmueller, A.; Nordgreen, T.; Karekla, M.; Haddouk, L.; Belmont, A.; Øverland, S.; Abi-Habib, R.; Bernaerts, S.; et al. Online consultations in mental healthcare during the COVID-19 outbreak: An international survey study on professionals' motivations and perceived barriers. *Internet Interv.* **2021**, *26*, 100405. [CrossRef]
20. Van Daele, T.; Karekla, M.; Kassianos, A.P.; Compare, A.; Haddouk, L.; Salgado, J.; Ebert, D.D.; Trebbi, G.; Bernaerts, S.; Van Assche, E.; et al. Recommendations for policy and practice of telepsychotherapy and e-mental health in Europe and beyond. *J. Psychother. Integr.* **2020**, *30*, 160–173. [CrossRef]
21. Kannampallil, T.M.J. Digital Translucence: Adapting Telemedicine Delivery Post-COVID-19. *Telemed. J. e-Health.* **2020**, *26*, 1120–1122. [CrossRef]
22. Shaw, S.; Wherton, J.; Vijayaraghavan, S.; Morris, J.; Bhattacharya, S.; Hanson, P.; Campbell-Richards, D.; Ramoutar, S.; Collard, A.; Hodkinson, I.; et al. Advantages and limitations of virtual online consultations in a NHS acute trust: The VOCAL mixed-methods study. *Health Serv. Deliv. Res.* **2018**, *6*. [CrossRef]
23. Moser, A.; Korstjens, I. Series: Practical guidance to qualitative research. Part 1: Introduction. *Eur. J. Gen. Pract.* **2017**, *23*, 271–273. [CrossRef]
24. Polit, D.F.; Beck, C.T. *Nursing Research: Generating and Assessing Evidence for Nursing Practice*, 10th ed.; Lippincott, Williams & Wilkins: Philadelphia, PA, USA, 2017.
25. Moser, A.; Korstjens, I. Series: Practical guidance to qualitative research. Part 3: Sampling, data collection and analysis. *Eur. J. Gen. Pract.* **2018**, *24*, 9–18. [CrossRef] [PubMed]
26. De Jonckheere, M.; Robinson, C.H.; Evans, L.; Lowery, J.; Youles, B.; Tremblay, A.; Kelley, C.; Sussman, J.B. Designing for Clinical Change: Creating an Intervention to Implement New Statin Guidelines in a Primary Care Clinic. *JMIR Hum. Factors* **2018**, *24*, e19. [CrossRef] [PubMed]
27. Goldsmith, L.J. Using Framework Analysis in Applied Qualitative Research. *Qual. Rep.* **2021**, *26*, 2061–2076. [CrossRef]
28. Gale, N.K.; Heath, G.; Cameron, E.; Rashid, S.; Redwood, S. Using the framework method for the analysis of qualitative data in multi-disciplinary health research. *BMC Med Res Methodol.* **2013**, *18*, 117. [CrossRef] [PubMed]
29. Furber, C. Framework analysis: A method for analyzing qualitative data. *AJM* **2010**, *4*, 97–100. [CrossRef]
30. Tong, A.; Sainsbury, P.; Craig, J. Consolidated criteria for reporting qualitative research (COREQ): A 32-item checklist for interviews and focus groups. *Int. J. Qual. Health Care* **2007**, *19*, 349–357. [CrossRef] [PubMed]
31. Donovan, C.L.; Poole, C.; Boyes, N.; Redgate, J.; March, S. Australian mental health worker attitudes towards cCBT: What is the role of knowledge? Are there differences? Can we change them? *Internet Interv.* **2015**, *2*, 372–381. [CrossRef]
32. Juhos, C.; Mészáros, J. Psychoanalytic psychotherapy and its supervision via videoconference: Experience, questions and dilemmas. *Am. J. Psychoanal.* **2019**, *79*, 555–576. [CrossRef]
33. Scharff, J.S. (Ed.) *Psychoanalysis Online: Mental Health, Teletherapy, and Training*; Routledge: London, UK, 2018.
34. Feijt, M.A.; de Kort, Y.A.; Bongers, I.M.; IJsselsteijn, W.A. Perceived Drivers and Barriers to the Adoption of eMental Health by Psychologists: The Construction of the Levels of Adoption of eMental Health Model. *J. Med. Internet Res.* **2018**, *20*, e153. [CrossRef]
35. Hedman, E.; Ljótsson, B.; Rück, C.; Bergström, J.; Andersson, G.; Kaldo, V.; El Alaoui, S. Effectiveness of Internet-based cognitive behaviour therapy for panic disorder in routine psychiatric care. *Acta Psychiatr. Scand.* **2013**, *128*, 457–467. [CrossRef]

36. Glueckauf, R.L.; Maheu, M.M.; Drude, K.P.; Wells, B.A.; Wang, Y.; Gustafson, D.J.; Nelson, E.L. Survey of psychologists' telebehavioral health practices: Technology use, ethical issues, and training needs. *Prof. Psychol. Res. Pract.* **2018**, *49*, 205–219. [CrossRef]
37. Cipolletta, S.; Mocellin, D. Online counseling: An exploratory survey of Italian psychologists' attitudes towards new ways of interaction. *Psychother. Res.* **2018**, *28*, 909–924. [CrossRef] [PubMed]
38. Tuna, B.; Avci, O.H. Qualitative analysis of university counselors' online counseling experiences during the COVID-19 pandemic. *Curr. Psychol.* **2023**, *42*, 8489–8503. [CrossRef] [PubMed]
39. Dores, A.R.; Geraldo, A.; Carvalho, I.P.; Barbosa, F. The Use of New Digital Information and Communication Technologies in Psychological Counseling during the COVID-19 Pandemic. *Int. J. Environ. Res. Public. Health* **2020**, *17*, 7663. [CrossRef]
40. Gangamma, R.; Walia, B.; Luke, M.; Lucena, C. Continuation of Teletherapy After the COVID-19 Pandemic: Survey Study of Licensed Mental Health Professionals. *JMIR Form. Res.* **2022**, *6*, e32419. [CrossRef] [PubMed]
41. Hardy, N.; Maier, C.; Gregson, T. Couple teletherapy in the era of COVID-19: Experiences and recommendations. *J. Marital. Fam. Ther.* **2021**, *47*, 225–243. [CrossRef]
42. Wester, S.R.; Vogel, D.L. Working with the masculine mystique: Male gender role conflict, counseling self-efficacy, and the training of male psychologists. *Prof. Psychol. Res. Pract.* **2002**, *33*, 370–376. [CrossRef]

Disclaimer/Publisher's Note: The statements, opinions and data contained in all publications are solely those of the individual author(s) and contributor(s) and not of MDPI and/or the editor(s). MDPI and/or the editor(s) disclaim responsibility for any injury to people or property resulting from any ideas, methods, instructions or products referred to in the content.

Article

Fatigue among Greek Parents of Children with Autistic Spectrum Disorder: The Roles of Spirituality and Social Support

Eugenia Halki, Maria Kapiri, Sotirios Plakas, Chrysoula Tsiou, Ourania Govina, Petros Galanis and Victoria Alikari *

Post Graduate Program "Management of Chronic Diseases- Neurosciences", Department of Nursing, University of West Attica, 12243 Athens, Greece; euhalki@gmail.com (E.H.); stkts23@gmail.com (M.K.); skplakas@uniwa.gr (S.P.); ctsiou@uniwa.gr (C.T.); ugovina@uniwa.gr (O.G.); pegalan@nurs.uoa.gr (P.G.)
* Correspondence: vicalikari@uniwa.gr

Abstract: The high demands of caring for and raising a child with autism spectrum disorder on a daily basis may lead parents to physical and mental fatigue. This study aimed to assess the effect of social support and spirituality on the fatigue of parents with children with autistic spectrum disorder. A cross-sectional study with a convenience sample was conducted in Schools of Special Education in Attica (Greece). The sample consisted of 123 parents who completed The Fatigue Assessment Scale (FAS), the Multidimensional Scale of Perceived Social Support (MSPSS), and the Functional Assessment of Chronic Illness Therapy Spiritual Well-Being Scale (FACIT Sp-12) to measure the levels of fatigue, social support, and spirituality, respectively. The Pearson correlation coefficient was used to investigate the relationship between the quantitative variables. To study the effect of social support and spirituality on fatigue, multivariable linear regression was applied. The mean age was 47.3 years old, 81.3% were women, and 38.9% stated "Close/Very close faith toward God". Higher levels of total MSPSS and FACIT Sp-12 were associated with lower total FAS (r = −0.50, p < 0.001 and r = −0.49, p < 0.001, respectively). Social support and spirituality were significant predictors of fatigue.

Keywords: autism spectrum disorder; fatigue; parents; social support; spirituality

1. Introduction

Caring for a child with autism spectrum disorder (ASD) is an extremely stressful experience, leading to a burdened daily life for both the parents and the rest of the family environment. The variety of problems that accompany ASD can cause a dramatic wave of changes in the lives of parents by affecting their emotional, social, and family lives in a multifaceted way. The high demands of raising a child with ASD lead to physical and mental fatigue for parents, as opposed to parents with children of normal development [1,2].

The perception of fatigue is characterized as multidimensional, subjective, and unpleasant, an experience that is difficult to define. This fact is attributed mainly to the subjective nature of the concept, and as a result, several different definitions and measurements arise [3]. One of the predominant emotions experienced by parents of children with ASD is complete exhaustion, which is not just related to the physical fatigue that a parent may feel from daily obligations but also to the inability to regulate autistic behavior [4]. Parents of children with ASD show higher levels of fatigue than parents of children with normal development. In cases where children have sleep disorders, nocturnal awakenings, and intense hyperactivity during the day, parents report severe symptoms of physical exertion, but also loss of control [5]. Fatigue experienced by parents of children with ASD is associated with high levels of stress [6], poor quality of sleep, inadequate social functioning, and poor physical and mental well-being [7]. In addition, maternal fatigue and stress can enhance children's problem behaviors and, in turn, increase the levels of fatigue that parents already feel [1]. According to the literature, it seems that mothers experience child behavior problems in a different way than fathers [8]. Mothers of children with ASD encountered higher levels of distress due to their child's behavior, care, anxiety, and inadequate communication abilities. Conversely, fathers are primarily impacted by distressing events unrelated to their child's disability, such as concerns regarding their professional trajectory or the family's financial stability [9].

The arrival of a child with ASD affects family relationships both between their own members and the wider social environment [10]. Parents believe that their experiences of raising a child with a developmental disorder are different from those of their relatives and friends who are raising normally developing children. Thus, they are differentiated from other parents and, therefore, feel lonely and isolated [11]. To overcome this problem, the parents' access to various social support resources is an extremely beneficial coping strategy against the stressful situations helping them to cope more successfully with the demands of their child's raising [12]. Support is provided by formal (e.g., the state or related organizations that aim to address the needs of the child with ASD and his family) and informal support resources (the wider family and friendly environment of the family [13]. The material help of family members may not be as important as their understanding of ASD and the acceptance of the child with ASD [14]. The perceived social support from various sources such as family or friends seems to be associated with lower levels of stress, and higher levels of quality of life, especially for mothers of children with ASD [15]. Therefore, it seems that social support has been associated with enhancing the mental and physical resilience of parents and consequently with improved and better quality of care for their child [16].

Spirituality is a multidimensional concept, which is difficult to define because of its different aspects. Quite often, the term spirituality is confused with religiosity. Religiosity is related to the acceptance of specific ritual practices and beliefs within an organized religion [17]. In contrast, spirituality is more as it constitutes a human phenomenon that potentially exists in all people and thus differs from religiosity. Essentially, spirituality is about a personal search within and outside of a religious context. This fact also explains that the spiritual life is not a privilege only for people who follow a religious doctrine [18]. The international literature emphasizes the importance of understanding parents' spiritual beliefs, values, and priorities as the cornerstone of compensating for the negative effects. Spirituality reflects relationships with ourselves, with other people, with God, and with nature [19], while at the same time being associated with a deep sense of peace and satisfaction [20]. Moreover, recent research has concluded that high levels of spirituality in parents of children with special educational needs or wider disabilities are strongly linked to improved dimensions of mental health. Spirituality strengthens them for coping with difficult psychosomatic situations in which they feel pressure under the weight of obligations, fear, anxiety, despair, shame, or even depression [21]. Through their involvement with faith, parents may draw strength to face adversity and adopt a more optimistic approach to life and they may come to experience relief from some of their emotional challenges through prayer [22]. Most parents, through spirituality, can reconsider their perceptions of their child's disability and turn it from a personal tragedy into a divine gift. They feel that the disability of their children is a blessing from God and that it was given to them by a higher power because of the parental skills they have [23].

As far as it is known, no previous research, not only in Greece but also worldwide, has studied these three variables in parents of children with ASD. Therefore, in order to fill the gap in the literature, the aim of this study was to explore the levels of fatigue, spirituality, and social support among parents of children with ASD. In addition, the relationship between these variables as well as the effect of spirituality, social support, and demographic characteristics on parents' fatigue was studied. According to the above literature, it was hypothesized that spirituality and social support would be significant predictors of fatigue.

2. Materials and Methods

This is a quantitative, descriptive, cross-sectional study conducted between September and November 2020. The cross-sectional nature of this study is supported by the literature among different populations [24–26].

The subjects of this study were parents of children with functioning autism who attend three Schools of Special Education (Secondary and High Schools) in Attica (the most populated county of Greece), Greece. The selection of this sample was based on the ease of access and approach of this population (convenience sampling) as the researchers are school nurses. The questionnaires were completed: (i) in the morning after the children were handed over to the teachers, and (ii) at noon while the parents were waiting for the finishing of school. Thus, the children could not see the questionnaires. Each parent was individually given a desk in a separate room where each parent could answer the questions without one parent being influenced by the other. The questionnaires were completed by one or both parents. The inclusion criteria were: (a) be parents of children with functional autism who were attending Schools of Special Education of Attica, (b) be able to read and understand the Greek language, (c) give consent to participate in this study, and (d) be time and space oriented. Parents with cognitive or psychological disorders, vision loss, and parents of children with other physical or mental disorders such as epilepsy, intellectual disability, and attention-deficit hyperactivity disorder were excluded from this study since these disorders are the subject of different studies. All 140 parents (both mothers and fathers) were recruited in this study of which 135 were eligible. Of these, 12 parents did not agree to take part in this study. Finally, 123 questionnaires were completed. The questionnaires were provided by the researchers who are school nurses. Each parent completed the questionnaires once.

The current study complied with the fundamental ethical principles governing the conduct of research. The permission to collect personal data was secured by the Institute of Educational Policy (http://iep.edu.gr/en/ accessed on 7 January 24) (Approval No: 50154/Δ3/30 April 2020). A meeting of the school teachers' association was held and after receiving positive written suggestions, the questionnaires were provided to the parents and were completed by the parents who wished to participate in this study. Written informed consent was approved by participants. The confidentiality of the information concerning the parents and students of the school was maintained. The parents were informed that the security and anonymity of the relevant material would be preserved and that the results would be used exclusively for the purposes of this research and only by the researchers.

To assess fatigue, social support, and spirituality, the following scales were used:

The Fatigue Assessment Scale (FAS) is structured by 10 items in a five-point Likert scale (1 = never to 5 = always) and examines the levels of perceived fatigue. The scores from the ten items were summed, with the total scores ranging from 10 to 50. For the extraction of the score, the answers of the participants were added. Participants with a score < 22 were classified as "non-fatigued", 22–34 as "fatigued" and 35–50 as "extremely fatigued". In this study, the total score was used (ranging from 10 to 50). Five questions are related to physical and five to mental fatigue [27]. It takes two minutes to complete. In addition, studies report the internal consistency and reliability of the FAS both in healthy (Cronbach's alpha 0.90) [27] and in patients (Cronbach's alpha 0.88) [28]. It has also been used among parents of children with ASD [1]. The psychometric properties of the Greek version have been tested in chronic disease patients with a Cronbach's alpha of 0.761 [29] and 0.825 [30].

The Multidimensional Scale of Perceived Social Support (MSPSS) [31] consists of 12 items, which are answered on a seven-point Likert scale (1 strongly disagree to 7 strongly agree). The tool evaluates three sources of social support: Family, Friends, and Significant Others. Each of the above sources is evaluated based on 4 items. The total score ranges between 1 and 7 and is obtained from the sum of the scores and divided by the number of items. The high score reflects higher levels of perceived social support. It is short, easy to use, and understandable even in low-educated populations. In addition, as reported in the research of Zimet et al. [31], the MSPSS shows good internal consistency in different groups of subjects. The scale has been used in Greek patients [32] and healthy populations [33] with very good internal consistency according to Cronbach's alpha (0.93) [34].

The Functional Assessment of Chronic Illness Therapy-Spiritual Well-Being Scale-12 non-illness (FACIT Sp-12) adapted to the general population is a self-administered questionnaire constructed in 1990 [35] as a short tool for assessing three domains of spirituality: Peace, Meaning of Life, and Faith. It is structured by 12 items on a five-point Likert scale (0 = not at all to 4 = a lot). The questions concern the period of the last 7 days. The total score is derived from the sum of the answers, with the highest scores indicating higher levels of spirituality. The tool has been translated into several languages, including Greek with a Cronbach's alpha of 0.77 [36].

Finally, data related to sociodemographic characteristics were recorded.

Categorical variables are described using absolute (*n*) and relative (%) frequencies, while quantitative variables are summarized by their mean, standard deviation, minimum, and maximum values. When exploring the association between two quantitative variables that exhibit a normal distribution, the Pearson correlation coefficient was utilized. We considered spirituality, social support, and demographic characteristics as the independent variables. Parents' fatigue was the dependent variable. First, we conducted bivariate analysis between the independent variables and the dependent variable. Then, variables with a *p*-value < 0.2 in the bivariate analysis were included in a multivariable linear regression model with fatigue scores as the dependent variables. We applied the backward stepwise method to identify statistically significant relationships ($p < 0.05$). In the multivariable models, we present unstandardized and standardized b coefficients, 95% confidence intervals, and *p*-values. Moreover, we performed one-way analysis of variance to investigate the impact of closeness to God with continuous variables. Due to limited numbers, we merged the categories "Not at all close faith toward God" and "Too little faith toward God" and the categories "Close faith toward God" and "Very close faith toward God". Statistical significance was set at the level of 0.05. Data analysis was applied using IBM SPSS 21.0 (Statistical Package for Social Sciences, SPSS Inc., Chicago, IL, USA).

3. Results

The study population included 123 participants. The mean age was 47.3 years, 81.3% were women, 77.2% were married, and 20 (18.6%) participants were married to each other. A percentage of 95.9% were Orthodox Christians and 38.9% stated that they feel "Close faith toward God"/Very close faith toward God". The sociodemographic characteristics of the parents are presented in Table 1.

Regarding the levels of fatigue, social support, and spirituality, the mean values of the three scales indicated moderate levels of total fatigue (mean 28.41, SD = 7.51), relatively high levels of total spirituality (mean 31.51, SD = 8.73), and very low levels of total social support (mean 5.16, SD = 1.12) (Table 2). Participants appeared to have experienced higher levels of physical fatigue (mean 20.81, SD = 5.80) compared to mental fatigue (mean 8.92, SD = 1.60). The majority evaluated positively the dimensions of spirituality and especially Peace (mean 12.91, SD = 3.01). The most important source of social support was Significant Others (mean 5.23, SD = 1.20).

As far as the correlations between the three variables are concerned, the results showed that both social support and spirituality were negatively associated with fatigue. Table 3 shows that higher levels of total FACIT Sp-12 were associated with lower levels of total fatigue (r = −0.49, $p < 0.001$). Also, higher levels of MSPSS were associated with lower levels of total FAS (r = −0.50, $p < 0.001$). Negative correlations were also observed between all the dimensions of FAS and all the dimensions of MSPSS and FACIT Sp-12. In addition, higher levels of total MSPSS were associated with higher levels of total FACIT Sp-12 (r = 0.51, $p < 0.001$). Also, positive correlations emerged between all the dimensions of MSPSS and all the dimensions of FACIT Sp-12.

Table 1. Participants' demographic characteristics.

	N	%
Gender		
Males	23	18.6
Females	100	81.3
Age *		47.3 (6.3)
Marital status		
Married (individuals)	75	60.9
Married (10) couples	20	16.2
Divorced	23	18.9
Unmarried	1	0.81
Widows	3	2.5
Children (either with ASD or not)		
1	33	26.8
2	72	58.5
>2	18	14.6
Educational level		
Secondary School	18	14.6
High School	52	42.2
University	32	26.0
MSc/Ph.D.	18	14.6
Employment status		
State employee	37	30.0
Private employee	49	39.8
Unemployed	21	17.0
Household	4	3.25
Retired	6	4.87
Freelance	5	4.2
Faith toward God		
Not at all close	4	3.25
Too little close	29	23.5
Little close	42	34.1
Close	12	9.75
Very close	36	29.2

* Mean (standard deviation).

Table 2. The descriptive characteristics of the scales.

Scales	Mean	SD *	Min	Max
FAS				
Physical Fatigue (theoretical range 5–25)	20.81	5.80	8	32
Mental Fatigue (theoretical range 5–25)	8.92	1.60	5	13
Total FAS (theoretical range 10–50)	28.41	7.51	11	43
MSPSS				
Significant Others (theoretical range 1–7)	5.23	1.20	1	7
Family (theoretical range 1–7)	5.12	1.31	1	7
Friends (theoretical range 1–7)	5.01	1.29	1	7
Total MSPSS (theoretical range 1–7)	5.16	1.12	1	7
FACIT Sp-12				
Peace (theoretical range 0–16)	12.91	3.01	3	16
Meaning of Life (theoretical range 0–16)	8.80	4.01	2	16
Faith (theoretical range 0–16)	9.89	3.91	1	16
Total FACIT Sp-12 (theoretical range 0–48)	31.51	8.73	10	46

* Standard Deviation.

Table 3. The correlations between fatigue, social support, and spirituality.

Scales	Physical Fatigue	Mental Fatigue	Total FAS	Significant Others	Family	Friends	Total MSPSS
Significant Others	−0.40 (<0.001)	−0.21 (0.02)	−0.46 (<0.001)		0.86 (<0.001)	0.62 (<0.001)	0.94 (<0.001)
Family	−0.41 (<0.001)	−0.29 (<0.001)	−0.47 (<0.001)			0.54 (<0.001)	0.91 (<0.001)
Friends	−0.38 (<0.001)	−0.24 (0.007)	−0.40 (<0.001)				0.81 (<0.001)
Total MSPSS	−0.45 (<0.001)	−0.28 (<0.001)	−0.50 (<0.001)				
Meaning of Life	−0.34 (<0.001)	−0.14 (0.1)	−0.38 (<0.001)	0.54 (<0.001)	0.47 (<0.001)	0.31 (<0.001)	0.50 (<0.001)
Peace	−0.55 (<0.001)	−0.31 (<0.001)	−0.56 (<0.001)	0.45 (<0.001)	0.56 (<0.001)	0.40 (<0.001)	0.53 (<0.001)
Faith	−0.21 (0.02)	−0.10 (0.2)	−0.24 (0.01)	0.22 (<0.001)	0.30 (0.01)	0.10 (0.5)	0.22 (0.01)
Total FACIT Sp-12	−0.46 (<0.001)	−0.24 (0.007)	−0.49 (<0.001)	0.49 (<0.001)	0.55 (<0.001)	0.32 (<0.001)	0.51 (<0.001)

Values are expressed as Pearson's correlation coefficient (p-value).

After bivariable analyses, statistical relationships emerged at the level of 0.20 ($p < 0.20$) between independent variables (spirituality, social support, and demographics) and total fatigue and its dimensions. For this reason, multivariable linear regressions were applied with total FAS and its dimensions as dependent variables and FACIT Sp-12, MSPSS as independent variables along with demographics. It is observed that Peace and support from Significant Others can positively affect total fatigue since higher levels of Peace were associated with a lower total FAS Score ($p < 0.001$) and higher levels of support from Significant Others were associated with a lower total FAS Score ($p = 0.008$). Also, gender (female) had a significant influence as mothers had a higher total FAS Score than fathers ($p = 0.001$) (Table 4). One-way analysis of variance confirmed that "Close faith toward God" was not related to total FAS ($p = 0.759$). The mean total FAS Score for those with "Not at all/Too little close faith toward God" was 29.21 (SD: 8.33), 28.20 (SD: 7.65) for those with "Little close faith toward God", and 27.95 (SD: 7.00) for those with "Close/Very close faith toward God".

Table 4. Multivariable linear regression analysis with total fatigue as the dependent variable and social support, spirituality, and demographic characteristics as independent variables.

Independent Variables	Standardized Coefficient Beta	Unstandardized Coefficient Beta	95% CI *		p-Value
			Lower	Upper	
Mothers compared to fathers	0.32	4.81	2.11	7.60	0.001
Peace	−0.43	−0.80	−1.14	−0.51	<0.001
Significant Others	−0.20	−1.35	−2.37	−0.46	0.008

The above variables explained 42% of the variability of total FAS. * Confidence interval.

In addition, investigating physical fatigue as dependent and FACIT Sp-12, MSPSS as independent variables, a positive effect on fatigue emerged since the higher levels of Peace were associated with lower physical fatigue ($p < 0.001$). Also, mothers experienced higher physical fatigue than fathers ($p = 0.002$) (Table 5). One-way analysis of variance confirmed that "Close faith toward God" was not related to physical fatigue ($p = 0.885$). The mean physical fatigue score for those with "Not at all/Too little close faith toward God" was 21.11 (SD: 6.36), 20.57 (SD: 5.90) for those with "Little close faith toward God", and 20.79 (SD: 5.49) for those with "Close/Very close faith toward God".

Table 5. Multivariable linear regression with physical fatigue as the dependent variable and social support, spirituality, and demographic characteristics as independent variables.

Independent Variables	Standardized Coefficient Beta	Unstandardized Coefficient Beta	95% CI *		p-Value
			Lower	Upper	
Mothers compared to fathers	0.24	4.30	1.61	6.90	0.002
Peace	−0.50	−0.71	−0.93	−0.41	<0.001

The above variables explained 37% of the variability of physical fatigue. * Confidence interval.

Similarly, the high level of social support from Family positively affects mental fatigue since an increase in support from Family was associated with an increase in the mental fatigue score ($p < 0.003$). A high educational level was associated with an increase in mental fatigue score ($p < 0.008$), and mothers experienced higher levels of mental fatigue than fathers ($p = 0.01$) (Table 6). One-way analysis of variance confirmed that "Close faith toward God" was not related to mental fatigue ($p = 0.810$). The mean mental fatigue score for those with "Not at all/Too little faith toward God" was 9.01 (SD: 1.72), 8.89 (SD: 1.80) for those with "Little faith toward God", and 8.81 (SD: 1.50) for those with "Close/Very close faith toward God".

Table 6. Multivariable linear regression with mental fatigue as the dependent variable and social support, spirituality, and demographic characteristics as independent variables.

Independent Variables	Standardized Coefficient Beta	Unstandardized Coefficient Beta	95% CI * Lower	95% CI * Upper	p-Value
Mothers compared to fathers	0.21	0.92	0.25	1.64	0.01
Educational level	0.20	0.34	0.08	0.51	<0.008
Family Support	−0.37	−0.36	−0.51	−0.10	0.003

The above variables explained 21% of the variability of mental fatigue. * Confidence interval.

Participants with a lower educational level and a higher "Close faith toward God" had higher scores of total FACIT Sp-12 ($\beta = -1.61$, CI: -2.60 to -0.51, $p = 0.005$ and $\beta = 2.50$, CI: 1.41 to 3.72, $p < 0.001$, respectively) (Table 7). One-way analysis of variance confirmed that "Close faith toward God" was related to total FACIT Sp-12 ($p < 0.001$). The mean total FACIT-Sp-12 Score for those with "Not at all/Too little close faith to God" was 27.01 (SD: 8.82), 30.90 (SD: 7.26) for those with "Little close faith toward God", and 35.17 (SD: 8.55) for those with "Close/very close faith toward God".

Table 7. Multivariable linear regression with total FACIT Sp-12 as the dependent variable and social support, and demographic characteristics as independent variables.

Independent Variables	Standardized Coefficient Beta	Unstandardized Coefficient Beta	95% CI * Lower	95% CI * Upper	p-Value
Educational level	−0.22	−1.61	−2.60	−0.51	0.005
Close faith toward God	0.43	2.50	1.41	3.72	<0.001

The above variables explained 18% of the variability of total FACIT Sp-12. * Confidence interval.

Regarding the differences between mothers and fathers, mothers scored higher (mean 29.65, SD: 6.83) on the total FAS than fathers (mean 22.96, SD: 6.84), ($p = 0.001$, Hedge's g = 0.99), higher on the physical fatigue scale (mean 21.61, SD: 5.55) than fathers (mean 17.00, SD: 5.82), ($p = 0.001$, Hedge's g = 0.83), and also higher on mental fatigue (mean 9.16, SD: 1.66) than fathers (mean 7.85, SD: 1.60) ($p = 0.001$, Hedge's g = 0.81).

4. Discussion

The current study was conducted among parents of children with ASD and investigated the effect of spirituality and social support on the levels of fatigue. This study is significant, as the lack of spirituality and social support may negatively affect parental fatigue leading to inadequate care for children with ASD [37].

According to the results, the parents experienced moderate levels of total fatigue and spirituality and very low levels of social support. Regarding fatigue, participants reported higher levels of physical fatigue and lower levels of mental fatigue. This finding is in line with the findings of the empirical study of Giallo et al. [1]. The moderate levels of parental fatigue in this study seem to be proportional to the severity of the cognitive and behavioral deficits of ASD considering that the sample of this study consisted of parents of children with functioning autism. In terms of spirituality, parents reported higher spirituality based on the dimensions of Peace, followed by Faith and Meaning of Life. Also, the dimension of Significant Others was the most important source of social support followed by Family and Friends. Nevertheless, other studies have identified Friends and Family as the most important sources of social support [38,39].

As far as the relationships between the three variables are concerned, it emerged that the higher total social support and its dimensions were associated with lower total fatigue and its dimensions. Similar findings were presented by Ardic [40], who observed a significant prevalence of exhaustion in parents receiving mitigated social support. In addition, as shown in other studies [37], the perceived social support received by parents of children with ASD appears to be associated with mental and physical well-being, resilience, and higher quality of life. Higher levels of social support were negatively associated with fatigue, stress, and depression in parents of children with ASD. Thus, these results reflect the importance of informal support networks, as an important strategy for dealing with the mental and physical effects of ASD [37].

Also, a negative correlation was found between fatigue and spirituality as the higher the spirituality levels the lower the fatigue levels. This finding is in line with the finding of a study [41] in which mothers of children with mental disabilities who took spiritual self-care training experienced a reduced burden of care. There is a sense that in the course of time, parents change the way they perceive their child's disorder and the world. It has been reported that parents of children with disabilities embrace a wide range of positive change, seek answers to questions such as the meaning and purpose of life [42], and acquire personal gifts such as strengthening religious beliefs and greater appreciation even for simpler things in life.

From the findings of this study, it seems that the higher total social support, support from Significant Others, Family, and Friends was associated with higher spirituality based on the dimensions of Meaning of Life, Peace, and Faith. In a previous study [43], the negative correlation between spirituality and social support was attributed to the fact that parents who experienced social isolation were more likely to seek spiritual support. In addition, spiritual pursuits were used more as a means of escape from the daily difficulties and burden of caring for a child with ASD. However, a positive correlation has been observed between social support and spirituality among different populations [44]. This relationship may be attributed to the fact that spiritual beliefs and religious behaviors encourage involvement in social support.

Concerning the effect of spirituality on fatigue levels, it was found that spirituality plays a significant positive role in mental and physical fatigue. Parents with higher levels of Meaning of Life, Peace, and Faith showed lower levels of total, physical and mental fatigue. Similarly, researchers [18] observed higher levels of resilience, sense of coherence, and adjustment in parents of children with ASD who had received some spiritual lessons. Similar results have been presented in previous studies [1,45], emphasizing the significant role of spiritual well-being in the improvement of various dimensions of the psychological sphere such as anxiety, lack of satisfaction, and depression. It seems that parents, through spirituality, face the problem with a positive attitude as they focus more on the positive dimensions and contributions of their child with ASD [46]. This fact may be able to alleviate perceived fatigue.

Regarding the effect of gender on fatigue levels, the present study shows that mothers experience more physical and mental fatigue than fathers. This finding seems to be consistent with other studies [47] which have shown that mothers experience the care of burden and symptoms of fatigue more often than fathers. In addition, according to Nacul et al. [48], fathers seem to be influenced more on a mental level, and women on a physical level. The strategies that parents apply in order to meet the requirements of the parental role differ between mother and father due to particular individual characteristics and differences in family circumstances. The intense fatigue among mothers is probably attributed to the mother's sense of guilt, the concern for the child's excessive dependence on the family, and the lack of resilience which leads to adjustment difficulties [49].

Finally, according to other results from the present study, it appears that the higher degree of religiosity and the low level of education had a positive effect on overall spirituality. Regarding religiosity, other studies [20] have suggested that engaging in metaphysical transcendence, spiritual beliefs, and prayer alleviates emotions, improves, and promotes the mental health of parents of children with ASD or other special educational needs.

The sample of this study (convenience sampling) came from schools in Attica; therefore, the generalization of the results may be subject to relevant restrictions. In addition, although the sample size was partially satisfactory, mothers appeared to be the vast majority of participants, which raises significant concerns about the representativeness of the sample. Also, the period of completing the questionnaires (COVID-19 pandemic) may have influenced the objectivity of the views expressed by the parents. However, we should note that the research process was not greatly affected by the COVID-19 pandemic as the special schools in Greece at that period operated in person and not online. Also, the cross-sectional nature of this study and the inability to establish a cause-and-effect relationship could be a limitation. In addition, another limitation of this study is that the researchers and participants knew each other, and therefore social desirability may have played an important role [50]. Future research is suggested that will include clinical data on children and their association with parental fatigue.

5. Conclusions

In conclusion, the present study recorded moderate levels of fatigue and spirituality but also low levels of social support for parents raising a child with ASD. Subsequently, significant negative correlations were observed between fatigue and social support, fatigue and spirituality, and a positive correlation between social support and spirituality. The effect of gender seems to be particularly important as mothers of children with ASD seem to experience fatigue to a greater extent than fathers. The results suggest that social support and spirituality help to reduce perceived fatigue and therefore strengthen the resilience of parents of children with ASD. However, the emphasis on personalized spiritual care remains an important dimension. School nurses can also encourage parents to express their spiritual beliefs and needs as well as their inclusion in organized groups or support and mutual aid networks between parents. The process of acquiring adjustment mechanisms that parents can use to manage the exhaustion caused by their child's stressful demands may be very useful.

Social policies that focus on psycho-educating parents about fatigue and its potential impact on their overall well-being, parenting skills, and caregiving responsibilities are recommended. In addition, implementing strategies to moderate the promotion of healthy behaviors and enhance opportunities for social support may also prove beneficial for parents.

Author Contributions: Conceptualization, V.A., M.K. and E.H.; methodology, V.A.; software, S.P. and P.G.; formal analysis, O.G.; investigation, M.K. and E.H.; data curation, E.H.; writing—original draft preparation, M.K. and E.H.; writing—review and editing, V.A.; supervision, V.A., C.T. and S.P.; project administration, V.A.; All authors have read and agreed to the published version of the manuscript.

Funding: This research received no external funding.

Institutional Review Board Statement: This study was conducted in accordance with the Declaration of Helsinki, and approved by the Ethics Committee of the Institute of Educational Policy (http://iep.edu.gr/en/ accessed on 7 January 2024) (Approval No: 50154/Δ3/30 April 2020) for studies involving humans.

Informed Consent Statement: Informed consent was obtained from all subjects involved in this study.

Data Availability Statement: The data presented in this study are available on request from the corresponding author. The data are not publicly available due to participants' confidentiality.

Conflicts of Interest: The authors declare no conflict of interest.

References

1. Giallo, R.; Wood, C.E.; Jellett, R.; Porter, R. Fatigue, wellbeing and parental self-efficacy in mothers of children with an autism spectrum disorder. *Autism* **2013**, *17*, 465–480. [CrossRef] [PubMed]
2. Begum, R.; Mamin, F.A. Impact of autism spectrum disorder on family. *Autism-Open Access* **2019**, *9*, 244. [CrossRef]
3. Beydoun, J.; Nasrallah, L.; Sabrah, T.; Caboral-Stevens, M. Towards a definition of caregiver fatigue: A concept analysis. *Adv. Nurs. Sci.* **2019**, *42*, 297–306. [CrossRef] [PubMed]
4. Kütük, M.Ö.; Tufan, A.E.; Kılıçaslan, F.; Güler, G.; Çelik, F.; Altıntaş, E.; Gökçen, C.; Karadağ, M.; Yektaş, Ç.; Mutluer, T.; et al. High depression symptoms and burnout levels among parents of children with autism spectrum disorders: A multi-center, cross-sectional, case-control study. *J. Autism Dev. Disord.* **2021**, *51*, 4086–4099. [CrossRef] [PubMed]
5. Benderix, Y.; Nordström, B.; Sivberg, B. Parents' experience of having a child with autism and learning disabilities living in a group home: A case study. *Autism* **2006**, *10*, 629–641. [CrossRef] [PubMed]
6. Miranda, A.; Mira, A.; Berenguer, C.; Rosello, B.; Baixauli, I. Parenting stress in mothers of children with autism without intellectual disability. Mediation of Behavioral Problems and Coping Strategies. *Front. Psychol.* **2019**, *10*, 464. [CrossRef]
7. Mihaila, I.; Hartley, S.L. Parental sleep quality and behavior problems of children with autism. *Autism* **2018**, *22*, 236–244. [CrossRef]
8. Seymour, M.; Wood, C.; Giallo, R.; Jellett, R. Fatigue, stress and coping in mothers of children with an autism spectrum disorder. *J. Autism Dev Disord.* **2013**, *43*, 1547–1554. [CrossRef]
9. Dabrowska, A.; Pisula, E. Parenting stress and coping styles in mothers and fathers of pre-school children with autism and Down syndrome. *J. Intellect. Disabil. Res.* **2010**, *54*, 266–280. [CrossRef]
10. Krieger, B.; Piškur, B.; Schulze, C.; Jakobs, U.; Beurskens, A.; Moser, A. Supporting and hindering environments for participation of adolescents diagnosed with autism spectrum disorder: A scoping review. *PLoS ONE* **2018**, *13*, e0202071. [CrossRef]
11. Ventola, P.; Lei, J.; Paisley, C.; Lebowitz, E.; Silverman, W. Parenting a child with ASD: Comparison of parenting style between ASD, anxiety, and typical development. *J. Autism Dev. Disord.* **2017**, *47*, 2873–2884. [CrossRef] [PubMed]
12. Vernhet, C.; Dellapiazza, F.; Blanc, N.; Cousson-Gélie, F.; Miot, S.; Roeyers, H.; Baghdadli, A. Coping strategies of parents of children with autism spectrum disorder: A systematic review. *Eur. Child Adolesc. Psychiatry* **2019**, *28*, 747–758. [CrossRef]
13. McIntyre, L.L.; Brown, M. Examining the utilisation and usefulness of social support for mothers with young children with autism spectrum disorder. *J. Intellect. Dev. Disabil.* **2018**, *43*, 93–101. [CrossRef]
14. Weiss, J.A.; Cappadocia, M.C.; MacMullin, J.A.; Viecili, M.; Lunsky, Y. The impact of child problem behaviors of children with ASD on parent mental health: The mediating role of acceptance and empowerment. *Autism* **2012**, *16*, 261–274. [CrossRef] [PubMed]
15. Hashir Ahammed, A.V. Quality of life, parental stress & perceived social support among parents of children with autism spectrum disorder. *Int. J. Indian Psychol.* **2021**, *9*, 358–374.
16. Ilias, K.; Cornish, K.; Kummar, A.S.; Park, M.S.; Golden, K.J. Parenting stress and resilience in parents of children with autism spectrum disorder (ASD) in Southeast Asia: A systematic review. *Front. Psychol.* **2018**, *9*, 280. [CrossRef]
17. Koenig, H.G.; King, D.E.; Carson, V.B. *Handbook of Religion and Health*, 2nd ed.; Oxford University Press: New York, NY, USA, 2012.
18. Arrey, A.E.; Bilsen, J.; Lacor, P.; Deschepper, R. Spirituality/Religiosity: A cultural and psychological resource among sub-saharan African migrant women with HIV/AIDS in Belgium. *PLoS ONE* **2016**, *11*, e0159488. [CrossRef]
19. Fradelos, E.C.; Tzavella, F.; Koukia, E.; Papathanasiou, I.V.; Alikari, V.; Stathoulis, J.; Panoutsopoulos, G.; Zyga, S. Integrating chronic kidney disease patient's spirituality in their care: Health benefits and research perspectives. *Mater. Socio Med.* **2015**, *27*, 354. [CrossRef]
20. Duarte, E.D.; Braga, P.P.; Guimarães, B.R.; da Silva, J.B.; Caldeira, S.A. Qualitative study of the spiritual aspects of parenting a child with Down Syndrome. *Healthcare* **2022**, *10*, 546. [CrossRef]
21. Pandya, S.P. Spirituality to build resilience in primary caregiver parents of children with autism spectrum disorders: A cross-country experiment. *Int. J. Dev. Disabil.* **2016**, *64*, 53–64. [CrossRef] [PubMed]
22. Willis, K.; Timmons, L.; Pruitt, M.; Schneider, H.L.; Alessandri, M.; Ekas, N.V. The relationship between optimism, coping, and depressive symptoms in hispanic mothers and fathers of children with autism spectrum. *Disorder. J. Autism Dev. Disord.* **2016**, *46*, 2427–2440. [CrossRef] [PubMed]
23. Salkas, K.; Magaña, S.; Marques, I.; Mirza, M. Spirituality in Latino families of children with autism spectrum disorder. *J. Fam. Soc. Work* **2016**, *19*, 38–55. [CrossRef]
24. Grossoehme, D.H.; Friebert, S.; Baker, J.N.; Tweddle, M.; Needle, J.; Chrastek, J.; Thompkins, J.; Wang, J.; Cheng, Y.I.; Lyon, M.E. Association of religious and spiritual factors with patient-reported outcomes of anxiety, depressive symptoms, fatigue, and pain interference among adolescents and young adults with cancer. *JAMA Netw. Open* **2020**, *3*, e206696. [CrossRef] [PubMed]
25. Szatkowska, K.; Sołtys, M. Perceived social support, spiritual well-being, and daily life fatigue in family caregivers of home mechanically ventilated individuals. *Rocz. Psychol.* **2019**, *21*, 53–68. [CrossRef]
26. Kazukauskiene, N.; Bunevicius, A.; Gecaite-Stonciene, J.; Burkauskas, J. Fatigue, social support, and depression in individuals with coronary artery disease. *Front. Psychol.* **2021**, *12*, 732795. [CrossRef] [PubMed]
27. Michielsen, H.J.; De Vries, J.; Van Heck, G.L. Psychometric qualities of a brief self-rated fatigue measure: The Fatigue Assessment Scale. *J. Psychosom. Res.* **2003**, *54*, 345–352. [CrossRef]
28. De Vries, J.; Michielsen, H.; Van Heck, G.L.; Drent, M. Measuring fatigue in sarcoidosis: The Fatigue Assessment Scale (FAS). *Br. J. Health Psychol.* **2004**, *9*, 279–291. [CrossRef]

29. Alikari, V.; Fradelos, E.; Sachlas, A.; Panoutsopoulos, G.; Lavdaniti, M.; Palla, P.; Giatrakou, S.; Stathoulis, J.; Babatsikou, F.; Zyga, S. Reliability and validity of the Greek version of "The Fatigue Assessment Scale". *Arch. Hell. Med.* **2016**, *33*, 231–238. Available online: https://www.mednet.gr/archives/2016-2/231abs.html (accessed on 23 December 2023).
30. Zyga, S.; Alikari, V.; Sachlas, A.; Fradelos, E.C.; Stathoulis, J.; Panoutsopoulos, G.; Georgopoulou, M.; Theophilou, P.; Lavdaniti, M. Assessment of fatigue in end stage renal disease patients undergoing hemodialysis: Prevalence and associated factors. *Med. Arch.* **2015**, *69*, 376–380. [CrossRef]
31. Zimet, G.D.; Powell, S.S.; Farley, G.K.; Werkman, S.; Berkoff, K.A. Psychometric characteristics of the Multidimensional Scale of Perceived Social Support. *J. Personal. Assess.* **1990**, *55*, 610–617.
32. Alexopoulou, M.; Giannakopoulou, N.; Komna, E.; Alikari, V.; Toulia, G.; Polikandrioti, M. The effect of perceived social support on hemodialysis patients' quality of life. *Mater. Socio Med.* **2016**, *28*, 338–342. [CrossRef]
33. Tzeletopoulou, A.; Alikari, V.; Krikelis, M.I.; Zyga, S.; Tsironi, M.; Lavdaniti, M.; Theofilou, P. Fatigue and perceived social support as predictive factors for aggressive behaviors among mental healthcare professionals. *Arch. Hell. Med.* **2019**, *36*, 792–799.
34. Tsilika, E.; Galanos, A.; Polykandriotis, T.; Parpa, E.; Mystakidou, K. Psychometric properties of the Multidimensional Scale of Perceived Social Support in Greek nurses. *Can. J. Nurs. Res.* **2018**, *51*, 23–30. [CrossRef]
35. Bredle, J.; Salsman, J.; Debb, S.; Arnold, B.; Cella, D. Spiritual well-being as a component of health-related quality of life: The functional assessment of chronic illness therapy—Spiritual well-being scale (FACIT-Sp). *Religions* **2011**, *2*, 77–94. [CrossRef]
36. Fradelos, E.C.; Tzavella, F.; Koukia, E.; Tsaras, K.; Papathanasiou, I.V.; Aroni, A.; Alikari, V.; Ralli, M.; Bredle, J.; Zyga, S. The translation, validation and cultural adaptation of Functional Assessment of Chronic Illness Therapy-Spiritual Well-Being 12 (facit-sp12) Scale in Greek Language. *Mater. Socio Med.* **2016**, *28*, 229. [CrossRef] [PubMed]
37. Marsack, C.N.; Samuel, P.S. Mediating effects of social support on quality of life for parents of adults with autism. *J. Autism Dev. Disord.* **2017**, *47*, 2378–2389. [CrossRef]
38. Paynter, J.; Davies, M.; Beamish, W. Recognizing the "forgotten man": Fathers' experiences in caring for a young child with autism spectrum disorder. *J. Intellect. Dev. Disabil.* **2018**, *43*, 112–124. [CrossRef]
39. Pepperell, T.A.; Paynter, J.; Gilmore, L. Social support and coping strategies of parents raising a child with autism spectrum disorder. *Early Child Dev. Care* **2018**, *188*, 1392–1404. [CrossRef]
40. Ardic, A. Relationship between parental burnout level and perceived social support levels of parents of children with autism spectrum disorder. *Int. J. Educ. Methodol.* **2020**, *6*, 533–543. [CrossRef]
41. Dindar, M.; Rahnama, M.; Afshari, M.; Moghadam, M.P. The effects of Spiritual Self-Care Training on caregiving strain in mothers of mentally retarded children. *J. Clin. Diagn. Res.* **2016**, *10*, QC01–QC05. [CrossRef]
42. Bernier, A.S.; McCrimmon, A.W. Attitudes and perceptions of Muslim parents toward their children with autism: A systematic review. *Rev. J. Autism Dev. Disord.* **2021**, *9*, 320–333. [CrossRef]
43. Gallagher, S.; Phillips, A.C.; Lee, H.; Carroll, D. The association between spirituality and depression in parents caring for children with developmental disabilities: Social support and/or last resort. *J. Relig. Health* **2015**, *54*, 358–370. [CrossRef] [PubMed]
44. Alorani, O.I.; Alradaydeh, M.T.F. Spiritual well-being, perceived social support, and life satisfaction among university students. *Int. J. Adolesc. Youth* **2018**, *23*, 291–298. [CrossRef]
45. Milgramm, A.; Corona, L.L.; Janicki-Menzie, C.; Christodulu, K.V. Community-based parent education for caregivers of children newly diagnosed with autism spectrum disorder. *J. Autism Dev. Disord.* **2022**, *52*, 1200–1210. [CrossRef] [PubMed]
46. Ekas, N.V.; Tidman, L.; Timmons, L. Religiosity/spirituality and mental health outcomes in mothers of children with autism spectrum disorder: The mediating role of positive thinking. *J. Autism Dev. Disord.* **2019**, *49*, 4547–4558. [CrossRef]
47. Picardi, A.; Gigantesco, A.; Tarolla, E.; Stoppioni, V.; Cerbo, R.; Cremonte, M.; Alessandri, G.; Lega, I.; Nardocci, F. Parental burden and its correlates in families of children with autism spectrum disorder: A multicentre study with two comparison groups. *Clin. Pract. Epidemiol. Ment. Health* **2018**, *14*, 143–176. [CrossRef]
48. Nacul, L.C.; Lacerda, E.M.; Campion, P.; Pheby, D.; Drachler, M.D.L.; Leite, J.C.; Poland, F.; Howe, A.; Fayyaz, S.; Molokhia, M. The functional status and well being of people with myalgic encephalomyelitis/chronic fatigue syndrome and their carers. *BMC Public Health* **2011**, *11*, 402. [CrossRef]
49. Marcinechová, D.; Záhorcová, L.; Lohazerová, K. Self-forgiveness, guilt, shame, and parental stress among parents of children with autism spectrum disorder. In *Current Psychology*; Springer: Berlin/Heidelberg, Germany, 2023; pp. 1–16.
50. Bernardi, R.A.; Nash, J. The importance and efficacy of controlling for social desirability response bias. *Ethics Behav.* **2023**, *33*, 413–429. [CrossRef]

Disclaimer/Publisher's Note: The statements, opinions and data contained in all publications are solely those of the individual author(s) and contributor(s) and not of MDPI and/or the editor(s). MDPI and/or the editor(s) disclaim responsibility for any injury to people or property resulting from any ideas, methods, instructions or products referred to in the content.

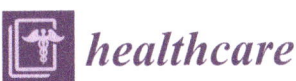 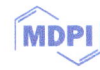

Systematic Review

Association between Organizational Support and Turnover Intention in Nurses: A Systematic Review and Meta-Analysis

Petros Galanis [1], Ioannis Moisoglou [2], Ioanna V. Papathanasiou [2,*], Maria Malliarou [2], Aglaia Katsiroumpa [1], Irene Vraka [3], Olga Siskou [4], Olympia Konstantakopoulou [5] and Daphne Kaitelidou [5]

1. Clinical Epidemiology Laboratory, Faculty of Nursing, National and Kapodistrian University of Athens, 11527 Athens, Greece; pegalan@nurs.uoa.gr (P.G.); aglaiakat@nurs.uoa.gr (A.K.)
2. Faculty of Nursing, University of Thessaly, 41500 Larisa, Greece; iomoysoglou@uth.gr (I.M.); malliarou@uth.gr (M.M.)
3. Department of Radiology, P. & A. Kyriakou Children's Hospital, 11527 Athens, Greece; irenevraka@yahoo.gr
4. Department of Tourism Studies, University of Piraeus, 18534 Piraeus, Greece; olsiskou@nurs.uoa.gr
5. Center for Health Services Management and Evaluation, Faculty of Nursing, National and Kapodistrian University of Athens, 11527 Athens, Greece; olympiak1982@hotmail.com (O.K.); dkaitelid@nurs.uoa.gr (D.K.)
* Correspondence: iopapathanasiou@uth.gr

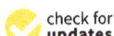

Citation: Galanis, P.; Moisoglou, I.; Papathanasiou, I.V.; Malliarou, M.; Katsiroumpa, A.; Vraka, I.; Siskou, O.; Konstantakopoulou, O.; Kaitelidou, D. Association between Organizational Support and Turnover Intention in Nurses: A Systematic Review and Meta-Analysis. *Healthcare* **2024**, *12*, 291. https://doi.org/10.3390/healthcare12030291

Academic Editors: Areti Stavropoulou and Sofia Koukouli

Received: 2 December 2023
Revised: 10 January 2024
Accepted: 18 January 2024
Published: 23 January 2024

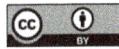

Copyright: © 2024 by the authors. Licensee MDPI, Basel, Switzerland. This article is an open access article distributed under the terms and conditions of the Creative Commons Attribution (CC BY) license (https://creativecommons.org/licenses/by/4.0/).

Abstract: Although recent studies suggest a negative relationship between organizational support and turnover intention among nurses, there has been no systematic review on this issue. The aim of this systematic review and meta-analysis was to synthesize and evaluate the association between organizational support and turnover intention in nurses. The review protocol was registered with PROSPERO (CRD42023447109). A total of eight studies with 5754 nurses were included. All studies were cross-sectional and were conducted after 2010. Quality was moderate in five studies and good in three studies. We found a moderate negative correlation between organizational support and turnover intention since the pooled correlation coefficient was −0.32 (95% confidence interval: −0.42 to −0.21). All studies found a negative correlation between organizational support and turnover intention ranging from −0.10 to −0.51. A leave-one-out sensitivity analysis showed that our results were stable when each study was excluded. Egger's test and funnel plot suggested the absence of publication bias in the eight studies. Subgroup analysis showed that the negative correlation between organizational support and turnover intention was stronger in studies in China and Australia than those in Europe. Organizational support has a moderate negative correlation with turnover intention in nurses. However, data regarding the impact of organizational support on turnover intention are limited. Moreover, our study had several limitations, and thus, we cannot generalize our results. Therefore, further studies should be conducted to assess the independent effect of organizational support on turnover intention in a more valid way. In any case, nursing managers should draw attention to organizational support by developing effective clinical practice guidelines for nurses so as to reduce turnover intention.

Keywords: organizational support; turnover intention; nurses; systematic review; meta-analysis

1. Introduction

Nurses, as frontline healthcare workers, are at the core of patient care delivery. They provide patients with the majority of care during their hospital stay, ensure the quality and safety of care, and contribute to patient satisfaction with it [1–3]. Ensuring the necessary resources for nursing staff is an essential prerequisite for providing quality nursing care [4]. However, over time, nurses' work environments have been characterized by nursing understaffing and inadequate organizational support [5,6]. The consequence of all the above is the occurrence of burnout among nurses, their lack of work engagement, and their intention to leave their profession [5,7,8]. The pandemic period of COVID-19 found healthcare systems struggling with the same organizational problems and weaknesses as the pre-COVID period [9]. During this period, the high workload and work intensity further burdened nurses, who were more likely to declare their intention to leave the profession [10].

Nurses' turnover constitutes, over time, a phenomenon that characterizes their profession. Nurses' turnover can be defined as voluntarily leaving a particular position and moving to another within the same organization or to another healthcare organization, or ultimately leaving the profession and choosing another profession [11]. The prevalence of nurses declaring their turnover intention was high before the pandemic, reaching over 40% [12], and remained high during the pandemic period [13]. Among healthcare workers, nurses report the highest intent to leave the job rate [14]. The main factors related to nurses' turnover intention are their working environment and, in particular, nursing staffing and the adequacy of resources [15,16]; stress related to work, to constant contact with patients and their relatives, and to conflicts with colleagues and supervisors [17]; organizational culture and fatigue [18]; shift work and organizational commitment [19]; and job dissatisfaction, burnout and depression [20–22].

After the COVID-19 pandemic, many nurses chose to stay in their jobs as it was difficult to change jobs due to the loss of many vacancies as an effect of the pandemic. As working conditions still remain difficult and nurses experience high rates of dissatisfaction and burnout [23], they choose quiet quitting, which is characterized by a decrease in their performance [24,25]. However, those who choose quiet quitting also report a high percentage of turnover intention [26]. Therefore, even the option of quiet quitting, which is a kind of defensive attitude of self-preservation for nurses in the demanding working environment, is not able to stop the tendency of nurses to leave the profession. For the factors associated with turnover intention, immediate solutions should be sought by the administrations of healthcare organizations worldwide as turnover intention is a strong determinant of actual turnover behavior [27,28].

Within the demanding and challenging work environment of healthcare delivery, a crucial factor influencing the turnover intention of nurses is the perceived organizational support they receive. According to the theory of perceived organizational support, employees believe that their work organization values their contribution and cares about their well-being [29]. In particular, perceived organizational support consists of organizational rewards, favorable job conditions, assistance to an employee to perform tasks efficiently and manage stressful situations, and support from the supervisor [30].

The benefits of organizational support are multifaceted, affecting nurses and their performance. When nurses receive organizational support, work engagement increases [7], nurses' innovative behavior is enhanced [31], they report greater affective commitment [32], the quality of care is improved, and nurses experience higher job satisfaction, psychological well-being, and lower burnout and anxiety [33–35]. The degree of organizational support received by nurses influences their intention to stay in the profession [36–39]. As there are already significant shortages of nurses worldwide, which are projected to continue until 2030 [40], halting the turnover phenomenon will help towards the availability of nurses and better staffing of healthcare services. Therefore, organizational support is an important tool for achieving this objective.

Among other organizational factors, recent studies found a negative relationship between organizational support and turnover intention among nurses [36,41,42]. However, to date, no systematic review has been published on the association between organizational support and turnover intention. Thus, the aim of this systematic review and meta-analysis was to synthesize and evaluate the relationship between organizational support and turnover intention among nurses.

2. Materials and Methods

The review protocol was registered with PROSPERO (CRD42023447109).

2.1. Search Methods

We searched PubMed, Medline, Scopus, Cinahl, Web of Science, and Cochrane from inception to 21 August 2023. We searched in all fields using the following strategy: ((nurses OR nursing OR nurse OR "nursing staff") AND ("organizational support" OR "organisational support")) AND ("turnover intention" OR intention OR "intent to leave" OR turnover OR "intent to quit" OR "intention to leave" OR "intention to quit"). The duration of the literature search of the studies by the authors lasted from 14 to 21 August 2023.

2.2. Selection Process

Our inclusion criteria were the following: (a) studies that included nurses working in clinical settings, (b) articles published in English, (c) studies that investigated the relationship between organizational support and turnover intention in nurses, and (d) studies that used valid instruments to measure organizational support and turnover intention. Organizational support is a broad term that can vary across different organizations and countries. In our review, we included studies that measured the perceived organizational support among nurses. In particular, perceived organizational support was defined as comprising nurses' overall perceptions and beliefs about how much organizations value and respect nurses' well-being and job satisfaction. We excluded meeting or conference abstracts, case reports, qualitative studies, reviews, meta-analyses, protocols, editorials, and letters to the Editor. Moreover, we excluded studies that measured nurses' intention to stay instead of intention to leave. Additionally, we excluded studies that simultaneously included nurses and other healthcare workers, so it was impossible to extract results only for nurses.

Applying the inclusion and exclusion criteria, two independent authors screened titles and abstracts of the records. Then, they screened the full texts of the records. A third senior author resolved all disagreements between the two independent authors.

2.3. Quality Appraisal

We used the Joanna Briggs Institute critical appraisal tools to assess the quality of studies included in our review [43]. All studies in our review were cross-sectional, and thus, we employed the Joanna Briggs Institute critical appraisal tool for this type of study. In particular, the Joanna Briggs Institute tool for cross-sectional studies comprises eight items. Higher scores indicate better quality. In particular, ≤3 is considered as having high-risk bias, 4–6 as having moderate-risk bias, and 7–8 as having low-risk bias. Two scholars performed the bias assessment.

2.4. Data Abstraction

Two scholars independently extracted the following data from each study: first author, year of publication, country, data collection time, percentage of females, age, sample size, study design, sampling method, clinical settings, assessment tools for organizational support and turnover intention, response rate, correlation coefficient between organizational support and turnover intention, unstandardized coefficient beta from linear regression models with turnover intention as the dependent variable, and p-values.

2.5. Synthesis

All studies presented correlation coefficients between organizational support and turnover intention while only two studies presented unstandardized coefficient betas. Thus, we performed meta-analysis for the correlation coefficients and not for unstandardized coefficient betas. In particular, we calculated the pooled correlation coefficient between organizational support and turnover intention and the 95% confidence interval (CI). Correlation coefficient between −0.1 and −0.29 indicates a small effect, between −0.3 and −0.49, a moderate effect, and higher than 0.49, a large effect [44]. Additionally, we assessed heterogeneity between studies by calculating the I^2 statistics and the p-value for the Hedges Q statistic. I^2 values higher than 75% indicate high heterogeneity while a p-value < 0.1 for the Hedges Q statistic indicates statistically significant heterogeneity [45]. Heterogeneity between studies was high, and thus, we applied the random effects model to calculate the pooled correlation coefficient. A leave-one-out sensitivity analysis was employed to estimate the influence of each study on the pooled correlation coefficient. A priori, we considered country, data collection time, percentage of females, sample size, quality of studies, and response rate as sources of heterogeneity. To examine heterogeneity, we performed subgroup analysis for categorical variables and meta-regression for continuous variables. We used Egger's test and funnel plot to estimate publication bias [46]. p-value < 0.05 for Egger's test and asymmetry of funnel plot indicate the presence of publication bias. We used OpenMeta [Analyst] to perform the meta-analysis [47]

3. Results

3.1. Identification and Selection of Studies

Figure 1 shows the flowchart of the literature search according to PRISMA guidelines. Initially, we identified a total of 10,354 records. After removal of duplicates, 9906 records were left. Then, we reviewed 21 records with relevant titles and abstracts. Finally, we included eight original research studies in our review and meta-analysis [36,41,42,48–52].

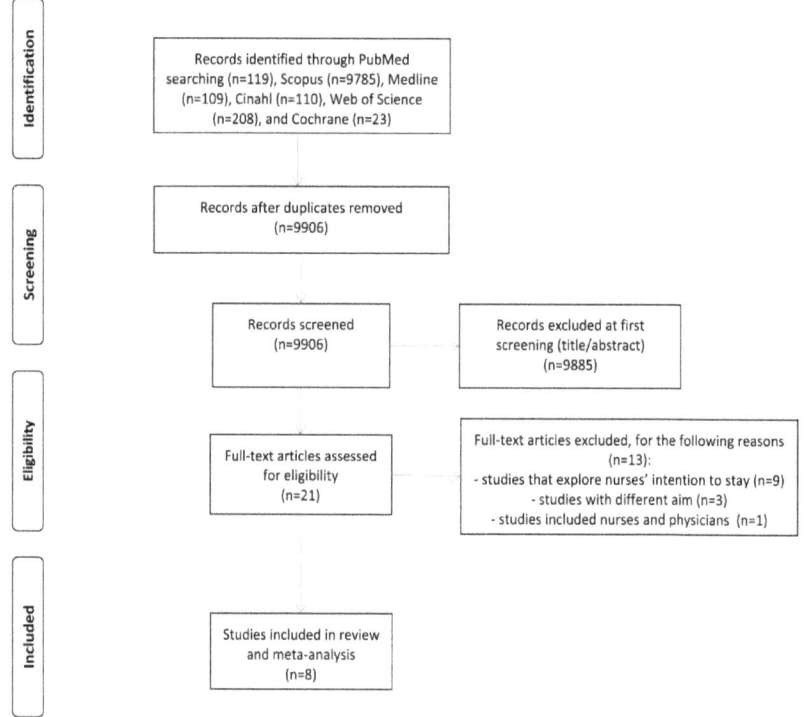

Figure 1. Flowchart of the systematic review.

3.2. Characteristics of the Studies

Table 1 shows the main characteristics of the eight studies included in our review. A total of 5754 nurses were included in our review and meta-analysis. The sample size in the included studies ranged from 242 nurses to 1761. Two studies had been conducted in Europe [48,51], two studies in China [41,42], two studies in Australia [49,52], one study in the USA [50], and one study in Egypt [36]. All studies were cross-sectional and had been conducted after 2010. The percentage of female nurses ranged from 79.0% to 96.6%. Seven studies used convenience samples while one study used a purposive sample [42]. All studies included nurses working in hospitals. Seven studies used the Survey of Perceived Organizational Support to measure organizational support while one study used the Perceived Organizational Support—Simplified Version Scale [42]. Three studies used the Turnover Intention Scale to measure turnover intention [36,41,42] while five studies used other self-developed scales that have been validated [48–52]. The response rate among studies ranged from 21.4% to 96.3%.

Table 1. Main characteristics of studies included in this systematic review.

Reference	Country	Data Collection Time	Females (%)	Age, Mean (SD)	Sample Size (n)	Study Design	Sampling Method	Clinical Settings	Assessment Tool for Organizational Support	Assessment Tool for Turnover Intention	Response Rate (%)	Correlation Coefficient (p-Value)
(Sheng et al., 2023) [41]	China	2020–2021	96.2	27.0 (3.9)	474	Cross-sectional	Convenience	Hospitals	SPOS	TIS	96.3	−0.27 (<0.01)
(Brunetto et al., 2016) [49]	Australia	2013	83.2	41–60 years: 64.8%	242	Cross-sectional	Convenience	Hospitals	SPOS	Eight-item scale	33.0	−0.25 (<0.01)
(Abou Hashish, 2017) [36]	Egypt	NR	NR	≤29 years: 47.2%; 30–40: 33.0%; ≥41: 19.8%	500	Cross-sectional	Convenience	Hospitals	SPOS	TIS	78.5	−0.10 (0.16)
(Shacklock et al., 2014) [52]	Australia	2010–2011	93.7	46.5 (10.4)	510	Cross-sectional	Convenience	Hospitals	SPOS	Three-item scale	31.5	−0.39 (<0.001)
(Liu et al., 2018) [42]	China	2016–2017	96.6	≤30 years: 51.1%; 31–50: 45.0%; ≥51: 3.9%	1761	Cross-sectional	Purposive	Hospitals	POS-SVS	TIS	85.2	−0.38 (<0.001)
(Filipova, 2011) [50]	USA	2010	94.0	44–53 years: 37.0%	656	Cross-sectional	Convenience	Hospitals	SPOS	Three-item scale	21.4	−0.51 (<0.001)
(Bobbio & Manganelli, 2015) [48]	Italy	2012	79.0	42.3 (8.1)	371	Cross-sectional	Convenience	Hospitals	SPOS	Three-item scale	41.0	−0.31 (<0.01)
(Galletta et al., 2011) [51]	France	2010	81.5	37.0 (7.9)	1240	Cross-sectional	Convenience	Hospitals	SPOS	Two-item scale	64.0	−0.20 (<0.001)

NR: not reported; POS-SVS: Perceived Organizational Support—Simplified Version Scale; SD: standard deviation; SPOS: Survey of Perceived Organizational Support; TIS: Turnover Intention Scale.

3.3. Quality Assessment

Supplementary Table S1 shows the quality of the studies included in our review. Quality was moderate in five studies [41,48,49,51,52] and good in three studies [36,42,50]. Failure to identify and eliminate confounding factors was the main threat to study quality.

3.4. Meta-Analysis

All studies reported a correlation coefficient between organizational support and turnover intention among nurses. The correlation coefficients and *p*-values for all studies are shown in Table 1. All studies found negative correlations between organizational support and turnover intention ranging from −0.10 [36] to −0.51 [50]. We found a statistically significant negative correlation since the pooled correlation coefficient was −0.32 (95% CI: −0.42 to −0.21, $p < 0.001$) (Figure 2). The overall correlation coefficient suggested a moderate negative correlation between organizational support and turnover intention. Heterogeneity between results was high ($I^2 = 93\%$, *p*-value for the Hedges Q statistic < 0.001).

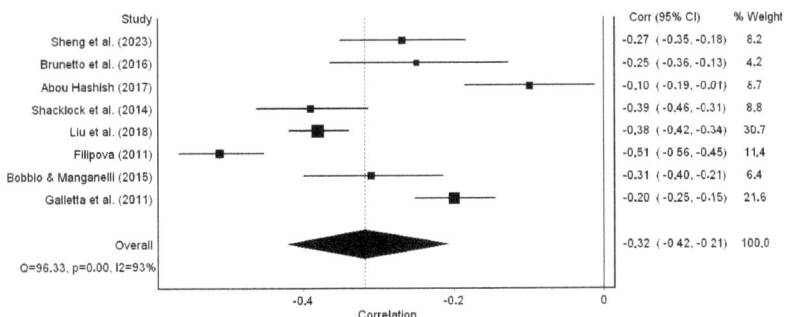

Figure 2. Forest plot of the eight studies included in this meta-analysis [36,41,42,48–52].

A leave-one-out sensitivity analysis showed that our results were stable when each study was excluded. In particular, the pooled correlation coefficient varied between −0.29 (95% CI: −0.41 to −0.16, $p < 0.001$), with Liu et al. [42] excluded, and −0.35 (95% CI: −0.46 to −0.23, $p < 0.001$), with Galletta et al. [51] excluded.

Egger's test (Egger bias = −1.43, 95% CI: −6.56 to 3.70, $p = 0.63$) and funnel plot (Figure 3) suggested the absence of publication bias in the eight studies.

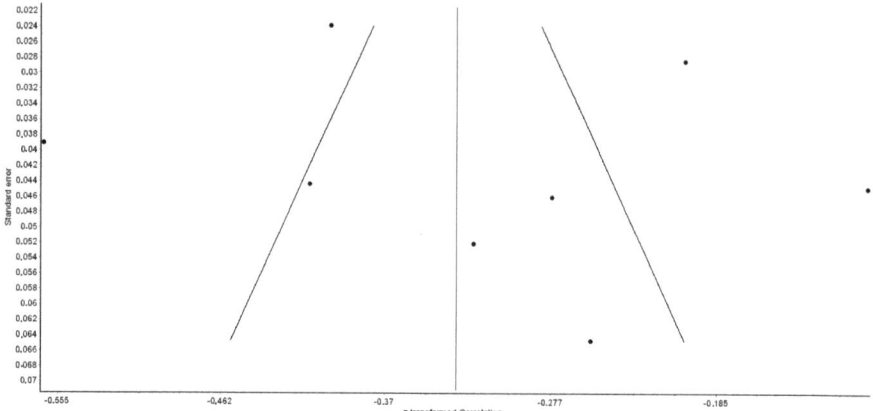

Figure 3. Funnel plot of the correlation coefficient between organizational support and turnover intention among nurses.

Subgroup analysis showed that the negative correlation between organizational support and turnover intention was stronger in studies in China (pooled r = −0.33, 95% CI: −0.81 to 0.41, $I^2 = 82\%$) and Australia (pooled r = −0.33, 95% CI: −0.87 to 0.57, $I^2 = 75\%$) than in studies in Europe (pooled r = −0.25, 95% CI: −0.76 to 0.45, $I^2 = 75\%$). Moreover, the negative correlation was stronger for studies with a low risk of bias (pooled r = −0.34, 95% CI: −0.73 to 0.22, $I^2 = 97\%$) than studies with a moderate risk of bias (pooled r = −0.28, 95% CI: −0.37 to −0.19, $I^2 = 76\%$).

Meta-regression showed that the pooled correlation coefficient was independent of the percentage of females (beta = −0.01, $p = 0.11$), data collection time (beta = 0.01, $p = 0.65$), sample size (beta = −0.00004, $p = 0.73$), and response rate (beta = 0.002, $p = 0.19$).

Only two studies had conducted multivariable analysis to estimate the independent effect of organizational support on nurses' turnover intention. Both of these studies found a negative association between organizational support and turnover intention. However, Liu et al. [42] found a statistically significant association (unstandardized coefficient beta = −0.012, $p < 0.01$) while Filipova [50] did not find a statistically significant association (unstandardized coefficient beta = −0.010, $p > 0.05$).

Moreover, only two studies investigated potential mediators of the relationship between organizational support and turnover intention. In particular, Filipova [50] found that organizational commitment completely mediated the negative relationship between organizational support and turnover intention while job satisfaction partially mediated this relationship. In a similar way, Shacklock et al. [52] found that job satisfaction partially mediated the negative relationship between organizational support and turnover intention. No studies investigated potential moderators of the relationship between organizational support and turnover intention.

4. Discussion

Our meta-analysis highlighted the moderate negative correlation between organizational support and turnover intention. Moreover, two studies found a negative association between organizational support and turnover intention after eliminating confounding [42,50]. Nurses' turnover intention has a significant impact on the functioning of healthcare organizations. This impact includes the understaffing of nursing departments from which nurses leave, the negative impact on nurses' mental health, the deterioration of patient safety (falls and medical errors), and patients' dissatisfaction with the healthcare services provided [53]. The impact also includes the waste of financial and other resources in recruiting new staff and training them to fully assume their duties [53,54]. As there are already serious safety problems in the provision of healthcare [55] and issues with the mental health of nurses [56], nurses' turnover intention seems to exacerbate the existing situation.

The decision of nurses to leave the profession is not a sudden decision but a process that goes through three stages [57]. In the first stage, the psychological, the employee through turnover-intention psychological responses to negative aspects of organization or job. He/she begins to feel dissatisfaction with his/her job, showing reduced commitment and attachment to his/her organization. In the second stage, the cognitive, turnover intention is defined as the final cognitive step leading to actual turnover. In the third stage, the behavioral, the employee now changes his/her behavior as, in addition to expressing his/her desire to leave, he/she loses enthusiasm and is late to work or even absent. A recent study in Greece, involving 629 nurses, showed that 60.9% of nurses choose quiet quitting [26]. Employees who choose this behavior reduce their effort, perform only highly necessary tasks, do not propose new ideas and practices, do not stay overtime, and do not come to work early. Their goal is to work only as much as necessary to avoid being fired. The study showed that nurses who opt for quiet quitting, in which they reduce their performance at work, are more likely to have high levels of turnover intention. Therefore, the factor that triggers turnover intention is the working environment of nurses, and the management of healthcare organizations should focus on improving it.

Even if nurses are dissatisfied with their work or experience burnout and report their turnover intention, organizational support can mitigate the effect of the two factors mentioned above on their turnover intention. Four studies showed the indirect, mediating role of organizational support on turnover intention through job satisfaction [42,49,51,52] and two studies showed the similar role through burnout [42,48]. Nurses report moderate levels of job satisfaction in primary healthcare settings and high levels of dissatisfaction in secondary ones [58,59]. Even now, in the post-COVID-19 era, as the workload has been reduced and the functioning of healthcare organizations has been normalized, nurses continue to show dissatisfaction at a higher rate than other healthcare professionals [23]. When nurses report increased satisfaction with their work, the likelihood of turnover intention is reduced [60]. The main organizational factor associated with increased job satisfaction is a good working environment, characterized by well-staffed nurses, adequate resources, reduced workload, satisfactory salaries and rewards, opportunities for development and promotion, recognition of the role of nurses, and effective supervision [61,62]. The aforementioned factors constitute the conceptual framework of perceived organizational support [30,63]. Therefore, ensuring and improving these factors constitutes a strong organizational support for nurses, which is directly linked to increasing their job satisfaction, and will indirectly reduce their turnover intention. In addition to job dissatisfaction, nurses also experience high rates of burnout. Before the COVID-19 pandemic, it is estimated that one out of three nurses reported being exhausted [64], and this rate increased to very high levels after the pandemic and its impact [23]. Burnout appears to be a strong predictor of nurses' turnover intention [65,66]. The effect of the way that nurses' work environments are organized and operated is also related to their burnout, in addition to their dissatisfaction. Factors such as low/inadequate nurse staffing levels, ≥ 12 h shifts, low autonomy, poor nurse–physician relationships, poor supervisor/leader support, job insecurity, and reduced opportunities for nurses to participate in hospital affairs make up the organizational factors that lead nurses to burnout [67,68]. During the COVID-19 pandemic, the extremely difficult and demanding working conditions combined with the organizational inefficiencies of the past resulted in a large proportion of nurses becoming burnt out [9]. Recognition of nurses' work, opportunities for development, and ensuring good working conditions through ongoing organizational support reduce nurses' burnout [69], increase trust in the organization [48,69], and ultimately reduce the chances of nurses' turnover intention being actualized [48].

Among studies in our review, Sheng et al. [41] found that high organizational support plays a mediating role in the relationship between nurses' practice environment and their well-being, which in turn is correlated to turnover intention [41]. The working environment and the demanding nature of nurses' work negatively affect their well-being [70], resulting in high rates of anxiety, depression, psychological stress, and post-traumatic stress disorder [71–73]. The more the well-being of nurses deteriorates, the higher the likelihood of turnover intention becomes [20,74]. Nurses often feel both weak and defenseless in the face of difficult situations, as in the case of the COVID-19 pandemic [75]. In these challenging and difficult times, the support they receive, either at the departmental level from their supervisors or at the organizational level, helps them cope with these difficulties and mitigates their impact on their well-being [75,76].

Additionally, Liu et al. found that violence in the nurses' workplace is a factor associated with an increase in turnover intention, while organizational support mediates the effect of violence on turnover intention [42]. Incidents of violence, both physical and verbal, have a high impact on nursing staff, with nurses in emergency departments almost all reporting being victims of violence [77,78]. Nurses are dissatisfied with their organization in terms of the prevention and management of violent incidents as well as their lack of training in dealing with such incidents [79]. The consequences of violent incidents affect the quality of care, employee performance, and nurses' mental health and the willingness to leave their jobs [78,80]. The consequences of violence, which even can lead to serious physical injury and death, make it imperative to protect nurses, who feel defenseless and vulnerable. When nurses receive organizational support and feel less vulnerability, their desire to leave their jobs is mitigated [81].

Moreover, Filipova found that increased nurses' commitment mediates the relationship between perceived organizational support and their intent to leave their jobs [50]. High commitment is an important factor influencing the quality of care and hospital performance [82]. A significant number of factors have been found to affect nurses' commitment, e.g., well-being, satisfaction, leadership and management style, and behavior and working environment [83]. When organizational support is low and nurses wish to leave their jobs, then, through organizational commitment, the negative effect of support on turnover intention is mitigated [84].

In summary, organizational support both directly and indirectly influences nurses' turnover intention. Through recognizing nurses' work, ensuring that nurses have the resources needed to provide care, and providing rewards and opportunities for improvement, the likelihood of nurses declaring their turnover intention is reduced. In particular, the management of healthcare organizations should aim to ensure adequate nursing staffing, monetary rewards, opportunities for promotion, and support from the supervisor. Also, organizational support reduces burnout and increases nurses' satisfaction. As nurses' satisfaction increases and burnout decreases, the percentage of nurses who report turnover intention decreases.

As the issue of turnover intention is complex, the management of healthcare organizations should also take into account and manage the other factors that can lead to turnover intention. These factors include job stress and fatigue, burnout, depression, organizational justice and culture, job prospect and stability, relationships with managers and colleagues, and the work environment [17,18,20–22,85].

5. Limitations

Our study has several limitations. First, the number of studies included in our review and meta-analysis is small. Moreover, the number of studies for subgroup analyses is even smaller. For example, there is only one study set in the USA and one study in Africa. Thus, the representativeness of our results is limited. Further studies in different countries, cultures, and settings should be conducted to obtain more valid results. Second, only two studies assessed the independent effect of organizational support on turnover intention in nurses by applying multivariable models. All studies estimated the correlation between organizational support and turnover intention. Thus, future studies should employ multivariable models to eliminate confounding in the relationship between organizational support and turnover intention. Moreover, we suggest that scholars explore the role of mediating or/and moderating variables since structural equation modeling enables us to perform mediation/moderation analysis in a valid way. Third, all studies included in our review were cross-sectional, and a causal relationship between organizational support and turnover intention cannot be established. Measuring organizational support and turnover intention at the same time may produce a spurious correlation. Thus, there is a need for longitudinal studies, which can further explain the relationship between organizational support and turnover intention. Fourth, seven studies used convenience samples, and only one study used a purposive sample. For example, nurses in all studies were mainly females. Therefore, selection bias is potential in our review. Further studies with more representative and stratified samples can add valuable evidence. Finally, we searched six major databases, applying the guidelines for systematic reviews, but it is still possible for us to have missed studies in our evaluation. For example, we did not include studies in non-English languages and grey literature.

6. Conclusions

Our meta-analysis suggests a moderate negative correlation between organizational support and turnover intention in nurses. In other words, nurses who have experienced more organizational support tend to be less likely to leave their jobs than those who have experienced less organizational support. As nursing understaffing characterizes a significant number of healthcare organizations and the shortage of nurses is a constant threat to health systems, the turnover intention of nurses may exacerbate the existing situation. This study highlighted the direct and indirect association between organizational support and turnover intention and, also, the specific characteristics of organizational support that should be strengthened by the administrations of healthcare organizations to reduce turnover intention. Our findings constitute an alarm for organizations, policy makers, and nursing managers to pay more attention to organizational support.

Supplementary Materials: The following supporting information can be downloaded at: https://www.mdpi.com/article/10.3390/healthcare12030291/s1, Table S1: Quality of studies included in the systematic review.

Author Contributions: Conceptualization, P.G.; methodology, P.G., I.M., M.M., I.V.P. and D.K.; software, P.G. and O.K.; validation, A.K., I.M., I.V., O.S. and O.K.; formal analysis, P.G., A.K. and I.V.; investigation, P.G., A.K., I.V., O.S. and O.K.; resources, P.G., I.M., M.M., I.V.P., A.K., I.V., O.S., O.K. and D.K.; data curation, I.M., M.M., I.V.P., A.K., I.V., O.S., O.K. and D.K.; writing—original draft preparation, P.G., I.M., A.K., I.V.P. and I.V.; writing—review and editing, P.G., I.M., M.M., I.V.P., A.K., I.V., O.S., O.K. and D.K.; supervision, P.G.; project administration, P.G. and D.K. All authors have read and agreed to the published version of the manuscript.

Funding: This research received no external funding.

Institutional Review Board Statement: Not applicable.

Informed Consent Statement: Not applicable.

Data Availability Statement: Our data are available from the corresponding author on reasonable request.

Conflicts of Interest: The authors declare no conflicts of interest.

References

1. Westbrook, J.I.; Duffield, C.; Li, L.; Creswick, N.J. How Much Time Do Nurses Have for Patients? A Longitudinal Study Quantifying Hospital Nurses' Patterns of Task Time Distribution and Interactions with Health Professionals. *BMC Health Serv. Res.* **2011**, *11*, 319. [CrossRef] [PubMed]
2. Kieft, R.A.M.M.; De Brouwer, B.B.J.M.; Francke, A.L.; Delnoij, D.M.J. How Nurses and Their Work Environment Affect Patient Experiences of the Quality of Care: A Qualitative Study. *BMC Health Serv. Res.* **2014**, *14*, 249. [CrossRef]
3. Karaca, A.; Durna, Z. Patient Satisfaction with the Quality of Nursing Care. *Nurs. Open* **2019**, *6*, 545. [CrossRef] [PubMed]
4. Sloane, D.M.; Smith, H.L.; McHugh, M.D.; Aiken, L.H. Effect of Changes in Hospital Nursing Resources on Improvements in Patient Safety and Quality of Care: A Panel Study. *Med. Care* **2018**, *56*, 1008. [CrossRef] [PubMed]
5. Lasater, K.B.; Aiken, L.H.; Sloane, D.M.; French, R.; Martin, B.; Reneau, K.; Alexander, M.; McHugh, M.D. Chronic Hospital Nurse Understaffing Meets COVID-19: An Observational Study. *BMJ Qual. Saf.* **2021**, *30*, 639–647. [CrossRef] [PubMed]
6. Robaee, N.; Atashzadeh-Shoorideh, F.; Ashktorab, T.; Baghestani, A.; Barkhordari-Sharifabad, M. Perceived Organizational Support and Moral Distress among Nurses. *BMC Nurs.* **2018**, *17*, 2. [CrossRef] [PubMed]
7. Gupta, V.; Agarwal, U.A.; Khatri, N. The Relationships between Perceived Organizational Support, Affective Commitment, Psychological Contract Breach, Organizational Citizenship Behaviour and Work Engagement. *J. Adv. Nurs.* **2016**, *72*, 2806–2817. [CrossRef]
8. Leone, C.; Bruyneel, L.; Anderson, J.E.; Murrells, T.; Dussault, G.; Henriques de Jesus, É.; Sermeus, W.; Aiken, L.; Rafferty, A.M. Work Environment Issues and Intention-to-Leave in Portuguese Nurses: A Cross-Sectional Study. *Health Policy* **2015**, *119*, 1584–1592. [CrossRef]
9. Galanis, P.; Vraka, I.; Fragkou, D.; Bilali, A.; Kaitelidou, D. Nurses' Burnout and Associated Risk Factors during the COVID-19 Pandemic: A Systematic Review and Meta-Analysis. *J. Adv. Nurs.* **2021**, *77*, 3286–3302. [CrossRef]
10. Falatah, R. The Impact of the Coronavirus Disease (COVID-19) Pandemic on Nurses' Turnover Intention: An Integrative Review. *Nurs. Rep.* **2021**, *11*, 787–810. [CrossRef]
11. Hayes, L.J.; O'Brien-Pallas, L.; Duffield, C.; Shamian, J.; Buchan, J.; Hughes, F.; Spence Laschinger, H.K.; North, N.; Stone, P.W. Nurse Turnover: A Literature Review. *Int. J. Nurs. Stud.* **2006**, *43*, 237–263. [CrossRef] [PubMed]
12. Labrague, L.J.; De los Santos, J.A.A.; Falguera, C.C.; Nwafor, C.E.; Galabay, J.R.; Rosales, R.A.; Firmo, C.N. Predictors of Nurses' Turnover Intention at One and Five Years' Time. *Int. Nurs. Rev.* **2020**, *67*, 191–198. [CrossRef] [PubMed]
13. Said, R.M.; El-Shafei, D.A. Occupational Stress, Job Satisfaction, and Intent to Leave: Nurses Working on Front Lines during COVID-19 Pandemic in Zagazig City, Egypt. *Environ. Sci. Pollut. Res.* **2021**, *28*, 8791–8801. [CrossRef] [PubMed]
14. Rotenstein, L.S.; Brown, R.; Sinsky, C.; Linzer, M. The Association of Work Overload with Burnout and Intent to Leave the Job Across the Healthcare Workforce During COVID-19. *J. Gen. Intern. Med.* **2023**, *38*, 1920–1927. [CrossRef] [PubMed]
15. Chen, H.; Li, G.; Li, M.; Lyu, L.; Zhang, T. A Cross-Sectional Study on Nurse Turnover Intention and Influencing Factors in Jiangsu Province, China. *Int. J. Nurs. Sci.* **2018**, *5*, 396–402. [CrossRef] [PubMed]
16. Bruyneel, A.; Bouckaert, N.; Maertens de Noordhout, C.; Detollenaere, J.; Kohn, L.; Pirson, M.; Sermeus, W.; Van den Heede, K. Association of Burnout and Intention-to-Leave the Profession with Work Environment: A Nationwide Cross-Sectional Study among Belgian Intensive Care Nurses after Two Years of Pandemic. *Int. J. Nurs. Stud.* **2023**, *137*, 104385. [CrossRef] [PubMed]
17. Lee, E.K.; Kim, J.S. Nursing Stress Factors Affecting Turnover Intention among Hospital Nurses. *Int. J. Nurs. Pract.* **2020**, *26*, e12819. [CrossRef]
18. Lee, E.; Jang, I. Nurses' Fatigue, Job Stress, Organizational Culture, and Turnover Intention: A Culture–Work–Health Model. *West J. Nurs. Res.* **2019**, *42*, 108–116. [CrossRef]
19. Arslan Yürümezoğlu, H.; Kocaman, G.; Mert Haydarİ, S. Predicting Nurses' Organizational and Professional Turnover Intentions. *Jpn. J. Nurs. Sci.* **2019**, *16*, 274–285. [CrossRef]
20. Pang, Y.; Dan, H.; Jung, H.; Bae, N.; Kim, O. Depressive Symptoms, Professional Quality of Life and Turnover Intention in Korean Nurses. *Int. Nurs. Rev.* **2020**, *67*, 387–394. [CrossRef]
21. Kim, H.; Kim, E.G. A Meta-Analysis on Predictors of Turnover Intention of Hospital Nurses in South Korea (2000–2020). *Nurs. Open* **2021**, *8*, 2406–2418. [CrossRef] [PubMed]
22. Labrague, L.J.; Gloe, D.S.; McEnroe-Petitte, D.M.; Tsaras, K.; Colet, P.C. Factors Influencing Turnover Intention among Registered Nurses in Samar Philippines. *Appl. Nurs. Res.* **2018**, *39*, 200–206. [CrossRef] [PubMed]
23. Galanis, P.; Moisoglou, I.; Katsiroumpa, A.; Vraka, I.; Siskou, O.; Konstantakopoulou, O.; Meimeti, E.; Kaitelidou, D. Increased Job Burnout and Reduced Job Satisfaction for Nurses Compared to Other Healthcare Workers after the COVID-19 Pandemic. *Nurs. Rep.* **2023**, *13*, 1090–1100. [CrossRef] [PubMed]
24. Galanis, P.; Katsiroumpa, A.; Vraka, I.; Siskou, O.; Konstantakopoulou, O.; Katsoulas, T.; Moisoglou, I.; Gallos, P.; Kaitelidou, D. Nurses Quietly Quit Their Job More Often than Other Healthcare Workers: An Alarming Issue for Healthcare Services. *Res. Sq.* **2023**; preprint. [CrossRef] [PubMed]
25. Galanis, P.; Katsiroumpa, A.; Vraka, I.; Siskou, O.; Konstantakopoulou, O.; Katsoulas, T.; Moisoglou, I.; Gallos, P.; Kaitelidou, D. The Influence of Job Burnout on Quiet Quitting among Nurses: The Mediating Effect of Job Satisfaction. *Res. Sq.* **2023**, preprint. [CrossRef]

26. Galanis, P.; Moisoglou, I.; Malliarou, M.; Papathanasiou, I.V.; Katsiroumpa, A.; Vraka, I.; Siskou, O.; Konstantakopoulou, O.; Kaitelidou, D. Quiet Quitting among Nurses Increases Their Turnover Intention: Evidence from Greece in the Post-COVID-19 Era. *Healthcare* **2024**, *12*, 79. [CrossRef] [PubMed]
27. Griffeth, R.W.; Hom, P.W.; Gaertner, S. A Meta-Analysis of Antecedents and Correlates of Employee Turnover: Update, Moderator Tests, and Research Implications for the next Millennium. *J. Manag.* **2000**, *26*, 463–488. [CrossRef]
28. Tett, R.P.; Meyer, J.P. Job Satisfaction, Organizational Commitment, Turnover Intention, and Turnover: Path Analyses Based on Meta-Analytic Findings. *Pers. Psychol.* **1993**, *46*, 259–293. [CrossRef]
29. Eisenberger, R.; Huntington, R.; Hutchison, S.; Sowa, D. Perceived Organizational Support. *J. Appl. Psychol.* **1986**, *71*, 500–507. [CrossRef]
30. Rhoades, L.; Eisenberger, R. Perceived Organizational Support: A Review of the Literature. *J. Appl. Psychol.* **2002**, *87*, 698–714. [CrossRef]
31. Qi, L.; Liu, B.; Wei, X.; Hu, Y. Impact of Inclusive Leadership on Employee Innovative Behavior: Perceived Organizational Support as a Mediator. *PLoS ONE* **2019**, *14*, e0212091. [CrossRef]
32. Sharma, J.; Dhar, R.L. Factors Influencing Job Performance of Nursing Staff: Mediating Role of Affective Commitment. *Pers. Rev.* **2016**, *45*, 161–182. [CrossRef]
33. Tang, Y.; Wang, Y.; Zhou, H.; Wang, J.; Zhang, R.; Lu, Q. The Relationship between Psychiatric Nurses' Perceived Organizational Support and Job Burnout: Mediating Role of Psychological Capital. *Front. Psychol.* **2023**, *14*, 1099687. [CrossRef] [PubMed]
34. Labrague, L.J.; De los Santos, J.A.A. COVID-19 Anxiety among Front-Line Nurses: Predictive Role of Organisational Support, Personal Resilience and Social Support. *J. Nurs. Manag.* **2020**, *28*, 1653–1661. [CrossRef] [PubMed]
35. Pahlevan Sharif, S.; Ahadzadeh, A.S.; Sharif Nia, H. Mediating Role of Psychological Well-Being in the Relationship between Organizational Support and Nurses' Outcomes: A Cross-Sectional Study. *J. Adv. Nurs.* **2018**, *74*, 887–899. [CrossRef] [PubMed]
36. Abou Hashish, E.A. Relationship between Ethical Work Climate and Nurses' Perception of Organizational Support, Commitment, Job Satisfaction and Turnover Intent. *Nurs. Ethics* **2017**, *24*, 151–166. [CrossRef]
37. Ma, Y.; Chen, F.; Xing, D.; Meng, Q.; Zhang, Y. Study on the Associated Factors of Turnover Intention among Emergency Nurses in China and the Relationship between Major Factors. *Int. Emerg. Nurs.* **2022**, *60*, 101106. [CrossRef]
38. Pahlevan Sharif, S.; Bolt, E.E.T.; Ahadzadeh, A.S.; Turner, J.J.; Sharif Nia, H. Organisational Support and Turnover Intentions: A Moderated Mediation Approach. *Nurs. Open* **2021**, *8*, 3615. [CrossRef]
39. Nei, D.; Snyder, L.A.; Litwiller, B.J. Promoting Retention of Nurses: A Meta-Analytic Examination of Causes of Nurse Turnover. *Health Care Manag. Rev.* **2015**, *40*, 237–253. [CrossRef]
40. Boniol, M.; Kunjumen, T.; Nair, T.S.; Siyam, A.; Campbell, J.; Diallo, K. The Global Health Workforce Stock and Distribution in 2020 and 2030: A Threat to Equity and "universal" Health Coverage? *BMJ Glob. Health* **2022**, *7*, 009316. [CrossRef]
41. Sheng, H.; Tian, D.; Sun, L.; Hou, Y.; Liu, X. Nurse Practice Environment, Perceived Organizational Support, General Well-Being, Occupational Burnout and Turnover Intention: A Moderated Multi-Mediation Model. *Nurs. Open* **2023**, *10*, 3828–3839. [CrossRef] [PubMed]
42. Liu, W.; Zhao, S.; Shi, L.; Zhang, Z.; Liu, X.; Li, L.; Duan, X.; Li, G.; Lou, F.; Jia, X.; et al. Workplace Violence, Job Satisfaction, Burnout, Perceived Organisational Support and Their Effects on Turnover Intention among Chinese Nurses in Tertiary Hospitals: A Cross-Sectional Study. *BMJ Open* **2018**, *8*, e019525. [CrossRef] [PubMed]
43. Dos Santos, W.M.; Secoli, S.R.; Püschel, V.A. de A. The Joanna Briggs Institute Approach for Systematic. *Rev. Lat. Am. Enfermagem.* **2018**, *26*, e3074.
44. Cohen, J. *Statistical Power Analysis for the Behavioral Sciences*, 2nd ed.; Academic Press: Cambridge, MA, USA, 2013; ISBN 1483276481.
45. Higgins, J.P.T.; Thompson, S.G.; Deeks, J.J.; Altman, D.G. Measuring Inconsistency in Meta-Analyses. *BMJ* **2003**, *327*, 557–560. [CrossRef] [PubMed]
46. Egger, M.; Smith, G.D.; Schneider, M.; Minder, C. Bias in Meta-Analysis Detected by a Simple, Graphical Test. *BMJ* **1997**, *315*, 629–634. [CrossRef] [PubMed]
47. Wallace, B.C.; Schmid, C.H.; Lau, J.; Trikalinos, T.A. Meta-Analyst: Software for Meta-Analysis of Binary, Continuous and Diagnostic Data. *BMC Med. Res. Methodol.* **2009**, *9*, 80. [CrossRef] [PubMed]
48. Bobbio, A.; Manganelli, A.M. Antecedents of Hospital Nurses' Intention to Leave the Organization: A Cross Sectional Survey. *Int. J. Nurs. Stud.* **2015**, *52*, 1180–1192. [CrossRef]
49. Brunetto, Y.; Rodwell, J.; Shacklock, K.; Farr-Wharton, R.; Demir, D. The Impact of Individual and Organizational Resources on Nurse Outcomes and Intent to Quit. *J. Adv. Nurs.* **2016**, *72*, 3093–3103. [CrossRef]
50. Filipova, A.A. Relationships Among Ethical Climates, Perceived Organizational Support, and Intent-to-Leave for Licensed Nurses in Skilled Nursing Facilities. *J. Appl. Gerontol.* **2010**, *30*, 44–66. [CrossRef]
51. Galletta, M.; Portoghese, I.; Penna, M.P.; Battistelli, A.; Saiani, L. Turnover Intention among Italian Nurses: The Moderating Roles of Supervisor Support and Organizational Support. *Nurs. Health Sci.* **2011**, *13*, 184–191. [CrossRef]
52. Shacklock, K.; Brunetto, Y.; Teo, S.; Farr-Wharton, R. The Role of Support Antecedents in Nurses' Intentions to Quit: The Case of Australia. *J. Adv. Nurs.* **2014**, *70*, 811–822. [CrossRef] [PubMed]
53. Bae, S.H. Noneconomic and Economic Impacts of Nurse Turnover in Hospitals: A Systematic Review. *Int. Nurs. Rev.* **2022**, *69*, 392–404. [CrossRef] [PubMed]

54. Roche, M.A.; Duffield, C.M.; Homer, C.; Buchan, J.; Dimitrelis, S. The Rate and Cost of Nurse Turnover in Australia. *Collegian* 2015, *22*, 353–358. [CrossRef]
55. Makary, M.A.; Daniel, M. Medical Error-the Third Leading Cause of Death in the US. *BMJ* 2016, *353*, i2139. [CrossRef] [PubMed]
56. Cranage, K.; Foster, K. Mental Health Nurses' Experience of Challenging Workplace Situations: A Qualitative Descriptive Study. *Int. J. Ment. Health Nurs.* 2022, *31*, 665–676. [CrossRef] [PubMed]
57. Takase, M. A Concept Analysis of Turnover Intention: Implications for Nursing Management. *Collegian* 2010, *17*, 3–12. [CrossRef]
58. Moisoglou, I.; Meimeti, E.; Arvanitidou, E.; Galanis, P.; Ntavoni, G.; Zavras, D. Job Satisfaction in Primary Health Care in Athens, Greece: A Pilot Study. *Int. J. Caring Sci.* 2021, *14*, 166–173.
59. Dilig-Ruiz, A.; MacDonald, I.; Demery Varin, M.; Vandyk, A.; Graham, I.D.; Squires, J.E. Job Satisfaction among Critical Care Nurses: A Systematic Review. *Int. J. Nurs. Stud.* 2018, *88*, 123–134. [CrossRef]
60. De Simone, S.; Planta, A.; Cicotto, G. The Role of Job Satisfaction, Work Engagement, Self-Efficacy and Agentic Capacities on Nurses' Turnover Intention and Patient Satisfaction. *Appl. Nurs. Res.* 2018, *39*, 130–140. [CrossRef]
61. Yasin, Y.M.; Kerr, M.S.; Wong, C.A.; Bélanger, C.H. Factors Affecting Nurses' Job Satisfaction in Rural and Urban Acute Care Settings: A PRISMA Systematic Review. *J. Adv. Nurs.* 2020, *76*, 963–979. [CrossRef]
62. Al Maqbali, M.A. Factors That Influence Nurses' Job Satisfaction: A Literature Review. *Nurs. Manag.* 2015, *22*, 30–37. [CrossRef] [PubMed]
63. Kurtessis, J.N.; Eisenberger, R.; Ford, M.T.; Buffardi, L.C.; Stewart, K.A.; Adis, C.S. Perceived Organizational Support: A Meta-Analytic Evaluation of Organizational Support Theory. *J. Manag.* 2015, *43*, 1854–1884. [CrossRef]
64. Gómez-Urquiza, J.L.; De la Fuente-Solana, E.I.; Albendín-García, L.; Vargas-Pecino, C.; Ortega-Campos, E.M.; Cañadas-De la Fuente, G.A. Prevalence of Burnout Syndrome in Emergency Nurses: A Meta-Analysis. *Crit. Care Nurse* 2017, *37*, e1–e9. [CrossRef] [PubMed]
65. Ran, L.; Chen, X.; Peng, S.; Zheng, F.; Tan, X.; Duan, R. Job Burnout and Turnover Intention among Chinese Primary Healthcare Staff: The Mediating Effect of Satisfaction. *BMJ Open* 2020, *10*, e036702. [CrossRef] [PubMed]
66. Shah, M.K.; Gandrakota, N.; Cimiotti, J.P.; Ghose, N.; Moore, M.; Ali, M.K. Prevalence of and Factors Associated with Nurse Burnout in the US. *JAMA Netw. Open* 2021, *4*, e2036469. [CrossRef] [PubMed]
67. Dall'Ora, C.; Ball, J.; Reinius, M.; Griffiths, P. Burnout in Nursing: A Theoretical Review. *Hum. Resour. Health* 2020, *18*, 41. [CrossRef] [PubMed]
68. Moisoglou, I.; Yfantis, A.; Tsioumna, E.; Galanis, P. The Work Environment of Haemodialysis Nurses and Its Mediating Role in Burnout. *J. Ren. Care* 2021, *47*, 133–140. [CrossRef] [PubMed]
69. Bobbio, A.; Bellan, M.; Manganelli, A.M. Empowering Leadership, Perceived Organizational Support, Trust, and Job Burnout for Nurses: A Study in an Italian General Hospital. *Health Care Manag. Rev.* 2012, *37*, 77–87. [CrossRef]
70. Chung, H.C.; Chen, Y.C.; Chang, S.C.; Hsu, W.L.; Hsieh, T.C. Nurses' Well-Being, Health-Promoting Lifestyle and Work Environment Satisfaction Correlation: A Psychometric Study for Development of Nursing Health and Job Satisfaction Model and Scale. *Int. J. Environ. Res. Public Health* 2020, *17*, 3582. [CrossRef]
71. Shen, X.; Zou, X.; Zhong, X.; Yan, J.; Li, L. Psychological Stress of ICU Nurses in the Time of COVID-19. *Crit. Care* 2020, *24*, 200. [CrossRef]
72. Tan, B.Y.Q.; Chew, N.W.S.; Lee, G.K.H.; Jing, M.; Goh, Y.; Yeo, L.L.L.; Zhang, K.; Chin, H.K.; Ahmad, A.; Khan, F.A.; et al. Psychological Impact of the COVID-19 Pandemic on Health Care Workers in Singapore. *Ann. Intern. Med.* 2020, *173*, 317–320. [CrossRef]
73. Maharaj, S.; Lees, T.; Lal, S. Prevalence and Risk Factors of Depression, Anxiety, and Stress in a Cohort of Australian Nurses. *Int. J. Environ. Res. Public Health* 2019, *16*, 61. [CrossRef] [PubMed]
74. Mirzaei, A.; Rezakhani Moghaddam, H.; Habibi Soola, A. Identifying the Predictors of Turnover Intention Based on Psychosocial Factors of Nurses during the COVID-19 Outbreak. *Nurs. Open* 2021, *8*, 3469–3476. [CrossRef] [PubMed]
75. Miller, J.; Young, B.; Mccallum, L.; Rattray, J.; Ramsay, P.; Salisbury, L.; Scott, T.; Hull, A.; Cole, S.; Pollard, B.; et al. "Like Fighting a Fire with a Water Pistol": A Qualitative Study of the Work Experiences of Critical Care Nurses during the COVID-19 Pandemic. *J. Adv. Nurs.* 2023, *80*, 237–251. [CrossRef] [PubMed]
76. Jung, H.; Jung, S.Y.; Lee, M.H.; Kim, M.S. Assessing the Presence of Post-Traumatic Stress and Turnover Intention Among Nurses Post–Middle East Respiratory Syndrome Outbreak: The Importance of Supervisor Support. *Workplace Health Saf.* 2020, *68*, 337–345. [CrossRef]
77. Byon, H.D.; Sagherian, K.; Kim, Y.; Lipscomb, J.; Crandall, M.; Steege, L. Nurses' Experience With Type II Workplace Violence and Underreporting During the COVID-19 Pandemic. *Workplace Health Saf.* 2021, *70*, 412–420. [CrossRef]
78. Li, N.; Zhang, L.; Xiao, G.; Chen, J.; Lu, Q. The Relationship between Workplace Violence, Job Satisfaction and Turnover Intention in Emergency Nurses. *Int. Emerg. Nurs.* 2019, *45*, 50–55. [CrossRef]
79. Ayasreh, I.R.; Hayajneh, F.A. Workplace Violence Against Emergency Nurses: A Literature Review. *Crit. Care Nurs. Q.* 2021, *44*, 187–202. [CrossRef]
80. Vento, S.; Cainelli, F.; Vallone, A. Violence Against Healthcare Workers: A Worldwide Phenomenon With Serious Consequences. *Front. Public Health* 2020, *8*, 570459. [CrossRef]

81. Cakal, H.; Keshavarzi, S.; Ruhani, A.; Dakhil-Abbasi, G. Workplace Violence and Turnover Intentions among Nurses: The Moderating Roles of Invulnerability and Organisational Support—A Cross-Sectional Study. *J. Clin. Nurs.* **2021**, preprint. [CrossRef]
82. Baird, K.M.; Tung, A.; Yu, Y. Employee Organizational Commitment and Hospital Performance. *Health Care Manag. Rev.* **2019**, *44*, 206–215. [CrossRef] [PubMed]
83. Vagharseyyedin, S. An Integrative Review of Literature on Determinants of Nurses' Organizational Commitment. *Iran. J. Nurs. Midwifery Res.* **2016**, *21*, 117. [CrossRef] [PubMed]
84. Albalawi, A.S.; Naughton, S.; Elayan, M.B.; Sleimi, M.T. Perceived Organizational Support, Alternative Job Opportunity, Organizational Commitment, Job Satisfaction and Turnover Intention: A Moderated-Mediated Model. *Organizacija* **2019**, *52*, 310–324. [CrossRef]
85. Sokhanvar, M.; Kakemam, E.; Chegini, Z.; Sarbakhsh, P. Hospital Nurses' Job Security and Turnover Intention and Factors Contributing to Their Turnover Intention: A Cross-Sectional Study. *Nurs. Midwifery Stud.* **2018**, *7*, 133–140.

Disclaimer/Publisher's Note: The statements, opinions and data contained in all publications are solely those of the individual author(s) and contributor(s) and not of MDPI and/or the editor(s). MDPI and/or the editor(s) disclaim responsibility for any injury to people or property resulting from any ideas, methods, instructions or products referred to in the content.

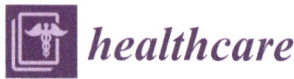

Article

Mental Healthcare through Cognitive Emotional Regulation Strategies among Prisoners

Younyoung Choi [1], Mirim Kim [2,*] and Jeongsoo Park [1]

1 Department of Psychology, Ajou University, Suwon 16499, Republic of Korea
2 BK21 FOUR R&E Center for Psychology, Korea University, Seoul 02841, Republic of Korea
* Correspondence: mirimkim@korea.ac.kr; Tel.: +82-2-3290-2558

Abstract: Prisoners are exposed to a deprived environment, which triggers mental illness and psychological problems. Abundant research has reported that mental illness problems, suicide, aggression, and violent behaviors occur in incarcerated people. Although the mental healthcare system for incarcerated people is emphasized, little research has been conducted due to their limited environment. In particular, the regulation of negative emotion is significantly associated with mental illness and anti-social and violent behaviors. However, mental healthcare through cognitive emotional regulation based on cognitive behavioral therapy has not been fully investigated. This study identified four different patterns in cognitive strategies for regulating negative emotions. Cognitive emotional regulation strategies (i.e., self-blame, other-blame, rumination, catastrophizing, putting into perspective, positive refocusing, positive reappraisal, acceptance, and refocus on planning) were examined and addressed their vulnerable psychological factors. We analyzed a total of 500 prisoners' responses to the cognitive emotional regulation questionnaire (CERQ) by latent class profiling analysis. A four-class model was identified based on the responses of CERQ. In addition, the significant effect of depression on classifying the four classes was found. Furthermore, differences in the average number of incarcerations were also shown across four classes. In conclusion, Class 2 (*Negative Self-Blamer*) uses dysfunctional/negative strategies that may place the group at a high risk of psychological disorder symptoms, including depression and post-traumatic stress. Class 3 (*Distorted Positivity*) uses positive/functional strategies but seems to utilize the positive strategies in distorted manners to rationalize their convictions. Class 1 (*Strong Blamer*) and Class 4 (*Moderator Blamer*) showed similar patterns focused on the "other-blame" strategy for regulating negative emotion, but they are at different levels, indicating that they attribute incarceration to external factors. These findings provide useful information for designing mental healthcare interventions for incarcerated people and psychological therapy programs for clinical and correctional psychologists in forensic settings.

Keywords: mental healthcare; mental illness; cognitive emotional regulation strategy; prisoners vulnerable social group; latent profiling analysis

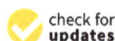

Citation: Choi, Y.; Kim, M.; Park, J. Mental Healthcare through Cognitive Emotional Regulation Strategies among Prisoners. *Healthcare* **2024**, *12*, 6. https://doi.org/10.3390/healthcare12010006

Academic Editors: Sofia Koukouli and Areti Stavropoulou

Received: 20 November 2023
Revised: 12 December 2023
Accepted: 17 December 2023
Published: 19 December 2023

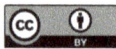

Copyright: © 2023 by the authors. Licensee MDPI, Basel, Switzerland. This article is an open access article distributed under the terms and conditions of the Creative Commons Attribution (CC BY) license (https://creativecommons.org/licenses/by/4.0/).

1. Introduction

Sykes's research [1] suggested that prisoners experience five types of deprivation in prison, including freedom, goods and services, sexual relations, autonomy, and security. Prisoners are socially isolated, receive poor-quality materials and services, are prohibited from contact with the opposite sex, and must passively follow the rules. The incarcerated environment can cause mental illnesses such as depression and anxiety and anti-social behaviors such as suicide, aggression, and violence. In fact, incarcerated people suffer from mental illness with maladaptive psychological characteristics such as anxiety and depression, as well as irrational beliefs and erroneous biases [2]. The Prison Policy Initiative (2022) reported that over 40% of people suffer from mental health disorders and experience subsequent depression and bipolar disorder due to the incarcerated environment [3,4]. In addition, the Prison Policy Initiative (2022) estimated that a prisoner is three times more likely to die from suicide than the general population [5].

The features of incarceration, such as disconnection from family, loss of autonomy, boredom and lack of purpose, and unpredictability of surroundings, are linked to negative mental health outcomes [6]. In addition, researchers at the University of Georgia found that people incarcerated from home were more likely to experience depression in 214 state prisons [7]. Furthermore, the number of incarcerations of offenders who were released from prison is significantly related to poor mental health in prison. Specifically, the number of incarcerations of offenders who suffer from poor mental health in prison is higher than in the general population [8,9]. However, research has also reported that prisoners have barriers to mental health treatment [10]. Mental healthcare and related professionals are rarely available in prisons. Furthermore, prisoners find it difficult to access mental healthcare in general [10].

The experience of continuous exposure to such an incarcerated environment evokes a variety of negative emotions. Mostly, negative emotions are the basis for triggering various mental illnesses and behavioral problems. Consequently, incarceration can worsen depression and last a long time after leaving prison [6]. In addition, the prison environment has various elements that cause distorted cognitive thinking. For example, Seo et al. [11] reported that murderers in prison possess distorted cognitive thinking processes, which lead to aggressive behaviors and suicidal thoughts. Although the mental healthcare system for incarcerated people is emphasized, few research studies have been conducted due to their limited environment. Previous research suggested that mental healthcare in terms of the ability to regulate negative emotions acts as a buffer for triggering various mental illnesses and behavioral problems such as suicidal behaviors, violence, depression, etc. [12–15]. Although prisoners' psychological problems due to the prison environment have been consistently reported as a major issue, negative emotions and distorted cognitive thinking processes among prisoners, have not been fully investigated. In addition, mental healthcare intervention regarding cognitive–emotional regulation has not been fully addressed.

Emotional regulation refers to the ability to manage one's emotional experiences and behaviors, particularly in situations of intense emotional arousal [16]. Emotion dysregulation is related to mental health, wherein negative emotions highly influence poor mental health. In addition, research found that trauma-exposed community individuals have shown a relationship between emotion dysregulation and mental health [17]. Furthermore, difficulties in regulating emotion have strong associations with the characteristics of psychopathy, including lack of empathy, impulsivity behaviors, and criminal tendencies [12–16].

Research has also reported that the characteristics of psychopathy are related to criminality and incarceration [16–20]. In a similar vein, Garofalo, Neumann, and Velotti [20] found that emotion dysregulation plays a significant mediation role in the association between psychopathy and aggressive behaviors. Preston and Anestis [21] also found that emotion dysregulation mediated the association between self-centered impulsivity traits of psychopathy and reactive aggression. In addition, Garofalo et al. [22] reported impairments in emotional regulation influence anger in both community and offender samples. Consequently, mental healthcare in forensic settings focus on correlational interventions and psychological therapy programs related to emotional regulation for reducing anti-social and aggressive behaviors [21].

Garnesfski, Kraaij, and Spinhoven [22] suggested that people choose internal or cognitive–emotional regulation methods as they grow. Therefore, cognitive strategies for regulating emotion may explain affective and cognitive mechanisms that underlie the externalizing and anti-social behaviors of adults. Garnefski, Kraaij, and Spinhoven [22] proposed a scale for CER (CERQ: Cognitive Emotion Regulation Questionnaire) in order to assess different types of cognitive strategies for regulating emotion under stressful events. Cognitive–emotional regulation (CER) refers to a cognitive process of managing emotions to deal with stressful events [22]. The CERQ measures nine types of CER strategies, including self-blame, other-blame, rumination, catastrophizing, putting into perspective, positive refocusing, positive reappraisal, acceptance, and refocusing on planning. These strategies are used for managing negative emotions in response to stressful or threatening events. In more detail, self-blame involves putting the blame on oneself for what has been experienced, while other-blame involves attributing the blame to the environment or others. Rumination is defined as repeatedly focusing on thoughts about the feelings associated with a negative event. Catastrophizing is characterized by thoughts that explicitly emphasize the severity of what has been experienced. Putting it into perspective involves downplaying the seriousness of the event and emphasizing its relative significance when comparing it to other events. Positive refocusing involves thinking about joyful and pleasant issues instead of the actual negative event. Positive reappraisal involves creating a positive meaning for the event in terms of personal growth. Lastly, acceptance is the act of accepting what has been experienced. Refocus on planning involves thoughts of resigning yourself to what has happened and reorganizing and making a plan about the events.

Abundant research regarding emotional regulation has reported robust associations with mental health. In addition, a feature of depressive disorder commonly includes cognitive changes that significantly influence the individual's function [23]. However, the identification of different types of cognitive strategies for regulating emotion under stressful situations among incarcerated people has not been fully investigated.

In addition, different patterns of cognitive strategies in emotional regulation may be related to the frequent anti-social behaviors and crimes. Therefore, the investigation regarding the association between different types of CER strategies can provide useful information for designing a mental health intervention and psychological therapy program for caring for mental illness among incarcerated people in forensic settings.

The Present Study

The main aim of this study is to identify different patterns of CER strategies among prisoners and to see how depressive disorder would impact the classifications of CER strategies. In addition, the study examines how much the different patterns can explain the number of incarcerations as the manifest variable of frequent anti-social behaviors. To achieve this, we first analyze the prisoners' responses to CERQ, which consists of nine different emotional strategies in response to negative events. Latent class profiling analysis is conducted to identify latent patterns of CER strategies. Afterward, Wald tests are used to examine the significant differences in the average number of incarcerations among the identified classes.

2. Method

2.1. Design and Setting

A total of 521 prisoners were selected from a prison in Pusan, South Korea, which has a moderate security level (S4). The psychological interviews were conducted by four doctoral-level clinical psychologists; basic psychiatric symptoms, including depression and anxiety, were evaluated for all participants. Additionally, a simple assessment of cognitive functioning, including memory, attention, concentration, and executive functioning, was conducted prior to the survey. Participants with severe cognitive impairment were excluded from the study. All participants were informed of the purpose and anonymity of the research. Each of the five prisoners conducted the survey in a privately blocked room. A USD 25 payment was provided to each participant. Finally, the responses of 500 prisoners were analyzed. This study received approval from the Human Subjects Review Committee at Donga University (2-1040709-AB-N-01-202001-BR-003-04).

2.2. Participant

After removing missing values and careless responses, 500 samples were analyzed in this study. The participants' basic demographic information and psychological characteristics were computed (Table 1). Their ages ranged from 16 to 75 years (Mean = 46.69,

SD = 11.59). The prisoners were incarcerated for a variety of convictions, including homicide (29.8%), violent offenses (15.4%), sexual violence offenses (30.0%), drug-related crimes (4.0%), property offenses (17.2%), and others (3.6%). Regarding education levels based on their last offense, 17.2% had only completed primary school (Year 6), 25.8% completed middle school, 44.0% finished senior high school, and 13.0% completed tertiary or above education. In terms of employment, 57% of the participants had a full-time job, 29% had a part-time job, and 14% were unemployed before being incarcerated. We also examined the basic psychological characteristics of the subjects, which were measured using the PHQ9 scale (Mean = 30.64, SD = 2.67).

Table 1. Demographic information and psychological characteristics of the participants.

Demographic Information	Categories	N	%
Criminals	Homicide	149	29.8
	Violent Offenses	77	15.4
	Sexual Violence Offenses	150	30.0
	Property Offenses	86	17.2
	Drug-Related Crimes	20	4.0
	Others	18	3.6
Years of Education	Below Primary School	12	2.4
	Primary School	73	14.6
	Middle School	133	26.6
	High School	221	44.2
	Above College	60	12
Job Status	Full-time Jobs	285	57.0
	Part-time Jobs	145	29.0
	Unemployed	70	14.0
Total		500	
		Mean	SD
Age		46.69	11.59
# of incarcerations		2.39	2.20
Depression	PHQ9	30.64	2.68

2.3. Measures

2.3.1. Cognitive Emotional Regulation Questionnaires

CER was assessed using the Korean version of the Cognitive Emotion Regulation Questionnaire (CERQ), which was validated by Ahn, Lee, and Joo [24]. The concept and CERQ were originally proposed by Garnefski and Kraaij [25]. The CERQ consists of 64 items measuring nine sub-factors of self-blame (SB), acceptance (ACP), rumination (RM), positive refocusing (PRF), positive reappraisal (PRA), putting into perspective (PIP), catastrophizing (CAT), blaming others (BO), and refocus on planning (ROP). Participants responded to each item on a five-point Likert scale ranging from 1 (Almost Never) to 5 (Almost Always). Cronbach's α of the total CERQ was 0.87. Cronbach's α of each sub-factor is presented on the diagonal of Table 2, along with correlation values on the off-diagonal.

2.3.2. Number of Incarcerations

The average number of incarcerations was 2.39 (Min = 1, Max = 15), as shown in Table 2.

Table 2. Correlations, mean, and standard deviation of cognitive emotion regulation strategies.

CER Strategy	1	2	3	4	5	6	7	8	9
Self-blame	0.80								
Acceptance	0.55 **	0.64							
Rumination	0.47 **	0.41 **	0.66						
Positive refocusing	0.28 **	0.33 **	0.19 **	0.75					
Positive reappraisal	0.26 **	0.47 **	0.29 **	0.48 **	0.74				
Putting into perspectives	0.23 **	0.40 **	0.23 **	0.38 **	0.64 **	0.59			
Catastrophizing	0.41 **	0.19 **	0.58 **	−0.02	−0.05	−0.08	0.78		
Blaming others	−0.27 **	−0.10 *	0.11 *	−0.06	0.09 *	0.13 **	0.17 **	0.74	
Refocus on planning	0.32 **	0.45 **	0.36 *	0.40 **	0.58 **	0.43 **	0.03	0.05	0.77
Mean	13.80	11.07	13.10	13.74	13.99	13.75	10.76	9.77	15.87
SD	3.78	2.55	3.20	3.47	3.55	3.04	3.99	3.40	3.05

Note. CER—cognitive emotional regulation; diagonal elements indicate Cronbach's α; ** $p < 0.01$; * $p < 0.05$.

2.4. Analysis Procedures

The analyses were conducted based on three main hypotheses in the current study. The first hypothesis posited that the responses of prisoners would be classified into different latent classes based on their cognitive–emotional regulation (CER) strategies. The second hypothesis is that depression, which is an important factor in mental health, would have an impact on the classification of the latent classes given CER strategies. Finally, the number of incarcerations would vary across the different latent classes of CER strategies. To test these hypotheses, we applied latent class profiling (LCP) analysis to the prisoners' responses to the CERQ and tested multinomial logistic regression to see the effect of depression on the classification of latent profiles. In addition, the Wald test was conducted to compare the four latent classes in terms of the average number of incarcerations. All analyses were conducted using *Mplus* 8.7 [26].

The LCP assumed unobservable latent sub-populations (i.e., latent classes) underlying the observed data [27]. In this study, we assumed that the prisoners had unique response patterns on CERQ, depending on the latent class to which they belonged. The LCP was based on the three-step method to lessen estimation bias resulting from the inclusion of the distal outcome (i.e., # of incarcerations) and to take the measurement error into account [28,29]. Therefore, two research models were analyzed in separate steps: (a) participants were classified into latent CER strategy classes based on their CERQ responses, and (b) differences in average number of incarcerations were examined across the latent classes.

3. Results

3.1. Identifying Latent Classes

Following Nylund et al.'s [30] recommendation, the bootstrap likelihood ratio test (BLRT) [31] and BIC [32] were used to decide the number of latent classes. BLRT assessed the improvement in model fit between neighboring class models by adding an additional class (i.e., comparison between $k - 1$ and k class models). If BLRT was significant, k classes would be preferred over the $k - 1$ classes. In BIC, a smaller value would indicate a better-fitting model for classification. We also considered each class size (i.e., the number of individuals in the class) and entropy as indicators of the model's fit. If a particular class had only a few assigned individuals, the model was not preferred due to interpretability issues. We evaluated the quality of classification based on entropy, counts of individuals in each class, and the meanings of the classification to avoid data-driven decision-making. The entropy, ranging from 0 to 1, would indicate a better classification as it increased, and enough class sizes are necessary for the interpretation [33]. Table 3 presents fit indices across diverse class models. Based on the above criteria, a four-class model was selected and used for further analysis. Although a five-class model had the smallest BIC and a significant BLRT, one of the classes had a small number of individuals ($n = 18$) contemplating the meaningful interpretation of the corresponding class [27,33]; therefore, we decided on the four-class model, considering its interpretable latent classes and adequate entropy value.

Table 3. Fit indices for identifying latent classes.

Fit Index	2 Classes	3 Classes	4 Classes	5 Classes
BIC	12319.27	12100.90	11937.32	11865.87
BLRT	625.19 **	280.52 **	225.72 **	133.59 **
Class sizes	143/357	22/242/236	36/45/188/231	18/105/224/47/106
Entropy	0.78	0.81	0.84	0.81

Note. ** $p < 0.01$.

Figure 1 displays the CERQ patterns of the four-class model, indicating the sub-factor scores, while Table 4 provides the corresponding demographic information for each class. Looking at Figure 1, we found that Class 1 and Class 4 have a particular characteristic of blaming others. These two groups had similar patterns but at different levels, in which Class 1 showed the use of a strategy exhibiting strong blame towards others, while Class 4 exhibited moderate blame towards others. Class 4 had a higher score of BO than Class 1, but Class 1 had the noticeably highest score of BO among other scores. On the other hand, Class 4 reported higher scores in other functional strategies than Class 1.

Class 2 consisted of a group of negative self-blamers. They were more likely to have CER strategies involving negative perspectives and less likely to blame others compared to other classes. Moreover, Class 2 reported higher scores in terms of dysfunctional strategies than the other classes.

Lastly, Class 3 represented a group exhibiting distorted positivity group. Participants in this class showed a similar pattern to Class 2 in terms of SB, ACP, and RM, but they had higher scores in PRF, PRA, PIP, and a lower score in CAT. Furthermore, both Class 3 and Class 4 reported higher scores in PRF, PRA, and PIP than in Class 2.

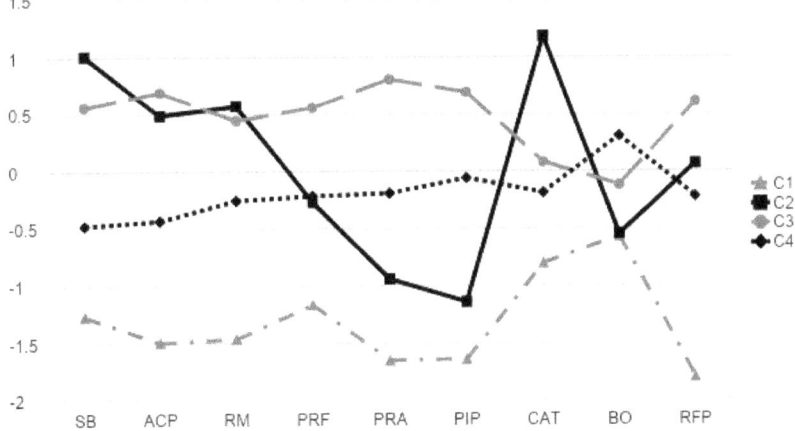

Figure 1. Cognitive emotion regulation scores across four classes. Note: SB—Self-blame; ACP—Acceptance; RM—Rumination; PRF—Positive refocusing; PRA—Positive reappraisal; PIP—Putting into perspectives; CAT—Catastrophizing; BO—Blaming others; RFP—Refocus on planning.

Table 4. Demographic information and psychological characteristics across classes.

Demographic Information	Categories	Class 1 Strong Blamer	Class 2 Negative Self-Blamer	Class 3 Distorted Positivity	Class 4 Moderate Blamer
		Frequency (%)			
Criminals	Homicide	11 (30.6)	23 (51.1)	51 (27.1)	64 (27.7)
	Violent Offenses	4 (11.1)	6 (13.3)	33 (17.6)	34 (14.7)
	Sexual Violence Offenses	16 (44.4)	12 (26.7)	42 (22.3)	80 (34.6)
	Property Offenses	3 (8.3)	2 (4.4)	38 (20.2)	43 (18.6)
	Drug-Related Crimes	-	1 (2.2)	14 (7.4)	5 (2.2)
	Others	2 (5.6)	1 (2.2)	10 (5.3)	5 (2.2)
Educational Years	Below Primary School	-	1 (2.2)	7 (3.7)	4 (1.7)
	Primary School	8 (22.2)	9 (20.0)	23 (12.2)	33 (14.3)
	Middle School	9 (25.0)	11 (24.4)	37 (19.7)	76 (32.9)
	High School	17 (47.2)	19 (42.2)	93 (49.5)	92 (39.8)
	Above College	2 (5.6)	5 (11.1)	27 (14.4)	26 (11.3)
Job Status	Full-time Jobs	21 (58.3)	28 (62.2)	111 (59.0)	125 (54.1)
	Part-time Jobs	9 (25.0)	9 (20.0)	53 (28.2)	67 (29.0)
	No Jobs	6 (16.7)	8 (17.8)	24 (12.8)	39 (16.9)
Total		36	45	188	231
		Mean (SD)			
Age		43.32 (12.46)	51.16 (11.30)	47.74 (10.46)	45.44 (12.12)
# of recidivism		2.22 (1.82)	1.71 (1.58)	2.49 (2.28)	2.46 (2.27)
Depression	PHQ9	29.94 (2.62)	31.49 (2.46)	30.35 (2.63)	30.83 (2.72)
Anxiety	STAI-S	37.75 (6.59)	40.56 (6.53)	42.97 (6.04)	40.37 (6.87)
	STAI-T	38.17 (7.63)	40.11 (6.03)	43.95 (5.70)	41.12 (6.38)

Taken together, individuals in Class 1 (strong blamers toward others) generally showed lower scores across all nine sub-factors compared to the other classes, with the highest BO sub-factor scores. Class 4 (moderate blamers to others) was similar to Class 1, but its scores on all sub-factors were higher than those of Class 1. In other words, people in C4 generally utilized all strategies. The other two classes, Class 2 and Class 3 had unique patterns. Although Class 2 had higher scores in all nine strategies than Class 1, the SB, ACP, RM, and CAT scores were higher than PRF, PRA, PIP, and BO. Notably, individuals in Class 2 had the highest CAT score among all the classes, indicating a greater tendency to employ negative strategies of SB, RM, and CAT. In addition, Class 2 showed a unique pattern with larger bumps compared to the other classes. Individuals within Class 2 had the highest scores of SB, RM, and CAT, reflecting negative perspectives towards the unpleasant situation in prison; however, they have sharp drops at PRF, PRA, and PIP related to the positive perspectives and BO. Class 3 generally used all strategies, with relatively higher use of ACP, PRF, PRA, PIP, and RFP and less use of CAT and BO, which represented negative/dysfunctional strategies. Although Class 3 employed relatively more adaptive emotional strategies than the other classes, considering the situation where prisoners were convicted and incarcerated, these strategies may not be truly adaptive emotional strategies but rather distorted positivity.

3.2. Multinomial Logistic Regression Analysis

Based on the literature [6,23], we considered depression as an important predictor to differentiate CER strategies and examined the effect of depression on the classification of the four classes using a multinomial logistic regression analysis. The results are presented in Table 5. As Class 2 was set as a reference class for the analysis, the regression effect indicates the extent to which the depressive disorder categorized the individuals into a specific latent class rather than into Class 2. The depression was a significant predictor to differentiate prisoners of Class 1/Class 3 from Class 2. The odds ratios for C1 and C3 were 0.80 and 0.85, respectively, indicating the decreased odds of classification into Class 1 and Class 3 by 20% and 15% compared to Class 2, when the level of depression increased.

Table 5. Multinomial logistic regression with depression.

Class Comparison	Estimate	S.E.	p-Value	Odds Ratio
Depression → C1	**−0.22**	0.09	0.01	**0.80**
Depression → C3	**−0.16**	0.06	0.01	**0.85**
Depression → C4	−0.08	0.06	0.10	0.91

Note. Reference class = C2; bold indicates significant test statistics.

3.3. Number of Incarcerations Comparisons across Classes

Given the four-class model, we investigated how the number of incarcerations varied across these classes, controlling the effect of depression. Table 6 presents the average number of incarcerations for each class: C1 (2.22); C2 (1.71); C3 (2.49); and C4 (2.46). Prisoners in Class 2, which was characterized by a higher level of CAT and a lower level of BO than the other classes, reported the lowest number of incarcerations. In addition, the proportion of first-time prisoners in Class 2 (71.1%) was the highest among the four classes: C1 (44.4%); C3 (45.2%); and C4 (50.2%). We conducted Wald tests to test statistical differences in the average number of incarcerations between classes and provided the test result in Table 6. As shown in the table, Class 2 showed statistically significant differences in the number of incarcerations compared to Class 3 and Class 4. The negative estimates for the Wald test indicate that the latter class had a higher number of incarcerations than the former; therefore, Class 3 and Class 4 had a higher average number of incarcerations than Class 2.

Table 6. Wald tests across latent classes for the number of incarcerations.

Class Comparison	Estimate	S.E.	p-Value
C1 vs. C2	0.50	0.38	0.18
C1 vs. C3	−0.27	0.34	0.43
C1 vs. C4	−0.24	0.34	0.48
C2 vs. C3	**−0.78**	0.29	0.01
C2 vs. C4	**−0.74**	0.28	0.01
C3 vs. C4	0.03	0.23	0.88

Note. Bold indicates significant test statistics.

The identified patterns of CER strategies in the current study explain the relatively lower number of incarcerations of Class 2 compared to Class 3 and Class 4. Class 3 had higher scores in PRF, PRA, and PIP but a lower score in CAT than Class 2. On the other hand, Class 4 had higher scores in PRF, PRA, PIP, and BO compared to Class 2, while they reported lower scores in SB, ACP, RM, and CAT. In conclusion, both classes commonly showed higher scores in PRF, PRA, and PIP, and a lower score in CAT. Therefore, the prisoners with more records of incarcerations reported higher scores in PRF, PRA, and PIP, and lower scores in CAT. However, the other comparisons were not statistically significant.

4. Discussion

The main aim of this study was to identify latent classes representing different patterns of CER strategies among prisoners and examine how these patterns explained incarcerations as an indicator of anti-social behaviors. Initially, we analyzed the prisoners' responses to CERQ, which consists of nine different strategies for regulating emotion in negative and stressful situations. LCP analysis was conducted to identify latent classes regarding different patterns of CER strategies, and the effect of depression on categorizing prisoners into specific latent classes was examined. Subsequently, Wald tests were used to examine whether the number of incarcerations varied across the latent classes and to see how the different CER strategies explained the incarcerations.

The present study identified four latent classes based on the scores of CER strategies. First, Class 2, referred to as "Negative Self-blamer," consisted of 45 prisoners, accounting for 9% of the total sample. This class was more likely to adopt negative/dysfunctional strategies (i.e., SB, RM, and CAT) for regulating emotion under stressful events. These individuals may blame themselves for incarceration, experience negative thoughts and emotions, and perceive their incarceration experiences negatively. Given the associations between negative/dysfunctional strategies and emotional dysregulation, depression, or post-traumatic stress [8,12], Class 2 may be at a high risk of psychological disorder symptoms. The current study found that Class 2 experienced a significantly lower number of incarcerations compared to Class 3 and Class 4, which reported higher scores in PRF, PRA, and PIP strategies. Previous research has indicated that anti-social and violent behaviors may occur as a means to cope with negative emotions [26]. Therefore, cautious interventions addressing psychological symptoms may help prevent suicide in prison and the likelihood of future incarceration within this group.

Second, Class 1 ($n = 36$) and Class 4 ($n = 231$) showed behavior referred to as "Moderate blamer toward others" and "Strong blamer toward others", respectively, and showed similar patterns of CER strategies focused on BO, but at different levels. These two classes accounted for 53.4% of the total sample, indicating that a significant proportion of prisoners attribute their anti-social behaviors or incarceration to external factors. This finding aligns with previous research showing a lack of self-criticism among a considerable number of prisoners [23]. It would be helpful to challenge their attribution and elicit self-directed behavioral changes in correction programs. Considering that placing high-risk and low-risk prisoners in the same group reduced program effects [27,28], it would be more effective to implement separate interventions in terms of emotional regulation patterns. In addition, the individuals in Class 1, with higher scores in BO and CAT and lower scores in the other sub-factors, were most likely to have low motivation to participate in correctional programs voluntarily. Therefore, behavioral approaches, such as contract agreements that enforce attendance through reduced control or incentives, may be helpful in increasing therapeutic effectiveness.

Third, Class 3 ($n = 188$) referred to as "Distorted Positivity," representing 37.6% of the total sample. This class used more positive/functional strategies, such as ACP, PRF, PRA, PIP, and RFP, compared to negative/dysfunctional strategies, such as CAT. Class 4 also reported a similar pattern to Class 3; both classes reported higher scores in PRF, PRA, and PIP compared to Class 1, as well as lower scores in CAT. However, Class 3 and Class 4 differed in terms of blame strategies; SB was more prevalent in Class 3, while BO was more prevalent in Class 4. Positive/functional strategies are generally helpful for psychological symptoms in the normal population. However, prisoners in Class 3 and Class 4 seemed to utilize these positive strategies in distorted manners to rationalize their convictions and crimes, given the statistically higher average number of incarcerations compared to Class 2. Although Class 3 and Class 4 experienced repeated incarcerations, they appeared to be well-adjusted in prison through their adaptive/functional emotional regulation skills.

5. Implications and Limitations

The findings of this study have several implications. First, to our knowledge, this is the first study to investigate different patterns of Cognitive–Emotional Regulation (CER) strategies among prisoners, providing insights into their intricate emotional and cognitive mechanisms for managing negative emotions. Moreover, recognizing the association between incarceration and poor mental health of offenders in prison [7], investigating patterns of emotional dysregulation as precursors to psychopathy [15,16,20,34,35], aggression [20,21], or depression [36,37] may serve as grounded evidence to develop rehabilitation intervention targeting mental health.

Second, given that the amalgamation of high-risk prisoners and low-risk prisoners in the same intervention group resulted in diminished effectiveness [38], our findings emphasize the importance of tailed interventions based on risk levels. Despite Class 2 (i.e., Negative Self-blamer) showing a lower incarceration rate compared to Class 3 and Class 4, this group is more susceptible to experiencing psychological disorder, potentially leading to suicide. One recent study suggests that self-blame is a more significant factor in predicting suicidal ideations than factors such as age, gender (male), and high perceived stress [39]. Moreover, while positive/functional strategies are typically recommended in normal populations for their psychological symptoms [40], our results indicate that Class 3, with higher use of adaptive emotional strategies, indicates repeatedly incarcerated for offenses. In addition, Class 1 indicates lower motivation to participate in correctional programs. Thus, recognizing each class suggests the necessity for different approaches intervening in each group.

Third, significantly different levels of incarceration across latent classes driven by CER strategies among prisoners highlight the importance of individual differences in CER when designing correction programs. Despite the general efficacy of cognitive–behavioral approaches in reducing criminal behaviors among offenders [41], research indicates differing responsiveness to interventions among offenders [38,42,43]. In terms of correctional intervention effectiveness, understanding how individuals regulate their emotions leading to incarceration can inform program design adjusting to specific cognitive and emotional processes. For example, improvement in terms of emotional and cognitive regulation at a different level was associated with juvenile recidivism [44]. Consequently, rehabilitation programs within prisons could benefit from personalized interventions imparting adaptive emotional regulation skills, with the aim of mitigating the risk of post-release anti-social behaviors. Thus, tailoring interventions to specific patterns regarding cognitive emotion strategies may enhance their effectiveness and reduce the risk of anti-social behaviors and recidivism.

Despite its contribution, this study has several limitations. First, the use of self-report measures may bring related bias and inaccuracy. Future research could benefit from incorporating objective measures or observational data to provide a comprehensive understanding of these strategies. Second, the sample in this study consisted of a specific group of prisoners, which limits the generalizability of the findings to other prisoners or contexts. Future studies with diverse prisoners or different contexts would strengthen and expand upon these results. Lastly, the cross-sectional study design prevents the establishment of causal relationships between CER and frequent anti-social behaviors. Further studies are needed to examine the temporal relations and predictive validity of these patterns in relation to reoffending behaviors.

Author Contributions: Conceptualization and data collection: Y.C.; methodology: M.K.; writing—original draft preparation: Y.C., M.K. and J.P. All authors listed have made a substantial, direct and intellectual contribution to the work. All authors have read and agreed to the published version of the manuscript.

Funding: This work was supported by the National Research Foundation of Korea (NRF) grant funded by the Korean government (MSIT) (NRF-2019R1F1A1061251) and BK21 FOUR R&E Center for Psychology at Korea University.

Institutional Review Board Statement: This study was approved on 18 March 2020 by the Institutional Review Board (IRB) at Human Subjects Review Committee at Donga University (approval No. 2-1040709-AB-N-01-202001-BR-003-04).

Informed Consent Statement: Informed consent was obtained from all subjects involved in the study.

Data Availability Statement: The derived data supporting the findings of this study are available from the corresponding author on request.

Conflicts of Interest: The authors declare that the research was conducted in the absence of any commercial or financial relationships that could be construed as a potential conflict of interest.

References

1. Sykes, G. The pains of imprisonment. In *The Society of Captives: A Study of a Maximum Security Prison*; Princeton University Press: Princeton, NJ, USA, 1958; pp. 63–78.
2. Mandracchia, J.T.; Morgan, R.D.; Garos, S.; Garland, J.T. Prisoner Thinking Patterns: An Empirical Investigation. *Crim. Justice Behav.* **2007**, *34*, 1029–1043. [CrossRef]
3. Katie, R.; Alexi, J. *Research Roundup: Incarceration Can Cause Lasting Damage to Mental Health*; Prison Policy Initiative: Northampton, MA, USA, 2021.
4. Wang, L. *Chronic Punishment: The Unmet Health Needs of People in State Prisons*; Prison Policy Initiative: Northampton, MA, USA, 2022.
5. Morgan, E.R.; Rivara, F.; Ta, M.; Crossman, D.; Jones, K.; Rowhani-Rahbar, A. Incarceration and subsequent risk of suicide: A statewide cohort study. *Suicide Life-Threat. Behav.* **2022**, *52*, 467–477. [CrossRef]
6. Stringer, H. Improving mental health for inmates. *Monit. Psychol.* **2019**, *50*, 46. Available online: https://www.apa.org/monitor/2019/03/mental-heath-inmates (accessed on 10 December 2023).
7. Bronson, J.; Berzofsky, M. *Indicators of Mental Health Problems Reported by Prisoners and Jail Inmates, 2011–2012*; U.S. Department of Justics Office of Justics, Programs Bureau of Justice Statistics: Washington, DC, USA, 2017.
8. Alexi, J.; Sawyer, W. *Arrest, Release, Repeat: How Police and Jails Are Misused to Respond to Social Problems*; Prison Policy Initiative: Northampton, MA, USA, 2019.
9. Wallace, D.; Wang, X. Does in-prison physical and mental health impact recidivism? *SSM Pop. Health* **2020**, *11*, 100569. [CrossRef]
10. Reingle Gonzalez, J.M.; Connell, N.M. Mental health of prisoners: Identifying barriers to mental health treatment and medication continuity. *Am. J. Public Health* **2014**, *104*, 2328–2333. [CrossRef]
11. Seo, J.H.; Kim, K.; Lee, K.; Kim, G. A study on linguistic and psychological characteristics and personality profiling in the writings of murders. *J. Korean Data Anal. Soc.* **2012**, *14*, 1355–1371.
12. Hare, R.D. *Hare Psychopathy Checklist-Revised*, 2nd ed.; Multi-Health Systems: Toronto, ON, Canada, 2003.
13. Hare, R.D.; Neumann, C.S. The PCL-R assessment of psychopathy: Development, structural properties, and new directions. In *Handbook of Psychopathy*; Patrick, C.J., Ed.; Guilford Press: New York, NY, USA, 2006; pp. 58–88.
14. Williams, K.M.; Paulhus, D.L.; Hare, R.D. Capturing the four-factor structure of psychopathy in college students via self-report. *J. Pers. Assess.* **2007**, *88*, 205–219. [CrossRef]
15. Hare, R.D. Psychopathy, affect and behavior. In *Psychopathy: Theory, Research and Implications for Society*; Cooke, D.J., Forth, A.E., Hare, R.D., Eds.; Kluwer: Dordrecht, The Netherlands, 1998; pp. 105–137.
16. Garofalo, C.; Neumann, C.S. Psychopathy and emotion regulation: Taking stock and moving forward. In *Routledge International Handbook of Psychopathy and Crime*; DeLisi, M., Ed.; Routledge: Abingdon, UK, 2018; pp. 58–79.
17. Coid, J.; Yang, M.; Ullrich, S.; Roberts, A.; Hare, R.D. Prevalence and correlates of psychopathic traits in the household population of Great Britain. *Int. J. Law Psychiatry* **2009**, *32*, 65–73. [CrossRef] [PubMed]
18. Hare, R.D.; Neumann, C.S. Psychopathy: Assessment and forensic implications. *Can. J. Psychiatry* **2009**, *54*, 791–802. [CrossRef] [PubMed]
19. Olver, M.E.; Neumann, C.S.; Wong, S.C.P.; Hare, R.D. The structural and predictive properties of the Psychopathy Checklist–Revised in Canadian Aboriginal and non-Aboriginal offenders. *Psychol. Assess.* **2013**, *25*, 167–179. [CrossRef] [PubMed]
20. Garofalo, C.; Neumann, C.S.; Velotti, P. Psychopathy and aggression: The role of emotion dysregulation. *J. Interpers. Violence* **2021**, *36*, NP12640–NP12664. [CrossRef] [PubMed]
21. Preston, O.C.; Anestis, J.C. The indirect relationships between psychopathic traits and proactive and reactive aggression through empathy and emotion dysregulation. *J. Psychopathol. Behav. Assess.* **2020**, *42*, 409–423. [CrossRef]
22. Garnefski, N.; Kraaij, V.; Spinhoven, P. Negative life events, cognitive emotion regulation and emotional problems. *Pers. Individ. Differ.* **2001**, *30*, 1311–1327. [CrossRef]
23. Weiss, N.H.; Forkus, S.R.; Contractor, A.A.; Dixon-Gordon, K.L. The interplay of negative and positive emotion dysregulation on mental health outcomes among trauma-exposed community individuals. *Psychol. Trauma Theory Res. Pract. Policy* **2020**, *12*, 219–226. [CrossRef] [PubMed]
24. Ahn, H.N.; Lee, N.; Joo, H. Validation of the cognitive emotion regulation questionnaire in a Korean population. *Korean J. Couns.* **2013**, *14*, 1773–1794. [CrossRef]
25. Garnefski, N.; Kraaij, V. The cognitive emotion regulation questionnaire. *Eur. J. Psychol. Assess.* **2007**, *23*, 141–149. [CrossRef]
26. Muthén, L.K.; Muthén, B.O. *Mplus User's Guide*, 8th ed.; Muthén & Muthén: Los Angeles, CA, USA, 2017.
27. Lubke, G.H.; Muthén, B. Investigating population heterogeneity with factor mixture models. *Psychol. Methods* **2005**, *10*, 21–39. [CrossRef]
28. Vermunt, J.K. Latent class modeling with covariates: Two improved three-step approaches. *Political Anal.* **2017**, *18*, 450–469. [CrossRef]
29. Wang, J.; Wang, X. *Structural Equation Modeling: Applications Using Mplus*, 2nd ed.; John Wiley & Sons: Hoboken, NJ, USA, 2019.
30. Nylund, K.L.; Asparouhov, T.; Muthén, B.O. Deciding on the number of classes in latent class analysis and growth mixture modeling: A Monte Carlo simulation study. *Struct. Equ. Model.* **2007**, *14*, 535–569. [CrossRef]
31. McLachlan, G.J.; Peel, D. *Finite Mixture Models*; Wiley: Hoboken, NJ, USA, 2004.
32. Schwartz, G. Estimating the dimension of a model. *Ann. Stat.* **1978**, *6*, 461–464. [CrossRef]

33. Jung, S.; Shin, M.; Lee, Y.R. An application of latent class analysis to classifying change trajectory of school achievement improvement of general high school and testing determinants of the classification. *J. Educ. Eval. Res.* **2015**, *28*, 1277–1299.
34. Garnefski, N.; Kraaij, V. Relationships between cognitive emotion regulation strategies and depressive symptoms: A comparative study of five specific samples. *Pers. Individ. Differ.* **2006**, *40*, 1659–1669. [CrossRef]
35. Zhou, J.; Witt, K.; Cao, X.; Chen, C.; Wang, X. Predicting reoffending using the Structured Assessment of Violence Risk in Youth (SAVRY): A 5-year follow-up study of male juvenile offenders in Hunan Province, China. *PLoS ONE* **2017**, *12*, e0169251. [CrossRef] [PubMed]
36. Ehring, T.; Tuschen-Caffier, B.; Schnulle, J.; Fisher, S.; Gross, J.J. Emotion regulation and vulnerability to depression: Spontaneous versus instructed use of emotion suppression and reappraisal. *Emotion* **2010**, *10*, 563. [CrossRef] [PubMed]
37. Walker, S.; Worrall, A. Life as a woman: The gendered pains of indeterminate imprisonment. *Prison. Serv. J.* **2000**, *132*, 27–37. [CrossRef]
38. Lipsey, M.W.; Cullen, F.T. The effectiveness of correctional rehabilitation: A review of systematic reviews. *Annu. Rev. Law Soc. Sci.* **2007**, *3*, 297–320. [CrossRef]
39. Okeke, A.O.; Obiora, A.; Ezeokaana, J.O.; Abamara, N.C. Age, gender, stress and self-blame as predictors of suicidal-ideation among prison inmates in South East Nigeria. *Soc. Sci. Res.* **2022**, *6*, 1.
40. Carl, J.R.; Soskin, D.P.; Kerns, C.; Barlow, D.H. Positive emotion regulation in emotional disorders: A theoretical review. *Clin. Psychol. Rev.* **2013**, *33*, 343–360. [CrossRef]
41. Pearson, F.S.; Lipton, D.S.; Cleland, C.M.; Yee, D.S. The effects of behavioral/cognitive-behavioral programs on recidivism. *Crime Delinq.* **2022**, *48*, 476–496. [CrossRef]
42. Antonowicz, D.H.; Ross, R.R. Essential components of successful rehabilitation programs for offenders. *Int. J. Offender. Ther. Comp. Criminol.* **1994**, *38*, 97–104. [CrossRef]
43. Gendreau, P. Offender rehabilitation: What we know and what needs to be done. *Crim. Justice Behav.* **1996**, *23*, 144–161. [CrossRef]
44. Docherty, M.; Lieman, A.; Gorden, B.L. Improvement in emotion regulation while detained predicts lower juvenile recidivism. *Youth Violence Juv. Justice* **2021**, *20*, 164–183. [CrossRef]

Disclaimer/Publisher's Note: The statements, opinions and data contained in all publications are solely those of the individual author(s) and contributor(s) and not of MDPI and/or the editor(s). MDPI and/or the editor(s) disclaim responsibility for any injury to people or property resulting from any ideas, methods, instructions or products referred to in the content.

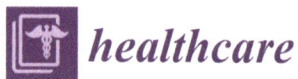

Article

Maternal Health Care Service Utilization in the Post-Conflict Democratic Republic of Congo: An Analysis of Health Inequalities over Time

Dieudonne Bwirire [1,*], Inez Roosen [1], Nanne de Vries [1], Rianne Letschert [2], Edmond Ntabe Namegabe [3] and Rik Crutzen [1]

1. Department of Health Promotion, CAPHRI Care and Public Health Research Institute, Faculty of Health, Medicine and Life Sciences, Maastricht University, 6229 HA Maastricht, The Netherlands; inez.roosen@maastrichtuniversity.nl (I.R.); nanne.devries@maastrichtuniversity.nl (N.d.V.); rik.crutzen@maastrichtuniversity.nl (R.C.)
2. Maastricht University, 6200 MD Maastricht, The Netherlands; r.letschert@maastrichtuniversity.nl
3. Faculté de Santé et Développement Communautaires, Université Libre des Pays des Grands Lacs (ULPGL), Goma 368, Democratic Republic of the Congo; ntabenamegabe2006@gmail.com
* Correspondence: d.bwirire@maastrichtuniversity.nl

Abstract: This study assessed inequality in maternal healthcare service utilization in the Democratic Republic of the Congo, using the Demographic and Health Surveys of 2007 and 2013–2014. We assessed the magnitude of inequality using logistical regressions, analyzed the distribution of inequality using the Gini coefficient and the Lorenz curve, and used the Wagstaff method to assess inequality trends. Women were less likely to have their first antenatal care visit within the first trimester and to attend more antenatal care visits when living in eastern Congo. Women in rural areas were less likely to deliver by cesarean section and to receive postnatal care. Women with middle, richer, and richest wealth indexes were more likely to complete more antenatal care visits, to deliver by cesarean section, and to receive postnatal care. Over time, inequality in utilization decreased for antenatal and postnatal care but increased for delivery by cesarean sections, suggesting that innovative strategies are needed to improve utilization among poorer, rural, and underserved women.

Keywords: maternal health care service utilization; trends; health inequalities; inequality measurement; post-conflict; Democratic Republic of Congo (DRC)

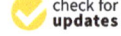

Citation: Bwirire, D.; Roosen, I.; de Vries, N.; Letschert, R.; Ntabe Namegabe, E.; Crutzen, R. Maternal Health Care Service Utilization in the Post-Conflict Democratic Republic of Congo: An Analysis of Health Inequalities over Time. *Healthcare* **2023**, *11*, 2871. https://doi.org/10.3390/healthcare11212871

Academic Editor: Ines Aguinaga-Ontoso

Received: 21 August 2023
Revised: 23 October 2023
Accepted: 26 October 2023
Published: 31 October 2023

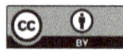

Copyright: © 2023 by the authors. Licensee MDPI, Basel, Switzerland. This article is an open access article distributed under the terms and conditions of the Creative Commons Attribution (CC BY) license (https://creativecommons.org/licenses/by/4.0/).

1. Introduction

The Alma-Ata Declaration of the World Health Organization (WHO) states that the existing gross inequalities in the health status of people are unacceptable and are, therefore, of common concern to all countries [1]. This establishes a standard of public commitment to make quality health care accessible for all [2]. The Alma-Ata Declaration was the forerunner of the Global Strategy for Health for All and the Sustainable Development Goals (SDGs). The SDGs are a collection of 17 interdependent global goals set by the United Nations (UN) General Assembly in 2015 for the year 2030. Specifically, SDG 3 is devoted to health, and one of its targets is to reduce the global maternal mortality rate to less than 70 per 100,000 live births by 2030 [3].

Improving maternal health is critical to fulfilling the aspiration to reach SDG 3 [4,5]. Significant progress is being made in improving millions of people's health [6], and some improvements have also been observed in maternal health. However, despite this progress, particularly in sub-Saharan Africa (SSA), the number of maternal deaths explained by a lack of access to and utilization of maternal health care services (MHCS) before, during, or after delivery [7] and socioeconomic inequality in health care use [8–10] are still high. The odds that a woman in SSA will die from complications related to pregnancy and childbirth is 1 n 20—an enormous difference from 1 in 6250 in the developed world [11]. Achievement of the 2030 SDGs is likely to be compromised if inequalities in health are not adequately addressed [12,13].

Countries that have experienced armed conflict often have the worst indicators of maternal mortality and very high levels of psychological impairment [14] and struggle to cope with the burden of diseases [15]. Often, there are significant health concerns, especially in maternal health care in these countries [16]. According to the United Nations (UN), efforts to improve maternal health are hindered by the presence of conflict, indicating that violence and instability can threaten governmental and international aid, further deterring health promotion [17]. While long-running conflicts have begun to decline or at least plateau, the underlying causes of many of these conflicts have not been addressed, and the potential for violence to flare up remains very real [18]. This can be observed in the Democratic Republic of the Congo (DRC), where many regions have known a series of destabilizing conflicts and wars [19]. This fragile environment may reinforce the existing cross-country maternal health inequities, particularly in the densely populated eastern regions [20]. According to the most recent Demographic and Health Survey (DHS 2013/2014), more than 200 ethnic groups live in the DRC, with the Bantu people as a large majority. The official language is French, and the capital city, Kinshasa, is the second-largest French-speaking city in the world. Four additional national languages are recognized: Kikongo, Lingala, Swahili, and Tshiluba. The majority of the country is Christian, mainly Catholic and Protestant. Despite a wealth of mineral resources, the DRC struggles with many socioeconomic problems, including high infant and maternal mortality rates, malnutrition, poor vaccination coverage, and lack of access to improved water sources and sanitation. Fertility remains high at more than five children per woman and is likely to remain high because of the low use of contraception and the cultural preference for larger families. Ongoing conflict, mismanagement of resources, and a lack of investment have resulted in food insecurity; almost 25% of children under the age of 5 were malnourished as of 2018. The overall coverage of basic public services—education, health, sanitation, and potable water—is very limited, with substantial regional and rural/urban disparities.

A limited number of studies have used all available Demographic and Health Surveys carried out in the DRC (EDS-RDC) datasets to examine the relationship between conflict and maternal healthcare service utilization in the DRC. We found one study by Ziegler et al. [21] that employed data from the 2007 and 2013–2014 EDS-RDC for this purpose. Of particular interest is that this study analyzed how predisposing, enabling, and need-based factors impact women's antenatal care (ANC) and skilled birth attendant (SBA) usage, drawing theoretical insights from Andersen's Behavioural Model of Health Care Utilization [22,23]. The study found that women in regions with extremely high levels of conflict were less likely to meet the WHO's ANC recommendations compared to those in regions with moderate levels of conflict, suggesting that conflict-affected countries require context-specific interventions if progress is to be made toward achieving SDG 3.1. In the present study, we will focus on the inequality trends in the utilization of ANC, delivery services, and postnatal care (PNC), presenting a cross-sectional perspective.

To review progress concerning inequality in the utilization of MHCS and expand the evidence base to understand the problem better, some countries have conducted studies such as the Demographic and Health Surveys (DHS) and Household Income Expenditure Surveys (HIES) [24,25]. Others have monitored health inequalities between regions [26]. Specifically for the DRC, where disparities in MHCS exist between different provinces [17], a comprehensive overview of the MHCS utilization in those populations that are completely left behind is imperative. Therefore, we intend to make a theoretical contribution to the literature on health inequality that would also be useful to scholars beyond the Democratic Republic of Congo. For this paper, health inequalities refer to differences in the distribution of a specific factor (such as health status, income, and opportunities) between different population groups, while health inequities, on the other hand, are inequalities in which the outcome is unnecessary and avoidable, as well as unjust and unfair [27].

Hypotheses and Aims of the Study

This study aims to assess health inequality trends in selected MHCS utilization variables in post-conflict DRC using publicly available DHS. Specifically, we address the following research questions (RQ):

RQ1. What is the magnitude of inequality in the utilization of MHCS in post-conflict DRC?

RQ2. What is the regional distribution of inequality in the utilization of MHCS in post-conflict DRC?

RQ3. What are the trends of inequalities in the utilization of MHCS in post-conflict DRC?

From these research questions, we further develop the following research hypotheses (H):

Hypothesis H1. *Health inequality in MHCS utilization has deteriorated in the DRC between 2007 and 2013–2014.*

Hypothesis H2. *There is an unequal distribution of MHCS utilization at the national, regional, or local level in the DRC. We assume that the western part of the country has better maternal health outcomes than the eastern part of the country.*

Hypothesis H3. *Between 2007 and 2013–2014, no progress has been made toward decreasing health inequalities.*

These hypotheses were examined following a preregistered analysis plan (available from https://doi.org/10.17605/OSF.IO/GVYUX accessed on 28 February 2020).

2. Material and Methods

2.1. Source of Data

Data on the utilization of MHCS from the DHS carried out in the DRC in 2007 and 2013–2014 were used in this study. The DHS is a periodic cross-sectional nationally representative household health survey based on a multi-stage cluster survey design funded by USAID (the U.S. Agency for International Development's) Bureau for Global Health. Relevant questions related to the utilization of MHCS were retrieved from the women's questionnaires of both waves, including women of reproductive age (15 to 49 years old) as the study population. Samples selected for enumeration are ensured to be representative and comparative across countries. For the DRC, the DHS involved a two-stage sampling procedure: first selecting the location and then selecting households per location at random. Within a household, respondents were selected by gender for the different questionnaire types. A respondent was included if he/she was a usual member of the household or had spent the night preceding the survey in the household. A random probability sample of households was designed to provide estimates of health, nutrition, water, environmental sanitation, and education at the national level for urban and rural areas and the 11 provinces. The objectives, organization, sample design, and questionnaires used in the DHS surveys are described elsewhere [28].

The global DHS project provided technical assistance in the design, implementation, and analysis of the survey (Monitoring and Evaluation to Assess and Use Results Demographic and Health Surveys: MEASURE DHS) of Macro International, Inc., Irvine, CA, USA.

This study follows the Strengthening the Reporting of Observational Studies in Epidemiology (STROBE) statement: guidelines for reporting observational studies [29]. Detailed descriptions of the application of the STROBE checklist can be found in Supplementary Materials File S1.

2.2. Data Collection Procedures

The current study used data from the two most recent rounds (2007 and 2013/2014) of the Congolese Demographic and Health Surveys (EDS-RDC).

The EDS-RDC I (1st wave) [30] was conducted from January to August 2007 using a 2-staged stratified cluster design. It provides data for a wide range of monitoring and impact evaluation indicators on maternal health in the DRC. A total of 9002 households were randomly selected, with a household response rate of 99.3%; 9995 women aged 15–49 were interviewed.

The EDS-RDC II (2nd wave) [31] was implemented from November 2013 to February 2014 using a multi-stage cluster sample survey. A total household sample of 18,360 was randomly selected, with a household response rate of 98.6%; 18,827 women aged 15–49 were interviewed.

Both surveys provide nationally representative maternal and child health estimates and basic demographic and health information [32]. All survey data are presented at both the national and sub-national levels. The latter is often, but not always, provinces or a group of provinces. All of the information collected is representative of the national level, the place of residence (urban and rural), and the level of each of the eleven administrative provinces at the time of the survey. The results also represent the level of each of the twenty-six new administrative provinces. All interviews were administered by the same company, using similar sampling designs and a standard set of questionnaires.

Ethics Approval and Consent to Participate

In this study, we made use of secondary DHS data from DRC. Therefore, our study did not require formal ethics approval. All ethics procedures were the responsibility of the institutions that either commissioned, funded, or carried out the original DHS surveys. The Institutional Review Board of Macro International, Inc. reviewed and approved the MEASURE Demographic and Health Surveys Project Phase II in compliance with the United States Department of Health and Human Services requirements for the "Protection of Human Subjects" (45 CFR 46). The 2007 and 2013–2014 EDS-RDC surveys were categorized under that approval. In addition, the study complied with the Maastricht University code of ethics for research in the social and behavioral sciences involving human participants, as well as with the national guidelines.

2.3. Variables of the Study

2.3.1. Outcome Variables

In this study, the selection of the primary outcome variables was guided by the framework of indicators proposed by the 'Countdown to 2030' global monitoring activities to track universal coverage for reproductive, maternal, newborn, and child health [33] and the WHO Global Reference List of 100 Core Health Indicators [34]. Notably, we examined a diverse set of MHCS utilization variables at different stages of the pregnancy, namely complete antenatal care (ANC), delivery, and postnatal care (PNC). We described the utilization of MHCS to the WHO requirements [35,36], which only consider it a positive pregnancy experience when women (1) receive at least one ANC visit during the first trimester of their pregnancy, (2) have at least eight ANC visits in total throughout their pregnancy, (3) are attended to at delivery by a skilled birth attendant (SBA), and (4) deliver in a health facility.

(1) Antenatal care (ANC), also known as prenatal care services, refers to the total number of women aged 15–49 with a live birth in the five years preceding the survey. In the survey, women were asked whether they had at least three visits for ANC checkups, received at least one TT injection, or underwent the following checkups and tests at least once during antenatal visits—weight, height, blood pressure, blood test, urine test—and whether they received information regarding pregnancy for the last birth during the five years preceding the survey. Undergoing a checkup was classified as timely if done within the first trimester; it was classified as late if done beyond the first trimester; the frequency of ANC visits was defined as adequate or inadequate as per the WHO recommendation—including four or more antenatal visits. This information was used to define full ANC in this study.

(2) Care during child delivery (safe delivery) is defined as the deliveries conducted either in a medical institution or at home assisted by a skilled person. The indicator provides information about births attended by skilled health personnel (percentage of births with skilled attendants and by place), institutional delivery (measured as the total number of interviewed women who had one or more live births delivered in a (private or public) health facility), and delivery by cesarean section (measured by the total number of live births to women aged 15–49 years delivered by caesarian section (C-section) in a health facility (private or public)). In the survey, women were asked where their children were born, who assisted during the deliveries, and many other delivery characteristics. This information was collected for the last five years preceding the survey.

(3) Postnatal care (PNC)—refers to the total number of women aged 15–49 with a last live birth in the last five years before the survey (regardless of the place of delivery). In the survey, women who had their last birth were asked "if they did have any checkups within 48 h after delivery?" and whether or not the "women underwent any health checkup by a health professional after delivery?" In this study, women who went for a checkup at any health facility within two weeks of delivery are considered to have used postnatal care services.

The majority of the selected outcome variables in this study are binary (yes or no) (e.g., Cesarean section, place of delivery, and professional health assistance during delivery), where 1 indicates the use of the service. Only two outcome variables, number of antenatal visits (0 = no antenatal visits, 1 = 1–3 visits, 2 = 4–7 visits, and 3 = 8 and more visits) and prenatal care received from (0 = no one, 1 = professional care, and 2 = traditional/non-professional care) were categorical variables consisting of three categories.

2.3.2. Independent Variables

At the national level, two independent variables were constructed: the survey year indicates whether a household participated in the DHS survey in 2007 or 2013/2014 as defined by DHS (0 = 2013/2014; 1 = 2007). We described the eastern DRC region (coded as 0) as centered on the North and South Kivu Provinces and nearby Orientale, Maniema, and Katanga. In this region, populations have been living with conflict and displacement for the past two decades due to many years of political and social crisis, and systems providing services for all aspects of life have been weakened. The western DRC region (coded as 1) includes the capital city (Kinshasa) and the provinces of Bandundu, Bas-Congo, Equateur, Kananga, Kasaï Oriental, and Kasaï Occidental, where the burden of the conflict has been less.

All variables that we used in this study are categorized as maternal health services and described in Supplementary Materials File S2.

2.3.3. Control Variables

The included control variables were selected to quantify each determinant's real contribution to inequality in that specific MHCS utilization variable, such as the type of place of residence of the respondent (living in urban or rural areas was included as dummy variable (2 = rural; 1 = urban); highest education level (a categorical variable was created based on the DRC school system, aggregating education levels as: no education (coded as 0), primary education (coded as 1), secondary education (coded as 2), and higher education (coded as 3); religion (a categorical variable was created using the codes and labels: 1 = catholic; 2 = protestant; 3 = salvation army; 4 = kimbanguist; 5 = other Christian; 6 = muslim; 7 = animist; 8 = no religion and 96 = other); ethnicity (a categorical variable was created using the codes and labels: 1 = bakongo north and south; 2 = bas-kasai and kwilu-kwango; 3 = cuvette centrale; 4 = ubangi and itimbiri; 5 = Uele lake albert; 6 = basele-kivu, Maniema and kivu; 7 = kasai, Katanga, Tanganyika; 8 = Lunda; 9 = pygmy; 96 = others); wealth index (identified five equal categories: poorest—coded as 1; poorer—coded as 2;

middle—coded as 3; richer—coded as 4; and richest—coded as 5), and respondents' current work status was included as a dummy variable (0 = no; 1 = yes) in the datasets.

2.4. Statistical Data Analysis

2.4.1. The Magnitude of Inequality (RQ1)

To document the true magnitude of inequality in health, data are required on (i) a measure of health (e.g., health status, health care, and other determinants, and the social and economic consequences of ill health) and (ii) a measure of social position or an 'equity stratifier' that defines strata in a social hierarchy (e.g., socioeconomic status, gender, ethnicity, and geographical area) [37]. We assessed the changes in the true magnitude of inequality in utilization of MHCS across different survey years (2007 and 2013–2014) and geographic regions (eastern vs. western of the DRC) using logistic regressions (dichotomous odds ratio (OR) and multinomial (relative risk ratio (RRR)), including previously discussed control variables. Dichotomous logistic regression was chosen for the binary dependent variables, and multinomial logistic regression for the categorical outcome variables. We used logistic regressions to check the adjusted effects of selected socioeconomic and demographic characteristics on the utilization of maternal healthcare services. Logistic regressions allow for the prediction of the relationship between the dependent and independent variables, taking into account multiple control variables. All the independent variables were verified for association with dependent variables at the bivariate level using chi-square tests. We considered $p \leq 0.05$ as the criterion for statistical significance. Logistic regression analysis results have been presented with 95% confidence intervals (95% CI).

2.4.2. Inequality Distribution (RQ2)

To analyze the distribution of inequality in each selected MHCS utilization variable and every region, we used the Gini coefficient (Gini) and the Lorenz curve. The Lorenz curve is a graphical representation of a function of the cumulative proportion of resources or services of ordered institutions mapped onto the corresponding cumulative proportion of their size. In a Lorenz curve diagram, an unequal distribution of inequality in the utilization of MHCS will loop further down and away from the 45-degree line. In contrast, a more equal distribution in the utilization of MHCS will move the line closer to the 45-degree line.

The Gini is defined as twice the area between the Lorenz curve and the diagonal. It reflects the ratio of the area between the Lorenz curve and the diagonal line to the whole area below the 45-degree line [38]. It ranges from zero (when there is no inequality = perfectly equal distribution) to one (most unequal = when all the population's health is concentrated in the hands of one person). We used the Gini as a critical measure of inequality for each selected MHCS utilization variable and every region separately (overall and for 2007 and 2013–2014 separately).

2.4.3. Inequality Trends (RQ3)

To investigate inequality trends in the MHCS utilization variables, we used the Wagstaff two group (2007 and 2013–2014 DHS and eastern and western regions) concentration indices (CI) comparison method (using STATA command conindex), which provides point estimates and standard errors of a range of concentration indices [39,40].

We used survey data to classify households into wealth quintiles based on ownership of household assets and housing characteristics. Wealth quintiles represent the relative socioeconomic position of a given country at a specific time rather than absolute wealth, all of which should be account considered when comparing wealth-related inequalities within countries. Thus, wealth quintiles are always a relative measure of how wealth is distributed within the population from the way the quintiles were calculated. For example, wealth quintiles calculated from a survey representative of one specific region of a country will only represent the distribution of wealth in that geographic region.

The DHS Wealth Index is based on the assumption that the possession of assets, services, and amenities is related to the relative economic position of the household in the country [41]. Based on the presence or absence of a large number of potential household assets, the DHS computes a continuous wealth index for each survey. The cut-off points in the wealth index at which to form the quintiles are calculated by obtaining a weighted frequency distribution of households, with the weight being the product of the number of de jure members of the household and the sampling weight of the household [37].

We finally calculated overall and group-specific CI. The CI is the most appropriate measure of health inequality because it meets the three basic requirements of a health inequality index, namely, (i) that it reflects the socioeconomic dimension of inequalities in health, (ii) that it reflects the experiences of the entire population, and (iii) that it is sensitive to changes in the distribution of the population across socioeconomic groups [42]. While the original application of CI was to study income inequality [43], economists have since extended the application of CI to study social inequality in health [42,44,45]. The CI quantifies the extent to which a health service coverage indicator is concentrated among the poorest or the richest. Subsequently, we adopted inference methods developed by Kakwani et al. [44] to test whether these indices are different from zero. We applied the inference test developed by Bishop et al. [46] to test for changes in the CI over time. To estimate the inequality in the utilization of MHCS to the economic condition of women, we fitted the concentration curves (CC). The CC plots shares of ANC, care during child delivery, and PNC against quintiles of the wealth index.

Data management and data analysis were performed by using STATA Version 12.0 (STATA Corp., College Station, TX, USA) and Distributive Analysis/Analyse Distributive (DAD) 4.4 [47].

3. Results

3.1. Characteristics of the Study Participants

Table 1 presents the descriptive characteristics of all respondents in the DRC by each survey year. It shows that in both survey waves, most respondents came from rural areas (60%), and the proportion of respondents from the western DRC decreased from 67% in 2007 to 62% in 2013–2014. The country's proportion of respondents with no education decreased from 21% in 2007 to 18% in 2013–2014, while the proportion of respondents with a higher education level slightly increased from 2.91% in 2007 to 2.98% in 2013–2014. Most of the respondents were working, and there was a further increase in the working population from 61% in 2007 to 68% in 2013–2014. The table shows that marital status changed significantly for the respondents living together; it increased from 9.8% in 2007 to 16.9% in 2013–2014, respectively. The country's dominant ethnic groups are located in the Kasai, Katanga, and Tanganyika (27%), followed by the Basele-Kivu, Maniema, Kivu (20%), and the Bas-Kasai and Kwilu-kwango (15%). Christianity is the most practiced religion (about 29% Catholic, 29% Protestant, and 35% other Christians).

Table 1. Descriptive characteristics of all respondents in the DRC by survey year (2007 and 2013–2014).

Variables	Overall	2007 DHS (N = 14.752)	2013–2014 DHS (N = 27.483)
	(%)	(%)	(%)
Place of residence			
Urban	40.3	47.91	36.26
Rural	59.7	52.09	63.74
Highest Education Level			
No education	18.96	21.08	17.83
Primary	38.51	37.8	38.88
Secondary	39.58	38.21	40.31
Higher	2.96	2.91	2.98
Region			
Kinshasa	12.04	16.67	9.58

Table 1. Cont.

Variables	Overall	2007 DHS (N = 14.752)	2013–2014 DHS (N = 27.483)
Bandundu	11.85	9.42	13.14
Bas-congo	5.81	7.3	5.02
Equateur	12.5	9.07	14.32
Kasai Occidental	7.59	7.27	7.76
Kasai Oriental	10.2	8.66	11.01
Katanga	10.83	9.25	11.66
Maniema	5.93	8.54	4.54
Nord-Kivu	6.84	8.16	6.13
Orientale	10.03	7.55	11.35
Sud-Kivu	6.38	8.07	5.49
Wealth Index			
Poorest	21.75	19.03	23.19
Poorer	19.09	17.64	19.87
Middle	19.05	18.38	19.41
Richer	18.76	20.17	18.01
Richest	21.35	24.78	19.53
Religion			
Catholic	29.14	29.67	28.86
Protestant	28.84	30.7	27.85
Salvation Army	0.24	0.36	0.18
Kimbanguist	3.07	3.23	2.99
Other Christian	34.74	32.33	36.02
Muslim	1.69	1.96	1.54
Animist	0.42	0.52	0.37
No religion	0.92	1.02	0.87
Bundu dia Kongo	0.08		0.12
Vuvamu	0.02		0.03
Other	0.65	0.13	0.93
.	0.19	0.08	0.25
Ethnicity			
Bakongo North and South	10.29	13.69	8.49
Bas-Kasai and Kwilu-Kwango	14.86	12.94	15.88
Cuvette Centrale	9.1	8.23	9.56
Ubangi and Itimbiri	9.81	6.29	11.68
Uele Lake Albert	7.34	4.85	8.66
Basele-k, man. and Kivu	19.75	25.12	16.9
Kasai, Katanga, Tanganika	26.88	26.76	26.95
Lunda	1.01	0.98	1.03
Pygmy	0.22	0.09	0.29
Foreign/non-Congolese	0.32		0.49
Others	0.25	0.71	0.01
.	0.16	0.33	0.07
Currently Working			
No	33.76	38	31.51
Yes	65.99	61.93	68.15

Table 1. Cont.

Variables	Overall	2007 DHS (N = 14.752)	2013–2014 DHS (N = 27.483)
.	0.25	0.07	0.35
Marital Status			
Never married	24.36	24.76	24.14
Married	51.54	56.03	49.15
Living together	14.5	9.86	16.96
Widowed	2.26	2.11	2.34
Divorced	1.94	1.72	2.06
Not living together	5.4	5.51	5.34

Data are presented as N and percentage. "." represents a missing/unknown subcategory.

3.2. The Magnitude of Inequality (RQ1)

The true magnitude of inequality in the socioeconomic and demographic characteristics of the study respondents on the utilization of MHCS is shown in Tables 2 and 3. The results indicate that there have been substantial gains in ANC, delivery, and PNC service utilization.

3.2.1. Antenatal Care (ANC)

The majority of women in the DRC received some kind of ANC services (Table 2). Overall, women living in eastern DRC were less likely to have their first ANC visit within the first trimester, less likely to have checkups (at least once) during ANC visits, and less likely to attend four or more ANC visits than those living in western Congo and meet adequate WHO requirements for ANC utilization. On the contrary, women living in western DRC were less likely to receive a check for height and to provide a blood sample. Women from rural areas were more likely to attend four or more ANC visits than those from urban areas. Women belonging to another religious category (other than Christians) were less likely to complete four or more ANC visits, and women with no religious affiliation were less likely to complete more than eight antenatal visits.

Compared to women from Bakongo North and South ethnic groups, women from Bas-Kasai and Kwilu-Kwango were eight-fold more likely to receive a check for weight and height but less likely to provide a blood sample and to receive TT immunization 2. Women from Cuvette Centrale were 14 times more likely to receive prenatal checks, six times for weight, but less likely to provide a blood sample. Women in Ubangi and Itimbiri were 11 times more likely to provide a urine sample; women in Uele Lake Albert were 35 times more likely to receive prenatal checks and 22 times for weight but less likely to provide a blood sample and to receive prenatal information about complications. Women from Basele-Kivu, Maniema, and Kivu were 16 times more likely to receive prenatal care, nine times for weight, and eight times for a urine sample, but less likely to provide a blood sample. Women from Kasai, Katanga, and Tanganyika were 24 times more likely to receive prenatal checks, 7 times more likely to receive a check for weight and urine samples, but less likely to provide blood samples and receive information regarding pregnancy complications. Women in the category other were 40 times more likely to receive prenatal care and prenatal check urine samples.

Compared to women in the poorest group, women in the poorer and middle groups were twice more likely to receive TT immunization 2 but less likely to receive a check of height. Women in the richer and the richest group were threefold to fourfold more likely to provide blood samples but less likely to receive a check for weight and blood pressure. Women with a secondary or higher level of education were twice as likely to receive TT immunization 2, nearly 24 times more likely to receive information regarding complications, and 2 to 60 times more likely to provide blood samples, but less likely to receive a check for weighing and blood pressure, compared to women with no education.

Table 2. Odds ratio of all selected maternal health variables by socio-demographic characteristics—logistic regression.

Variables	Delivery					Antenatal Care						Postnatal Care		
	Everbirth-Csection	Lastbirth-Csection	Number	Weighed	Height	Blood Pressure	Urine Sample	Blood Sample	Tetainjectbp2	Receivedinfo-regcompl	Receivedpost-natcheckup	Visitedhealth-faclast12months
	odds ratio	odds ratio	odds ratio	odds ratio	odds ratio	odds ratio	odds ratio	odds ratio	odds ratio	odds ratio	odds ratio	odds ratio
Base = Eastern Congo												
Western Congo	1025	1236	1444	1277	1163	1476	3.745 ***	0.623 **	0.841	0.751	0.997	1009
	(0.707–1.487)	(0.886–1.725)	(0.715–2.916)	(0.647–2.521)	(0.298 ***)*	(0.780–2.794)	(1.593–8.805)	(0.400–0.971)	(0.509–1.387)	(0.501–1.126)	(0.837–1.187)	(0.905–1.126)
Base = 2013–2014												
2007	0.793 **	0.823	0.921	1252	0.794	1061	1006	0.949	0.758	0.373 ***	13.06 ***	0.836 ***
	(0.655–0.959)	(0.676–1.001)	(0.527–1.609)	(0.787–1.992)	(0.393–1.604)	(0.737–1.527)	(0.566–1.785)	(0.713–1.262)	(0.539–1.066)	(0.282–0.493)	(7.255–23.51)	(0.777–0.899)
Base = Catholic												
Protestant	0.920	0.819	1005	0.792	1163	0.873	0.705	1270	1035	1201	1032	1046
	(0.720–1.176)	(0.632–1.060)	(0.517–1.952)	(0.461–1.359)	(0.594–2.280)	(0.561–1.359)	(0.361–1.375)	(0.900–1.793)	(0.695–1.541)	(0.855–1.686)	(0.890–1.197)	(0.953–1.148)
Kimbanguist	0.404 ***	0.357 ***	1745	0.204 **	0.145	0.877	0.527	1634	0.820	0.952	0.484 ***	0.811
	(0.221–0.740)	(0.184–0.693)	(0.511–5.959)	(0.0466–0.895)	(0.0181–1.162)	(0.381–2.018)	(0.0634–4.376)	(0.717–3.725)	(0.353–1.905)	(0.485–1.871)	(0.338–0.693)	(0.653–1.008)
Other Christians	0.781 **	0.743 **	1269	0.896	1663	0.806	0.572	1173	1221	0.829	0.783 ***	1033
	(0.619–0.984)	(0.578–0.955)	(0.604–2.666)	(0.507–1.584)	(0.831–3.327)	(0.519–1.252)	(0.295–1.107)	(0.826–1.666)	(0.802–1.860)	(0.591–1.164)	(0.676–0.906)	(0.945–1.130)
Muslim	0.544	0.543	2.753	1570	0.187	0.254	1163	1264	3033	0.600	0.840	0.907
	(0.287–1.033)	(0.274–1.074)	(0.882–8.601)	(0.550–4.482)	(0.0194–1.802)	(0.0350–1.837)	(0.138–9.828)	(0.467–3.426)	(0.698–13.18)	(0.159–2.259)	(0.527–1.340)	(0.692–1.190)
Animist	0.529	0.574	4291			1015		1419	1603	2043	0.926	1421
	(0.0861–3.254)	(0.0938–3.512)	(0.646–28.50)			(0.190–5.428)		(0.396–5.081)	(0.435–5.904)	(0.533–7.832)	(0.438–1.956)	(0.888–2.272)
No religion	0.517	0.462		0.254		0.567	2172	3.945 **	1554	1215	0.802	1024
	(0.167–1.601)	(0.118–1.810)		(0.0481–1.339)		(0.109–2.949)	(0.479–9.852)	(1.146–13.58)	(0.380–6.350)	(0.418–3.530)	(0.485–1.326)	(0.692–1.513)
Other	1137	1124	1571	3.293	2679	0.889		0.341	0.661	1154	0.551 ***	0.960
	(0.472–2.741)	(0.436–2.900)	(0.291–8.483)	(0.824–13.16)	(0.719–9.983)	(0.183–4.324)		(0.0820–1.416)	(0.185–2.356)	(0.401–3.319)	(0.357–0.852)	(0.697–1.321)
Base = Bakongo North and South												
Bas-Kasai and Kwilu-Kwngo	0.595 ***	0.493 ***	8.754	7.987 ***	7.777 **	0.641	3430	0.475 **	0.425 **	0.650	1.267 **	0.985
	(0.410–0.863)	(0.341–0.713)	(1.879–33.95)	(1.315–45.98)		(0.307–1.340)	(0.766–15.37)	(0.259–0.870)	(0.187–0.966)	(0.380–1.111)	(1.001–1.604)	(0.866–1.122)
Cuvette Centrale	0.560 **	0.463 ***	13.85 **	5.978 **	1653	1284	2920	0.380 ***	0.593	0.951	0.582 ***	1.321 ***
	(0.335–0.936)	(0.265–0.809)	(1.559–123.1)	(1.146–31.19)	(0.244–11.22)	(0.565–2.920)	(0.560–15.22)	(0.188–0.767)	(0.250–1.407)	(0.477–1.893)	(0.440–0.771)	(1.128–1.548)

Table 2. *Cont.*

Variables	Delivery		Antenatal Care								Postnatal Care	
	Everbirth-Csection	Lastbirth-Csection	Number	Weighed	Height	Blood Pressure	Urine Sample	Blood Sample	Tetanijectbp2	Receivedinforegcompl	Receivedpostnatcheckup	Visitedhealth-faclast12months
	odds ratio	odds ratio	odds ratio	odds ratio	odds ratio	odds ratio	odds ratio	odds ratio	odds ratio	odds ratio	odds ratio	odds ratio
Ubangi and Itimbiri	0.535 ***	0.435 ***	6162	1044	2512	0.981	11.64 ***	0.537	0.840	0.631	0.435 ***	1.335 ***
	(0.362–0.791)	(0.285–0.665)	(0.680–55.83)	(0.222–4.909)	(0.417–15.14)	(0.465–2.068)	(2.791–48.53)	(0.285–1.014)	(0.355–1.991)	(0.351–1.135)	(0.338–0.560)	(1.158–1.541)
Uele Lake Albert	1360	1434	34.34 ***	21.52 ***	1027	1389	0.401	0.167 ***	0.487	0.395 **	0.806	1022
	(0.806–2.294)	(0.855–2.404)	(3.445–342.3)	(4.270–108.5)	(0.127–8.335)	(0.481–4.013)	(0.0333–4.820)	(0.0752–0.369)	(0.174–1.367)	(0.187–0.834)	(0.590–1.101)	(0.842–1.240)
Basele-k, man. And Kivu	2.111 ***	2.372 ***	16.19 **	9.505 ***	4289	1286	7.827 **	0.215 ***	0.490	0.675	1143	1.433 ***
	(1.322–3.371)	(1.548–3.636)	(1.623–161.6)	(1.968–45.90)	(0.694–26.51)	(0.479–3.455)	(1.463–41.88)	(0.103–0.449)	(0.193–1.246)	(0.342–1.329)	(0.854–1.531)	(1.215–1.690)
Kasai, Katanga, Tanganika	0.630 ***	0.611 ***	23.73 ***	7.352 ***	3202	1463	6.586 ***	0.219 ***	0.504	0.515 **	0.675 ***	1.235 ***
	(0.447–0.888)	(0.432–0.863)	(2.773–203.0)	(1.781–30.36)	(0.557–18.42)	(0.739–2.895)	(1.577–27.51)	(0.123–0.393)	(0.229–1.107)	(0.308–0.859)	(0.536–0.849)	(1.096–1.393)
Lunda	1486	1618	4774	1703	0.600	0.375	1265	1.407	0.768	0.462	1102	1.712 ***
	(0.649–3.400)	(0.693–3.777)	(0.239–95.49)	(0.755–33.42)	(0.0410–8.780)	(0.0744–1.893)	(0.389–4.121)	(0.959–2.064)	(0.148–3.983)	(0.120–1.774)	(0.608–1.998)	(1.205–2.432)
Other	0.458	0.523	39.47 ***	1088	5772		41.64 ***	0.214	1728	0.491	0.705	1083
	(0.166–1.266)	(0.189–1.444)	(2.957–526.8)	(0.124–23.40)	(0.375–88.82)		(4.806–360.8)	(0.0407–1.124)	(0.178–16.74)	(0.133–1.816)	(0.371–1.342)	(0.737–1.592)
Base = Urban												
Rural	0.788	0.755 **	1232	1088	1478	1.897 ***	0.717	0.631 **	0.541 **	0.721	0.641 ***	0.884 **
	(0.610–1.018)	(0.579–0.985)	(0.569–2.668)	(0.551–2.147)	(0.706–3.091)	(1.173–3.068)	(0.337–1.524)	(0.440–0.904)	(0.333–0.880)	(0.500–1.038)	(0.547–0.751)	(0.794–0.984)
Base = Poorest												
Poorer	1013	1156	0.678	0.885	0.752	0.910	0.938	1.407	1.547 **	1078	1112	1.130 **
	(0.729–1.407)	(0.813–1.644)	(0.375–1.224)	(0.517–1.514)	(0.351–1.609)	(0.575–1.438)	(0.433–2.032)	(0.959–2.064)	(1.007–2.377)	(0.751–1.549)	(0.947–1.306)	(1.011–1.264)
Middle	1170	1301	0.823	0.988	0.420 **	0.885	1144	1.407	1.691 **	1220	1.236 **	1090
	(0.838–1.634)	(0.913–1.854)	(0.464–1.459)	(0.554–1.762)	(0.194–0.911)	(0.555–1.413)	(0.558–2.346)	(0.972–2.037)	(1.086–2.632)	(0.846–1.759)	(1.049–1.457)	(0.973–1.221)
Richer	1.755 ***	1.726 ***	0.298 **	0.468	0.965	0.599	0.601	2.710 ***	1325	1372	1.401 ***	1.125
	(1.244–2.477)	(1.217–2.447)	(0.112–0.790)	(0.216–1.011)	(0.432–2.156)	(0.350–1.026)	(0.224–1.615)	(1.753–4.189)	(0.794–2.213)	(0.887–2.122)	(1.156–1.697)	(0.988–1.281)
Richest	1.711 ***	1.757 ***	0.105 **	0.143 **	0.436	0.394 **	0.709	4.180 ***	1294	1218	1.824 ***	1126
	(1.173–2.497)	(1.183–2.610)	(0.0179–0.623)	(0.0247–0.825)	(0.107–1.772)	(0.166–0.935)	(0.213–2.361)	(2.254–7.749)	(0.613–2.731)	(0.709–2.091)	(1.444–2.304)	(0.971–1.306)
Base = no—currently not working												

Table 2. *Cont.*

Variables	Delivery			Antenatal Care							Postnatal Care	
	Everbirth-Csection	Lastbirth-Csection	Number	Weighed	Height	Blood Pressure	Urine Sample	Blood Sample	Tetainjectbp2	Receivedinfo-regcompl	Receivedpost-natcheckup	Visitedhealth-faclast12months
	odds ratio	odds ratio	odds ratio	odds ratio	odds ratio	odds ratio	odds ratio	odds ratio	odds ratio	odds ratio	odds ratio	odds ratio
Yes—currently working	0.956	1027	1192	1626	0.612	0.831	0.931	1045	0.789	1007	0.894	1.502 ***
	(0.769–1.189)	(0.826–1.277)	(0.672–2.114)	(0.909–2.908)	(0.341–1.101)	(0.564–1.225)	(0.498–1.741)	(0.761–1.436)	(0.538–1.158)	(0.756–1.341)	(0.786–1.017)	(1.393–1.621)
Base = no education												
Primary education level	0.827	0.799	1070	0.861	1225	0.854	1185	1128	1184	0.827	1.170 **	1.202 ***
	(0.624–1.098)	(0.597–1.069)	(0.615–1.862)	(0.511–1.450)	(0.648–2.316)	(0.562–1.297)	(0.558–2.518)	(0.806–1.578)	(0.802–1.747)	(0.591–1.157)	(1.006–1.359)	(1.084–1.332)
Secondary education level	1083	1043	0.410 **	0.327 ***	0.711	0.833	0.834	2.231 ***	1.702 **	1322	1.574 ***	1.309 ***
	(0.788–1.487)	(0.760–1.431)	(0.195–0.862)	(0.161–0.665)	(0.293–1.726)	(0.500–1.387)	(0.357–1.944)	(1.492–3.336)	(1.041–2.783)	(0.885–1.974)	(1.326–1.869)	(1.167–1.468)
Higher education level	1.669	1.860 **				0.0750 **		59.56 ***	4726	23.93 ***	3.805 ***	1.584 ***
	(0.937–2.973)	(1.033–3.352)				(0.00841–0.669)		(6.627–535.2)	(0.514–43.43)	(3.161–181.2)	(2.247–6.443)	(1.284–1.955)
Constant	0.0823 ***	0.0633 ***	0.00429 ***	0.0150 ***	0.0353 ***	0.181 ***	0.00660 ***	2.838 **	10.85 ***	2.956 ***	1216	0.310 ***
	(0.0450–0.150)	(0.0350–0.114)	(0.000318–0.0580)	(0.00210–0.107)	(0.00401–0.311)	(0.0559–0.585)	(0.000916–0.0475)	(1.120–7.189)	(3.345–35.17)	(1.219–7.168)	(0.834–1.773)	(0.247–0.389)
Observations	16.609	16.592	2.163	2.164	2.146	2.184	2.11	2.198	2.169	2.173	11.37	28.643

*** $p < 0.01$, ** $p < 0.05$.

Table 3. Relative risk ratio on categorical variables—multinomial regressions.

Variables	Number Antenatal Visits				Prenatal Care Received from	
	No Visits	1–3 Visits	4–7 Visits	8 or More Visits	Professional Care	Traditional Care
	Relative Risk Ratio	Relative Risk Ratio	Relative Risk Ratio	Relative Risk Ratio	Relative Risk Ratio	Relative Risk Ratio
Base = Eastern Congo						
Western Congo		1.577	2.372 ***	1290	1.746 **	5.205 ***
		(0.953–2.609)	(1.406–4.002)	(0.381–4.372)	(1.099–2.775)	(2.124–12.76)
Base = 2013–2014						
2007		0.734	0.711	1010	0.784	0.565
		(0.497–1.082)	(0.475–1.064)	(0.427–2.389)	(0.543–1.133)	(0.257–1.240)

Table 3. Cont.

Variables	Number Antenatal Visits				Prenatal Care Received from		
	No Visits	1–3 Visits	4–7 Visits	8 or More Visits	Base = No One	Professional Care	Traditional Care
Base = Catholic							
Protestant		0.919	0.926	0.422		0.839	1156
		(0.566–1.494)	(0.565–1.518)	(0.139–1.280)		(0.525–1.341)	(0.432–3.092)
Kimbanguist		0.707	0.437	0.185		0.519	0.427
		(0.304–1.647)	(0.181–1.055)	(0.0246–1.387)		(0.233–1.156)	(0.0809–2.254)
Other Christians		0.876	0.882	0.604		0.870	0.662
		(0.544–1.410)	(0.543–1.432)	(0.209–1.747)		(0.551–1.373)	(0.256–1.710)
Muslim		0.396	0.454	0 ***		0.290 **	4015
		(0.107–1.457)	(0.115–1.794)	(0–0)		(0.0859–0.979)	(0.612–26.34)
Animist		0.347	1441	0 ***		0.714	0.730
		(0.0394–3.060)	(0.111–18.79)	(0–0)		(0.0851–5.982)	(0.0373–14.27)
No religion		0.240 **	0.263 **	0.0250 ***		0.233 ***	0 ***
		(0.0779–0.737)	(0.0841–0.824)	(0.00236–0.265)		(0.0894–0.607)	(0–0)
Other		0.700	0.158 ***	0 ***		0.348 **	1477
		(0.265–1.850)	(0.0422–0.592)	(0–0)		(0.132–0.918)	(0.284–7.694)
Base = Bakongo North and South							
Bas-Kasai and Kwilu-Kwango		0.916	1097	0.813		1034	3614
		(0.335–2.504)	(0.395–3.047)	(0.0694–9.514)		(0.385–2.772)	(0.552–23.68)
Cuvette Centrale		0.313 **	0.819	9.33		0.568	3118
		(0.116–0.847)	(0.301–2.228)	(0.862–100.9)		(0.222–1.455)	(0.519–18.72)
Ubangi and Itimbiri		0.553	0.789	4036		0.668	1078
		(0.204–1.495)	(0.287–2.169)	(0.375–43.48)		(0.256–1.741)	(0.133–8.756)
Uele Lake Albert		0.861	1631	3714		1083	17.07 **
		(0.258–2.873)	(0.462–5.750)	(0.245–56.40)		(0.342–3.431)	(1.890–154.1)
Basele-k, man. And Kivu		2387	4.415 **	8997		3.028 **	13.41 **
		(0.775–7.352)	(1.378–14.15)	(0.650–124.5)		(1.024–8.952)	(1.595–112.7)
Kasai, Katanga, Tanganika		0.483	0.618	4430		0.560	1912
		(0.194–1.202)	(0.243–1.574)	(0.475–41.29)		(0.231–1.354)	(0.319–11.44)
Lunda		1000	2222	33.47 **		1602	0 ***
		(0.210–4.757)	(0.473–10.43)	(1.741–643.4)		(0.382–6.718)	(0–1.07 × 10⁻¹⁰)

Table 3. *Cont.*

Variables	Number Antenatal Visits				Prenatal Care Received from		
	No Visits	1–3 Visits	4–7 Visits	8 or More Visits	Base = No One	Professional Care	Traditional Care
Other		0.531	0.741	0 ***		0.572	4955
		(0.0966–2.921)	(0.114–4.812)	(0–0)		(0.110–2.984)	(0.247–99.41)
Base = Urban							
Rural		0.719	0.690	3.636 **		0.726	2.576
		(0.404–1.281)	(0.390–1.222)	(1.207–10.95)		(0.425–1.242)	(0.976–6.798)
Base = Poorest							
Poorer		0.941	1300	1851		1169	0.769
		(0.608–1.457)	(0.829–2.037)	(0.646–5.303)		(0.777–1.760)	(0.340–1.741)
Middle		1.699 **	1.928 **	2317		1.959 ***	0.387
		(1.046–2.761)	(1.158–3.210)	(0.747–7.193)		(1.231–3.116)	(0.144–1.040)
Richer		1342	1.928 **	0.825		1.585	1365
		(0.753–2.395)	(1.075–3.458)	(0.142–4.795)		(0.932–2.695)	(0.509–3.657)
Richest		0.684	1970	7.077 **		1257	2451
		(0.233–2.010)	(0.683–5.682)	(1.225–40.90)		(0.455–3.478)	(0.492–12.22)
Base = no—currently not working							
Yes—currently working		1029	1129	0.571		1060	1749
		(0.677–1.565)	(0.747–1.705)	(0.221–1.477)		(0.719–1.562)	(0.802–3.814)
Base = no education							
Primary education level		1.481	1.752 ***	1594		1.512 **	3.554 ***
		(0.995–2.205)	(1.149–2.671)	(0.604–4.209)		(1.037–2.204)	(1.567–8.061)
Secondary education level		3.285 ***	5.633 ***	3.828 **		4.497 ***	4.643 ***
		(1.769–6.100)	(3.039–10.44)	(1.152–12.72)		(2.476–8.165)	(1.647–13.09)
Higher education level		2674	3784	32.45 **		3646	0 ***
		(0.234–30.59)	(0.416–34.44)	(1.435–733.6)		(0.411–32.35)	(0–0)
Constant		3.441 *	1081	0.0111 ***		4.264 **	0.00446 ***
		(0.919–12.88)	(0.277–4.222)	(0.000571–0.215)		(1.228–14.81)	(0.000293–0.0677)
Observations	2.537	2.537	2.537	2.537	2.568	2.568	2.568

Relative risk measures the association between the exposure and the outcome. Robust ci in parentheses (figures in brackets show 95 percent confidence intervals). *** $p < 0.01$, ** $p < 0.05$, * $p < 0.1$.

3.2.2. Delivery

Women were found to be assisted during child delivery. In general, they were more likely to receive professional and traditional delivery care when living in western DRC than in eastern DRC. Compared to 2013/2014, women were nearly 0.8 times less likely to deliver by C-section in 2007. Compared to urban areas, women in rural areas were nearly 0.7 times less likely to have their last birth by C-section. Compared to women in the poorest wealth index group, women in the richer and the richest wealth index groups were nearly two times more likely to deliver by C-section. Women with a higher education level were nearly two times more likely to have their last birth by C-section compared to women with no educational background.

Compared to Christians, Kimbanguist women, as women with other religious affiliations, were less likely to deliver by C-section. Women from Bas-Kasai and Kwilu-Kwango, Cuvette Centrale, Ubangi and Itimbiri, Kasai, Katanga, and Tanganyika ethnic groups were less likely to deliver by C-section compared to women from Bakongo ethnic group. Women from Basele-Kivu, Maniema, and Kivu were nearly 2 to 3 times more likely to deliver by C-section.

3.2.3. Postnatal Care (PNC)

Inequality was present during the utilization of PNC. In general, women who visited a health facility received a checkup from a health professional after delivery. Women in rural areas were less likely to receive PNC and less likely to visit a health facility in the last 12 months compared to women in urban areas. Compared to 2013–2014, women were nearly 13 times more likely to get a postnatal checkup but less likely to visit a health facility in the last 12 months than in 2007. Compared to Christians, Kimbanguists and other Christian women were less likely to receive PNC.

Compared to women from the Bakongo North and South ethnic groups, women from Bas-Kasai and Kwilu-Kwango were more likely to receive postnatal checkups. Women were more likely to visit a health facility in the last 12 months in Cuvette Centrale, Ubangi and Itimbiri, Basele-Kivu, Maniema, Kasai, Katanga, Tanganyika, and Lunda but less likely to receive a postnatal checkup. Women in the richer and the richest groups were most likely to receive PNC compared to women in the poorest group. Women who are working were most likely to visit a health facility in the last 12 months, compared to women who are currently not working. Women with a primary, a secondary, or a higher level of education were most likely to receive a postnatal checkup, visit a health facility in the last 12 months, and most likely to receive information regarding the complication, respectively.

Table 3 presents the results of the multinomial regression analysis for the categorical outcome variables.

3.2.4. Number of Antenatal Visits

Women were more than twice as likely to complete four to seven antenatal visits when living in the western DRC compared to the eastern DRC. Women from rural areas were four times more likely to attend eight or more antenatal visits than those from urban areas. Women belonging to another religious category (other than Christians) and women with no religious affiliation were less likely to complete more than eight antenatal visits.

Compared to women from Bakongo North and South ethnic groups, women from Basele-Kivu, Maniema, and Kivu were more than four times more likely to complete 4–7 antenatal visits, and women from Lunda were 33 times more likely to complete more than eight antenatal visits. However, women from Cuvette Centrale were less likely to complete 1–3 antenatal visits.

Compared to women with the poorest wealth index, women with middle, richer, and richest wealth indexes were two and seven times more likely to complete more than eight antenatal visits. Women with primary, secondary, or higher education were 2 to 6 times or 33 times more likely to complete more than eight antenatal visits compared to women with no education.

3.2.5. Prenatal Care Received

Women were twice as likely to receive professional prenatal care and nearly five times more likely to receive traditional prenatal care when living in western DRC than in eastern DRC. Women practicing Islam and women with no religious affiliation were less likely to receive professional prenatal care.

Compared to women from Bakongo North and South ethnic groups, women from Basele-Kivu, Maniema, and Kivu were three times and 14 times more likely to receive professional and traditional prenatal care, respectively. Women from Uele Lake Albert were nearly 17 times more likely to receive traditional prenatal care.

Compared to women with the poorest wealth index, women with the middle wealth index were twice as likely to receive professional and traditional prenatal care. Women with primary or secondary education were more likely to receive professional and traditional prenatal care than women without education.

3.3. Inequality Distribution (RQ2)

Table 4 presents the Gini coefficients for each selected MHCS utilization variable between the regions (western vs. eastern DRC) and between the years of the surveys (2007 vs. 2013–2014). It shows that the Gini varied between 0.10 and 0.98, indicating the presence of inequality in both regions and over time, but also considerable heterogeneity between those. Overall, enormous inequality could be observed in prenatal care for (urine samples (0.98), followed by prenatal check number (whether or not having ANC during pregnancy) (0.94); and in delivery by C-sections (every birth (0.91); and last birth by C-section (0.93)). On the contrary, more equality could be observed in the received prenatal care (i.e., number of antenatal visits, TT immunization, received pregnancy information) and in the received postnatal care (i.e., received postnatal checkups and assistance during delivery).

Table 4. Gini coefficients for all selected maternal variables.

All Selected Variables	Eastern DRC			Western DRC		
	Overall	2007	2013/14	Overall	2007	2013/14
Cesarean-section						
Ever birth C-section	0.91	0.94	0.90	0.96	0.96	0.96
Last birth C-section	0.93	0.95	0.92	0.97	0.96	0.97
Prenatal care						
Prenatal check_no	0.94	0.93	0.94	0.95	0.95	0.95
Received prenatal care	0.17	0.24	0.13	0.15	0.14	0.15
Prenatal check weighed	0.89	0.88	0.88	0.93	0.92	0.94
Prenatal check height	0.93	0.97	0.91	0.97	0.97	0.98
Prenatal check blood pressure	0.84	0.83	0.84	0.82	0.82	0.81
Prenatal check urine sample	0.98	0.97	0.99	0.94	0.95	0.94
Prenatal check blood sample	0.45	0.45	0.45	0.42	0.42	0.42
Tetanus injections	0.18	0.24	0.15	0.17	0.19	0.17
Received pregnancy information	0.45	0.61	0.39	0.51	0.67	0.43
Postnatal Care						
Received postnatal checkup	0.48	0.04	0.49	0.51	0.13	0.52
Visited health facilities in the last 12 months	0.62	0.66	0.61	0.64	0.67	0.62
Assistance during delivery	0.15	0.17	0.14	0.16	0.17	0.15

Between 2007 and 2013–2014, data show an overall increase in the Gini for C-sections—particularly in western DRC, where a slight increase was observed in the last birth by C-section (from 0.96 to 0.97)—and for prenatal care from 0.94 to 0.95 in whether or not having ANC during pregnancy, from 0.89 to 0.93 in weight. Similarly, an increase from 0.93 to 0.94 in whether or not having ANC during pregnancy) and from 0.97 to 0.99 for urine samples was observed in eastern DRC. Overall, there was a decrease in the Gini for received prenatal care for tetanus injections and received pregnancy information in eastern DRC but an increase in the Gini for a received postnatal checkup in both geographic regions.

Supplementary Materials File S3 displays the Lorenz curves for each MHCS utilization variable separately. The Lorenz curves are relatively far from the line of equality, suggesting a high degree of inequality in the selected MHCS variables. The most significant degree of inequality was observed for prenatal checks for urine samples, whether or not having ANC during pregnancy, height, weight, blood pressure, and C-sections, while the smallest degree of inequality was observed for received prenatal care (i.e., blood samples, TT immunization, the number of antenatal visits, and received pregnancy information), received postnatal checkups, assistance during delivery, and visited the health facilities in the last 12 months.

3.4. Inequality Trends (RQ3)

The current analysis found inequality in the utilization of ANC, delivery, and PNC services in DRC—a summary of all results from this analysis is in Table 5.

3.4.1. Antenatal Care (ANC)

Significant differences were found in ANC service utilization between the regions (CI 0.03 in western DRC vs. 0.10 in eastern DRC) and between the years of the surveys. However, patterns of inequality remained relatively consistent for prenatal check numbers, weight, height, and prenatal check blood pressure in both regions. More specifically, in western DRC, a slight decrease could be observed in the CI for the prenatal care received, for prenatal check for a blood sample, and received pregnancy information. No changes could be observed in the CI for tetanus injections and the number of ANC visits. However, in eastern DRC, a slight decrease could be observed in the CI for the prenatal check for height, received pregnancy information, and the number of ANC visits, but a slight increase in tetanus injections. No changes could be observed in the CI for prenatal care received urine sample check and prenatal check blood sample.

3.4.2. Delivery

Between 2007 and 2013–2014, we found a decrease in the CI for delivery by C-section. Particularly in eastern DRC, a decrease could be observed in the CI for both every birth and the last birth by C-section at the same time, while the CI for delivery by C-section remained relatively consistent in western DRC.

3.4.3. Postnatal Care (PNC)

Overall, it could be observed that there was a decrease in the CI for received postnatal checkups and visited health facilities in the last 12 months but a slight increase in the CI for assistance during delivery between 2007 and 2013–2014. For instance, in western DRC, we found a decrease in the CI for the three postnatal variables (received postnatal checkup, visited health facilities in the last 12 months, and assistance during delivery). In eastern DRC, the same trend could be observed in only two variables (received postnatal checkup and visited health facilities in the last 12 months); a slight increase could be observed in assistance during delivery.

Table 5. Concentration indices by selected maternal variables, by survey year (2007 vs. 2013–2014), and by geographic regions (western vs. eastern) of the DRC.

All Selected Variables	2007				2013/14				Western Congo				Eastern Congo			
	Group 0 = Eastern Congo	Group 1 = Western Congo	Socioeconomic Inequality in the Health Variable	Statistical Significance Between the 2 Groups in the Socioeconomic Inequality	Group 0 = Eastern Congo	Group 1 = Western Congo	Socioeconomic Inequality in the Health Variable	Statistically Significance between the 2 Groups in the Socioeconomic Inequality	CI	PeriodSurvey = 0 (2013/2014)	PeriodSurvey = 1 (2007)	Test for Stat. Significant Differences	CI	PeriodSurvey = 0 (2013/2014)	PeriodSurvey = 1 (2007)	Test for Stat. Significant Differences
Delivery																
Ever C-section	0.67	0.68	0.68	0.97	0.65	0.68	0.67	0.89	0.68	0.68	0.68	0.97	0.65	0.65	0.67	0.97
Last birth C-section	0.68	0.69	0.68	1.00	0.66	0.69	0.68	0.82	0.69	0.69	0.69	0.94	0.66	0.66	0.68	0.87
Prenatal care																
Prenatal care received	0.47	0.85	0.63	0.47	0.53	0.67	0.59	0.75	0.73	0.67	0.85	0.80	0.52	0.53	0.47	0.83
Prenatal check number	0.67	0.68	0.68	0.97	0.68	0.68	0.68	0.92	0.68	0.68	0.68	0.87	0.67	0.68	0.67	0.91
Prenatal check weighed	0.64	0.67	0.66	0.90	0.65	0.67	0.67	0.82	0.67	0.67	0.67	0.88	0.65	0.65	0.64	0.95
Prenatal check height	0.69	0.69	0.69	0.98	0.66	0.69	0.68	0.54	0.69	0.69	0.69	0.93	0.67	0.66	0.69	0.55
Prenatal check blood pressure	0.59	0.59	0.59	0.71	0.61	0.58	0.59	0.90	0.58	0.58	0.59	0.86	0.60	0.61	0.59	0.74
Prenatal check urine sample	0.69	0.68	0.69	0.53	0.70	0.67	0.68	0.46	0.68	0.67	0.68	0.67	0.70	0.70	0.69	0.91
Prenatal check blood sample	0.22	0.29	0.26	0.44	0.21	0.24	0.23	0.58	0.26	0.24	0.29	0.79	0.21	0.21	0.22	0.27
Tetanus injections	0.53	0.58	0.56	0.88	0.62	0.59	0.60	0.74	0.59	0.59	0.58	0.93	0.60	0.62	0.53	0.67
Received pregnancy information	0.29	0.31	0.31	0.02	0.26	0.21	0.23	0.71	0.03	0.21	0.31	0.24	0.10	0.26	0.29	0.01
Number antenatal visits	0.49	0.11	0.31	0.91	0.13	0.12	0.12	0.72	0.11	0.12	0.11	0.63	0.23	0.13	0.49	0.75
Postnatal care																
Received postnatal checkup	0.70	0.65	0.66	0.49	0.09	0.02	0.03	0.28	0.01	0.02	0.65	0.00	0.10	0.09	0.70	0.00
Visited health facilities in the last 12 months	0.37	0.38	0.37	0.93	0.25	0.30	0.28	0.37	0.33	0.30	0.38	0.71	0.29	0.25	0.37	0.83
Assistance during delivery	0.40	0.49	0.46	0.88	0.49	0.46	0.47	0.88	0.47	0.46	0.49	0.97	0.46	0.49	0.40	0.78

4. Discussion

This study assessed inequality trends during the utilization of MHCS in post-conflict DRC. While continuous improvements in the utilization of MHCS were found at different stages of pregnancy, several aspects remain inequitable. Moreover, our study found important variations in the utilization of MHCS by geographic region, socioeconomic households, and survey years, shedding light on disparities that need to be addressed. These variations were investigated, and the key results are discussed next.

On the magnitude of inequality, both the odds and the relative risk ratios revealed some degree of inequality during the utilization of MHCS. In the DRC, inequalities could be observed between the western and eastern regions, the poorest and richest socioeconomic groups, and between 2007 and 2013–2014. When zooming in on the levels of utilization of MHCS, the study indicates that these were higher in western compared to eastern DRC; in rural compared to urban areas; among Christians compared to other religious affiliations; in women with a primary, secondary, or higher level of education compared to women with no education; in women from the richer and the richest wealth index; and 2013–2014 as compared to 2007. Our finding that the magnitude of inequality in MHCS utilization is substantial in the DRC is not coincidental. Strong regional inequalities in health have been previously observed within and among countries [48–51]. In Afghanistan, for instance, one study comparing various provinces based on the severity of conflict showed that the mean coverage of ANC, facility delivery, and SBA was significantly lower for severe conflict provinces when compared to minimal conflict provinces—suggesting that there are notable disparities between provinces [52].

These findings are essential in the context of DRC because the magnitude of inequality in MHCS utilization may be related to the decade-long armed conflict in the country. They put forward the need for designing appropriate programs that aim to increase MHCS utilization, particularly for women belonging to lower economic strata, those belonging to other religious affiliations than Christians, and those living in eastern and rural areas who were less likely to meet the WHO's requirements of a positive pregnancy experience.

The logistic and multivariate regressions show that ethnicity continues to influence the utilization of MHCS, mainly in the country's dominant ethnic groups. These findings suggest that there is a consistent pattern of disparities among the different ethnic groups that have been lagging, suggesting that ethnicity could have an essential role in program effectiveness. These findings are consistent with previous studies showing that ethnicity influenced the utilization of maternal health services [53–55]. Specifically for the DRC, ethnicity plays a vital role in the acquisition, maintenance, and distribution of wealth [56]—which may influence the utilization of the MHCS.

Over time, inequality in the distribution of MHCS was present in both regions. Total inequality was present in ANC and delivery by C-sections, while some degree of equality could be observed in the received PNC. A few studies have looked at the regional distribution of health indicators within a single country and found that substantial differences among subareas were apparent [57,58], suggesting that inequitable distributions of healthcare services across geographic locations may result in poor or underutilization of MHCS. However, further breakdowns in the distribution of MHCS utilization are needed to explain the differences between subareas. For the DRC, this finding is fundamental because it gives directions for identifying subareas of relatively high need for MHCS utilization.

Regarding inequality trends, a decrease in the utilization of prenatal and postnatal checks and professional assistance during delivery could be observed in respondents from rural areas. This finding suggests that rural locations also accounted for the observed decrease in the utilization of MHCS and is consistent with previous studies showing that utilization of MHCS is lowest in rural areas [59], and the risk of maternal mortality is highest amongst women in rural areas [60].

In this study, we found that the highest educational attainment level was positively associated with utilizing ANC, delivery, and PNC. These findings are consistent with results from previous studies in post-conflict settings showing that maternal education level is a critical aspect in the utilization of MHCS [50,61–63]. For the DRC, the few available studies cannot explain whether the association between maternal education and maternal healthcare utilization could be attributed to other factors. Given that SDGs are interdependent, ensure healthy lives, and promote well-being for all, it is only possible if other SDGs, such as SDG 1 (ending poverty), SDG 4 (improving access to education), and SDG 5 (guaranteeing gender equity), among others [64,65], are achieved. The DRC could meet SDG 3.1 (reduce the global maternal mortality ratio to less than 70 per 100,000 live births by 2030) by funding maternal health services and education and developing and maintaining a supportive monitoring process—as both are needed.

Wealth was identified as a significant factor influencing the utilization of MHCS in the DRC. For instance, women with a high wealth index had a higher chance of completing adequate ANC visits and receiving delivery care. Moreover, being currently employed or unemployed also revealed a relation to MHCS utilization. Also, being employed increased the possibility of visiting health facilities in the last 12 months, while being unemployed decreased professional as well as non-professional assistance during delivery. Our findings are consistent with findings from another study conducted in Ghana, Senegal, and Sierra Leone, showing that women with lower wealth did not benefit from the positive effects of the policy reform (e.g., removing user fees) to access facility-based delivery services [66].

We find that each variable of MHCS utilization presents a different pattern, and some variables of MHCS utilization may be more sensitive than others. For example, a decrease could be observed in received postnatal checkups, visited health facilities in the last 12 months, and assistance during delivery in both regions in the DRC. Poorer women or women residing in the eastern DRC have higher levels of inequality in the utilization of MHCS as compared to the richest women or women residing in the western DRC. These findings show persistent patterns of inequality among regional women's groups and are consistent with previous studies showing a strong positive relationship between wealth and health [42,67–69], suggesting that the higher the wealth status of women, the higher their likelihood of seeking appropriate MHCS.

Within-country variations are products of complex socioeconomic factors, showing that no single measure of equality can capture all disparities. In this regard, there might be other factors to consider in future research, such as post-war country status, political orientation, history of dictatorship, and human rights that are not included in the DHS dataset but would highlight more about the influence of maternal healthcare services distribution and utilization in the DRC.

From a policy perspective, our findings provide valuable guidance for policymakers and stakeholders working towards improving MHCS utilization in the DRC and similar contexts.

Strengths and Limitations

Population-representative data on health status and its determinants are a critical need in the post-conflict context [70]. The use of recent and high-quality data is especially preferable when analyzing maternal healthcare service utilization for data-driven decision-making. However, in several African countries (including the DRC), no national health survey data have been available for several decades. The DHS has several important advantages that make it particularly useful as a programming tool in post-conflict environments.

A major strength of this study is that the DHS produces high-quality data, which is representative of the sub-national regions [32] and provides much-needed data on health service utilization [71]. Given the general lack of primary data in post-conflict settings, we strongly believe that these DHS data are still the most reliable data source that could be used to analyze maternal health service utilization. For these reasons, we used the two most recent DHS data collected in 2007 and 2013–2014 as the primary source of data to assess inequality trends in the utilization of MHCS in the DRC. Since the study uses a high-quality DHS database, the findings are reliable for decision making. Moreover, the

DHS creates a unique opportunity to investigate the levels and trends in socioeconomic inequalities in maternal health variables at a scale that was never possible in the past. We were able to disaggregate the DHS data of key health services indicators to assess geographic and socioeconomic characteristics of MHCS utilization. However, given that this analysis is based on secondary data, several limitations to this study must be considered. Firstly, both surveys only included women aged 15–49 years. Knowing the correct age is critical for identifying at-risk women and ascertaining age-specific and age-adjusted risks of maternal mortality. Respondents in DHS surveys are sampled in such a way that the survey sample represents the population (women aged 15–49) of the country. However, the data on siblings are collected from respondents aged 15–49 only, which, by the study design, truncates the siblings in extreme age groups in the reproductive period. For example, a respondent of age 15 is unlikely to have a sibling above age 45, and similarly, a respondent of 49 is unlikely to have a sibling below 20. As a result, the siblings in the age range below 20 or above 45 may not be captured adequately from the DHS survey respondents. Therefore, it is difficult to assess age truncation or underreporting of adult sisters in these two extreme age groups from sibling survival history data [72]. As such, the surveys excluded women below the age of 15 years as well as women above 49 years (and thus, study findings cannot be generalized outside of the sampled population). Because there might be an issue in terms of using MHCS under 15 years, we believe this age range represents women of reproductive age, which is required for our study. Secondly, all the health measures in DHS are collected based on a self-report or proxy report except for height and weight and a few other outcomes, such as anemia. Misclassification biases can occur. Often, its magnitude is also unknown, making correction difficult. For these reasons, we tried to interpret individual-level data more carefully, especially when making causal interpretations. Thirdly, an appropriate variable for work status could have been measured by checking "work status during pregnancy" and "marital status during pregnancy"; however, those variables are not available. Finally, all information collected in DHS surveys (except for weight, height measurements, and vaccination data) is subject to reporting and recall biases that can arise from the recall period or sampling approach. However, a detailed evaluation of DHS data has shown that these data are reasonably well-reported [71], and appropriate strategies are embedded into the design of DHS data collection tools that address recall bias.

5. Conclusions and Recommendations

The purpose of this study was to assess inequality trends during the utilization of MHCS in post-conflict DRC. Although it could be argued that there has been a declining trend for some variables from 2007 to 2013–2014, several factors, such as place of residence, ethnicity, education level, religious affiliation, wealth index, and year of survey, were associated with inequality in the utilization of ANC, delivery care, and PNC. Thus, to reduce inequalities in the utilization of MHCS in the DRC, innovative strategies targeting these factors are needed at the regional, subnational, and national levels. Building on our research questions, three key messages emerged from the current analysis: First, substantial gains have been observed in the utilization of ANC, delivery, and PNC services. Second, for some variables, the CCs are far from the line of equality, and the CI are different from zero, suggesting a pro-urban, pro-wealthier, and pro-western DRC distribution. To meet WHO requirements, all women in the DRC should receive at least one ANC visit during the first trimester of their pregnancy, increase to eight ANC visits in total throughout their pregnancy, be attended to at delivery by an SBA, and deliver in a health facility. Third, the current analysis found inequality in the utilization of ANC, delivery, and PNC services in DRC. Trend analyses indicate that region, ethnic group, the place of residence of women, the wealth index, and the level of education of women influence MHCS utilization to some extent. For the DRC, this evidence should serve as a foundation for designing targeted interventions aiming to reduce inequality in MHCS utilization. At the same time, understanding the multiplicity of factors that influence the utilization of MHCS is key to the development of interventions that will work in reducing maternal mortality.

Further research is needed to shed light on the eastern–western and rural–urban differences in not only MHCS utilization but also in the differential factors with significant influence on ANC, delivery, and PNC. Qualitative research on barriers to the utilization of MHC services among poorer, rural, and underserved women is needed to gain insight into inequality trends during the utilization of MHCS in post-conflict settings.

Supplementary Materials: The following supporting information can be downloaded at: https://www.mdpi.com/article/10.3390/healthcare11212871/s1, File S1: STROBE; File S2: Description of all variables (maternal health services); File S3: Lorenz curves for each MHCS. Table S1: Descriptive characteristics of all respondents in the DRC by survey year; Table S2: Odds ratio by socio-demographic characteristics-Logistic regression; Table S3: Relative Risk Ratio on categorical variables—OMultinomial regressions; Table S4: Gini coefficients for all selected maternal health variables; Table S5: Concentration indices by maternal health variables and by survey year 2007 and 2013–2014.

Author Contributions: D.B., I.R. and R.C. conceived the article and prepared the methodology; I.R. and D.B. carried out the data analysis; R.C., N.d.V., E.N.N. and R.L. supervised and validated. D.B. prepared the initial draft of the manuscript, which was revised and approved by all authors. All authors have read and agreed to the published version of the manuscript.

Funding: This research received no external funding.

Institutional Review Board Statement: Permission to use the data in this study was approved by the international ICF, which is a part of the DHS program (DHS 2015). The original ethical clearance for these surveys was obtained by the institutional review board from the ICF/DHS program. Institutional Review Board Findings Form ICF IRB-MACRO project number 31406.00.002.12. Further information about the ethical review is available on the website: https://dhsprogram.com/Methodology/Protecting-the-Privacy-of-DHS-SurveyRespondents.cfm (accessed on 1 September 2019).

Informed Consent Statement: Informed consent was obtained by DHS from all subjects involved in the study.

Data Availability Statement: This study used datasets available from USAID's Demographic and Health Survey (DHS) program. After registration on the website, datasets can be downloaded and used via the DHS program website: https://dhsprogram.com/data/new-user-registration.cfm (accessed on 21 April 2023).

Acknowledgments: The authors would like to thank the DHS program for providing the EDS-RDC datasets. Special thanks to Thomas F. Monaghan for his valuable comments on the statistical analysis plan and Katie Ward for useful comments on an earlier draft of this manuscript.

Conflicts of Interest: The authors declare no conflict of interest.

Abbreviations

ANC	Antenatal care
C-section	Cesarean section
CC	Concentration curve
CI	Concentration indices
95% CI	Confidence interval
DHS	Demographic and health survey
DRC	Democratic Republic of Congo
EDS-RDC	Demographic and Health Surveys (DHS) carried out in the Democratic Republic of Congo
HIES	Household income expenditure survey
ICF International	A global consulting and digital services provider that implements the DHS Program
MHCS	Maternal health care services
OR	Odds ratio

PNC	Postnatal care
SDG	Sustainable development goal
RRR	Relative risk ratio
SBA	Skilled birth attendant
SSA	sub-Saharan Africa
USAID	The United States Agency for International Development
WHO	World Health Organization

References

1. World Health Organization. Declaration of Alma-Ata. In Proceedings of the International Conference on Primary Health Care, Alma-Ata, Kazakhstan, 6–12 September 1978; p. 3.
2. Lee, M.-S. The principles and values of health promotion: Building upon the Ottawa charter and related WHO documents. *Korean J. Health Educ. Promot.* **2015**, *32*, 1–11. [CrossRef]
3. World Health Organization; UNICEF. *A Vision for Primary Health Care in the 21st Century: Towards Universal Health Coverage and the Sustainable Development Goals*; World Health Organization: Geneva, Switzerland, 2018; p. 64.
4. World Health Organization. *Trends in Maternal Mortality 2000 to 2017: Estimates by WHO, UNICEF, UNFPA, World Bank Group and the United Nations Population Division*; World Health Organization: Geneva, Switzerland, 2019; p. 16.
5. Novignon, J.; Ofori, B.; Tabiri, K.G.; Pulok, M.H. Socioeconomic inequalities in maternal health care utilization in Ghana. *Int. J. Equity Health* **2019**, *18*, 1–11. [CrossRef] [PubMed]
6. ECOSOC; UN. *Special Edition: Progress towards the Sustainable Development Goals Report of the Secretary-General*; Advanced Unedited Version; United Nations: New York, NY, USA, 2019.
7. Tey, N.-P.; Lai, S.-l. Correlates of and barriers to the utilization of health services for delivery in South Asia and Sub-Saharan Africa. *Sci. World J.* **2013**, *2013*, 423403. [CrossRef] [PubMed]
8. Alam, N.; Hajizadeh, M.; Dumont, A.; Fournier, P. Inequalities in maternal health care utilization in sub-Saharan African countries: A multiyear and multi-country analysis. *PLoS ONE* **2015**, *10*, e0120922. [CrossRef] [PubMed]
9. Arsenault, C.; Jordan, K.; Lee, D.; Dinsa, G.; Manzi, F.; Marchant, T.; Kruk, M. Equity in antenatal care quality: An analysis of 91 national household surveys. *Lancet Glob. Health* **2018**, *6*, e1186–e1195. [CrossRef]
10. Goli, S.; Nawal, D.; Rammohan, A.; Sekher, T.; Singh, D. Decomposing the socioeconomic inequality in utilization of maternal health care services in selected countries of South Asia and sub-Saharan Africa. *J. Biosoc. Sci.* **2018**, *50*, 749–769. [CrossRef]
11. United Nations. *Millennium Development Goals Report*; United Nations: New York, NY, USA, 2012; p. 72.
12. United Nations. *World Economic and Social Survey 2013: Sustainable Development Challenges*; United Nations: New York, NY, USA, 2013.
13. Smith, M.J. Health Equity in Public Health: Clarifying our Commitment. *Public Health Ethics* **2014**, *8*, 173–184. [CrossRef]
14. Rubenstein, L. *Post-Conflict Health Reconstruction: New Foundations for US Policy Working Paper Washington*; United States Institute of Peace: Washington, DC, USA, 2009; p. 62.
15. Institute of Development Studies. Universal Health Coverage and Development. Available online: https://www.ids.ac.uk/news/universal-health-coverage-and-focus-on-long-term-development/ (accessed on 29 March 2021).
16. Jones, G.A.; Rodgers, D. The World Bank's World Development Report 2011 on conflict, security and development: A critique through five vignettes. *J. Int. Dev.* **2011**, *23*, 980–995. [CrossRef]
17. Zhang, T.; Qi, X.; He, Q.; Hee, J.; Takesue, R.; Yan, Y.; Tang, K. The Effects of Conflicts and Self-Reported Insecurity on Maternal Healthcare Utilisation and Children Health Outcomes in the Democratic Republic of Congo (DRC). *Healthcare* **2021**, *9*, 842. [CrossRef]
18. Institute for Economics and Peace. *Global Peace Index 2020: Measuring Peace in a Complex World*; Institute for Economics and Peace: Sydney, Austraria, 2020; p. 107.
19. Muraya, J.; Ahere, J. *Perpetuation of Instability in the Democratic Republic of the Congo: When the Kivus Sneeze, Kinshasa Catches a Cold*; Occasional Paper Series; ACCORD: Umhlanga Rocks, South Africa, 2014; Volume 2014, pp. 1–46.
20. Southall, D. Armed conflict women and girls who are pregnant, infants and children; a neglected public health challenge. What can health professionals do? *Early Hum. Dev.* **2011**, *87*, 735–742. [CrossRef]
21. Ziegler, B.R.; Kansanga, M.; Sano, Y.; Kangmennaang, J.; Kpienbaareh, D.; Luginaah, I. Antenatal care utilization in the fragile and conflict-affected context of the Democratic Republic of the Congo. *Soc. Sci. Med.* **2020**, *262*, 113253. [CrossRef] [PubMed]
22. Andersen, R.; Newman, J.F. Andersen and Newman framework of health services utilization. *J. Health Soc. Behav.* **1995**, *36*, 1–10. [CrossRef] [PubMed]
23. Andersen, R.M. Revisiting the behavioral model and access to medical care: Does it matter? *J. Health Soc. Behav.* **1995**, *36*, 1–10. [CrossRef]
24. Corsi, D.J.; Neuman, M.; Finlay, J.E.; Subramanian, S. Demographic and health surveys: A profile. *Int. J. Epidemiol.* **2012**, *41*, 1602–1613. [CrossRef] [PubMed]
25. Misu, F.; Alam, K. Comparison of inequality in utilization of maternal healthcare services between Bangladesh and Pakistan: Evidence from the demographic health survey 2017–2018. *Reprod. Health* **2023**, *20*, 43. [CrossRef] [PubMed]

26. Hosseinpoor, A.R.; Bergen, N.; Barros, A.J.; Wong, K.L.; Boerma, T.; Victora, C.G. Monitoring subnational regional inequalities in health: Measurement approaches and challenges. *Int. J. Equity Health* **2016**, *15*, 18. [CrossRef]
27. Bwirire, D.; Crutzen, R.; Ntabe Namegabe, E.; Letschert, R.; de Vries, N. Health inequalities in post-conflict settings: A systematic review. *PLoS ONE* **2022**, *17*, e0265038. [CrossRef]
28. Measure DHS. *Demographic and Health Survey Interviewer's Manual*; ICF International: Calverton, MD, USA, 2012; p. 126.
29. Von Elm, E.; Altman, D.G.; Egger, M.; Pocock, S.J.; Gøtzsche, P.C.; Vandenbroucke, J.P.; Initiative, S. The Strengthening the Reporting of Observational Studies in Epidemiology (STROBE) Statement: Guidelines for reporting observational studies. *Int. J. Surg.* **2014**, *12*, 1495–1499. [CrossRef]
30. Ministère du Plan; Macro International. *Enquête Démographique et de Santé République Démocratique du Congo 2007*; Macro International Inc.: Calverton, MD, USA, 2008; p. 499.
31. Ministère du Plan et Suivi de la Mise en Oeuvre de la Révolution de la Modernité; Ministère de la Santé Publique. *Deuxième Enquête Démographique et de Santé en République Démocratique du Congo (EDS-RDC II 2013–2014)*; Measure DHS, ICF International: Rockville, MD, USA, 2014; p. 678.
32. ICF Macro. DHS Methodology. Available online: https://dhsprogram.com/Methodology/Survey-Types/DHS-Methodology.cfm (accessed on 1 September 2019).
33. Boerma, T.; Requejo, J.; Victora, C.G.; Amouzou, A.; George, A.; Agyepong, I.; Barroso, C.; Barros, A.J.; Bhutta, Z.A.; Black, R.E. Countdown to 2030: Tracking progress towards universal coverage for reproductive, maternal, newborn, and child health. *Lancet* **2018**, *391*, 1538–1548. [CrossRef]
34. World Health Organization. *Global Reference List of 100 Core Health Indicators*; World Health Organization: Geneva, Switzerland, 2015; p. 136.
35. World Health Organization. *WHO Recommendations on Antenatal Care for a Positive Pregnancy Experience*; World Health Organization: Geneva, Switzerland, 2016; p. 172.
36. World Health Organization. *New Guidelines on Antenatal Care for a Positive Pregnancy Experience*; World Health Organization: Geneva, Switzerland, 2016; Available online: https://www.who.int/news/item/07-11-2016-new-guidelines-on-antenatal-care-for-a-positive-pregnancy-experience (accessed on 18 November 2022).
37. World Health Organization. *Health Inequities in the South-East Asia Region: Selected Country Case Studies*; WHO Regional Office for South-East Asia: New Delhi, India, 2009; p. 138.
38. Zhang, T.; Xu, Y.; Ren, J.; Sun, L.; Liu, C. Inequality in the distribution of health resources and health services in China: Hospitals versus primary care institutions. *Int. J. Equity Health* **2017**, *16*, 1–8. [CrossRef]
39. Wagstaff, A.; Van Doorslaer, E.; Watanabe, N. On decomposing the causes of health sector inequalities with an application to malnutrition inequalities in Vietnam. *J. Econom.* **2003**, *112*, 207–223. [CrossRef]
40. O'Donnell, O.; O'Neill, S.; Van Ourti, T.; Walsh, B. Conindex: Estimation of concentration indices. *Stata J.* **2016**, *16*, 112–138. [CrossRef] [PubMed]
41. Rutstein, S.O.; Johnson, K. *The DHS Wealth Index, DHS Comparative Reports No. 6*; ORC Macro: Calverton, MD, USA, 2004; p. 77.
42. Wagstaff, A.; Paci, P.; van Doorslaer, E. On the measurement of inequalities in health. *Soc. Sci. Med.* **1991**, *33*, 545–557. [CrossRef]
43. Lambert, P.J. The distribution and redistribution of income. In *Current Issues in Public Sector Economics*; Springer: London, UK, 1992; pp. 200–226. [CrossRef]
44. Kakwani, N.; Wagstaff, A.; Van Doorslaer, E. Socioeconomic inequalities in health: Measurement, computation, and statistical inference. *J. Econ.* **1997**, *77*, 87–103. [CrossRef]
45. Van Doorslaer, E.; Wagstaff, A.; Bleichrodt, H.; Calonge, S.; Gerdtham, U.-G.; Gerfin, M.; Geurts, J.; Gross, L.; Häkkinen, U.; Leu, R.E. Income-related inequalities in health: Some international comparisons. *J. Health Econ.* **1997**, *16*, 93–112. [CrossRef] [PubMed]
46. Bishop, J.A.; Formby, J.P.; Zheng, B. Inference tests for Gini-based tax progressivity indexes. *J. Bus. Econ. Stat.* **1998**, *16*, 322–330.
47. Duclos, J.; Araar, A.; Fortin, C. *DAD: A Software for Distributive Analyses*; MIMAP Programme, International Development Research Centre, Government of Canada, and CIRPÉE Université Laval: Québec, QC, Canada, 2006; p. 21.
48. Ogundele, O.J.; Pavlova, M.; Groot, W. Inequalities in reproductive health care use in five West-African countries: A decomposition analysis of the wealth-based gaps. *Int. J. Equity Health* **2020**, *19*, 1–20. [CrossRef]
49. Yourkavitch, J.; Burgert-Brucker, C.; Assaf, S.; Delgado, S. Using geographical analysis to identify child health inequality in sub-Saharan Africa. *PLoS ONE* **2018**, *13*, e0201870. [CrossRef]
50. Bhandari, T.R.; Sarma, P.S.; Kutty, V.R. Utilization of maternal health care services in post-conflict Nepal. *Int. J. Women's Health* **2015**, *7*, 783. [CrossRef]
51. Ali, B.; Debnath, P.; Anwar, T. Inequalities in utilisation of maternal health services in urban India: Evidences from national family health survey—4. *Clin. Epidemiol. Glob. Health* **2021**, *10*, 100672. [CrossRef]
52. Mirzazada, S.; Padhani, Z.A.; Jabeen, S.; Fatima, M.; Rizvi, A.; Ansari, U.; Das, J.K.; Bhutta, Z.A. Impact of conflict on maternal and child health service delivery: A country case study of Afghanistan. *Confl. Health* **2020**, *14*, 38. [CrossRef] [PubMed]
53. Umar, A.; Kennedy, C.; Tawfik, H. Female economic empowerment as a significant factor of social exclusion on the use of antenatal and natal services in Nigeria. *MOJ Women's Health* **2017**, *5*, 217–220. [CrossRef]
54. Pandey, J.P.; Dhakal, M.R.; Karki, S.; Poudel, P.; Pradhan, M.S. *Maternal and Child Health in Nepal: The Effects of Caste, Ethnicity, and Regional Identity: Further Analysis of the 2011 Nepal Demographic and Health Survey*; Nepal Ministry of Health and Population, New ERA, and ICF International: Kathmandu, Nepal, 2013; p. 58.

55. Goland, E.; Hoa, D.T.P.; Målqvist, M. Inequity in maternal health care utilization in Vietnam. *Int. J. Equity Health* **2012**, *11*, 1–8. [CrossRef] [PubMed]
56. Schatzberg, M.G. Ethnicity and Class at the Local Level: Bars and Bureaucrats in Lisala, Zaire. *Comp. Politics* **1981**, *13*, 461–478. [CrossRef]
57. Fang, P.; Dong, S.; Xiao, J.; Liu, C.; Feng, X.; Wang, Y. Regional inequality in health and its determinants: Evidence from China. *Health Policy* **2010**, *94*, 14–25. [CrossRef]
58. Abolhallaje, M.; Mousavi, S.M.; Anjomshoa, M.; Beigi Nasiri, A.; Seyedin, H.; Sadeghifar, J.; Aryankhesal, A.; Rajabi Vasokolaei, G.; Beigi Nasiri, M. Assessing health inequalities in Iran: A focus on the distribution of health care facilities. *Glob. J. Health Sci.* **2014**, *6*, 285–291. [CrossRef]
59. Mekonnen, Y.; Mekonnen, A. *Utilization of Maternal Health Care Services in Ethiopia*; Ethiopian Health and Nutrition Research Institute: Calverton, MD, USA, 2002; p. 25.
60. Bongaarts, J. *Trends in Maternal Mortality: 1990 to 2015*; World Bank Group and the United Nations Population Division: Geneva, Switzerland, 2016; p. 16.
61. Chi, P.C.; Bulage, P.; Urdal, H.; Sundby, J. A qualitative study exploring the determinants of maternal health service uptake in post-conflict Burundi and Northern Uganda. *BMC Pregnancy Childbirth* **2015**, *15*, 18. [CrossRef]
62. Badiuzzaman, M.; Murshed, S.M.; Rieger, M. Improving maternal health care in a post conflict setting: Evidence from Chittagong Hill tracts of Bangladesh. *J. Dev. Stud.* **2020**, *56*, 384–400. [CrossRef]
63. Yaya, S.; Uthman, O.A.; Bishwajit, G.; Ekholuenetale, M. Maternal health care service utilization in post-war Liberia: Analysis of nationally representative cross-sectional household surveys. *BMC Public Health* **2019**, *19*, 28. [CrossRef]
64. Waage, J.; Yap, C.; Bell, S.; Levy, C.; Mace, G.; Pegram, T.; Unterhalter, E.; Dasandi, N.; Hudson, D.; Kock, R. Governing the UN Sustainable Development Goals: Interactions, infrastructures, and institutions. *Lancet Glob. Health* **2015**, *3*, e251–e252. [CrossRef]
65. Yaya, S.; Ghose, B. Global inequality in maternal health care service utilization: Implications for sustainable development goals. *Health Equity* **2019**, *3*, 145–154. [CrossRef] [PubMed]
66. McKinnon, B.; Harper, S.; Kaufman, J.S. Who benefits from removing user fees for facility-based delivery services? Evidence on socioeconomic differences from Ghana, Senegal and Sierra Leone. *Soc. Sci. Med.* **2015**, *135*, 117–123. [CrossRef] [PubMed]
67. Lorentzen, P.; McMillan, J.; Wacziarg, R. Death and development. *J. Econ. Growth* **2008**, *13*, 81–124. [CrossRef]
68. Aghion, P.; Howitt, P.; Murtin, F. *The Relationship between Health and Growth: When Lucas Meets Nelson-Phelps*; National Bureau of Economic Research: Cambridge, MA, USA, 2010.
69. Davidson, R.; Kitzinger, J.; Hunt, K. The wealthy get healthy, the poor get poorly? Lay perceptions of health inequalities. *Soc. Sci. Med.* **2006**, *62*, 2171–2182. [CrossRef] [PubMed]
70. Drapcho, B.; Mock, N. DHS and Conflict in Africa: Findings from a Comparative Study and Recommendations for Improving the Utility of DHS as a Survey Vehicle in Conflict Settings. Citeseer. 2000. Available online: www.certi.org/publications/policy/dhs-8.pdf (accessed on 18 January 2023).
71. Ties Boerma, J.; Sommerfelt, A.E. Demographic and health surveys (DHS): Contributions and limitations. *World Health Stat. Q.* **1993**, *46*, 222–226.
72. Ahmed, S.; Li, Q.; Scrafford, C.; Pullum, T.W. *DHS Methodological Reports No. 13: An Assessment of DHS Maternal Mortality Data and Estimates*; ICF International: Rockville, MD, USA, 2014; p. 156.

Disclaimer/Publisher's Note: The statements, opinions and data contained in all publications are solely those of the individual author(s) and contributor(s) and not of MDPI and/or the editor(s). MDPI and/or the editor(s) disclaim responsibility for any injury to people or property resulting from any ideas, methods, instructions or products referred to in the content.

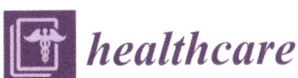

Article

Use of Advance Directives in US Veterans and Non-Veterans: Findings from the Decedents of the Health and Retirement Study 1992–2014

Ho-Jui Tung [1],* and Ming-Chin Yeh [2]

[1] Department of Health Policy and Community Health, Jiann-Ping Hsu College of Public Health, Georgia Southern University, P.O. Box 8015, Statesboro, GA 30460-8015, USA
[2] Nutrition Program, Hunter College, City University of New York, New York, NY 10065, USA
* Correspondence: htung@georgiasouthern.edu; Tel.: +1-912-478-1342; Fax: +1-912-478-0171

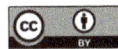

Citation: Tung, H.-J.; Yeh, M.-C. Use of Advance Directives in US Veterans and Non-Veterans: Findings from the Decedents of the Health and Retirement Study 1992–2014. *Healthcare* **2023**, *11*, 1824. https://doi.org/10.3390/healthcare11131824

Academic Editors: Sofia Koukouli and Areti Stavropoulou

Received: 16 May 2023
Revised: 13 June 2023
Accepted: 20 June 2023
Published: 22 June 2023

Copyright: © 2023 by the authors. Licensee MDPI, Basel, Switzerland. This article is an open access article distributed under the terms and conditions of the Creative Commons Attribution (CC BY) license (https://creativecommons.org/licenses/by/4.0/).

Abstract: Evidence shows that older patients with advance directives such as a living will, or durable power of attorney for healthcare, are more likely to receive care consistent with their preferences at the end of life. Less is known about the use of advance directives between veteran and non-veteran older Americans. Using data from the decedents of a longitudinal survey, we explore whether there is a difference in having an established advance directive between the veteran and non-veteran decedents. Data were taken from the Harmonized End of Life data sets, a linked collection of variables derived from the Health and Retirement Study (HRS) Exit Interview. Only male decedents were included in the current analysis (N = 4828). The dependent variable, having an established advance directive, was measured by asking the proxy, "whether the deceased respondent ever provided written instructions about the treatment or care he/she wanted to receive during the final days of his/her life" and "whether the deceased respondent had a Durable Power of Attorney for healthcare?" A "yes" to either of the two items was counted as having an advance directive. The independent variable, veteran status, was determined by asking participants, "Have you ever served in the active military of the United States?" at their first HRS core interview. Logistic regression was used to predict the likelihood of having an established advance directive. While there was no difference in having an advance directive between male veteran and non-veteran decedents during the earlier follow-up period (from 1992 to 2003), male veterans who died during the second half of the study period (from 2004 to 2014) were more likely to have an established advance directive than their non-veteran counterparts (OR = 1.24, $p < 0.05$). Other factors positively associated with having an established advance directive include dying at older ages, higher educational attainment, needing assistance in activities of daily living and being bedridden three months before death, while Black decedents and those who were married were less likely to have an advance directive in place. Our findings suggest male veterans were more likely to have an established advance directive, an indicator for better end-of-life care, than their non-veteran counterparts. This observed difference coincides with a time when the Veterans Health Administration (VHA) increased its investment in end-of-life care. More studies are needed to confirm if this higher utilization of advance directives and care planning among veterans can be attributed to the improved access and quality of end-of-life care in the VHA system.

Keywords: veterans; living will; durable power of attorney for healthcare; advance directives; advanced care planning; Veterans Health Administration

1. Introduction

Advances in medical technologies (e.g., chemotherapy, tube-feeding, and ventilators) have made dying an increasingly prolonged and "medicalized" process [1]. In many cases, these life-sustaining treatments may prolong the lives of patients with terminal illnesses, but not necessarily enhance the quality of their lives. Dying patients may go through invasive, costly, and futile interventions in acute care settings [2] that are incongruent with the characteristics of quality end-of-life care both patients and families prefer [3]. Advance directives are care planning tools, introduced as a solution to improve the quality of end-of-life care [4] and they can take the form of a living will or durable power of attorney for healthcare (DPAHC). Patients can document their treatment preferences, along with a variety of end-of-life choices, when they are still capable of making decisions.

Evidence indicates that advance care planning (ACP) is less likely to take place in hospitals and intensive care units, where timely transitions to palliative care could be slowed and a patient's preferences might not be honored sometimes [5]. Although there are reports on the limitations, regarding the efficacy and effectiveness of advance directives in clinical practices [1,6]. Studies have found that the use of ACP is associated with better transitions to palliative care and more use of hospice where patient-centered care is honored [7–9]. Considered an important indicator of better planning for end-of-life care, several systematic review articles also conclude that the use of ACP is associated with other positive outcomes, such as dying in preferred place, reducing invasive and futile treatments, and achieving some characteristics of "good death" [10–13]. It has been recognized that advance directives are not a panacea to all the problems in end-of-life care. Instead, they should serve as the starting point for ongoing communication between patients, surrogates, and health professionals [14].

Empirical research on the use of ACP has identified a variety of factors associated with the use of ACP, including age, race/ethnicity, socioeconomic status (SES), psychological, religious, and attitudinal factors [1]. Racial and ethnic disparities have been heavily investigated and significant racial disparities in the use of ACP are identified [15,16], where African Americans are less likely to have an established advance directive than their white counterparts. Significant differences in the use of advance directives are also found among patients with different terminal illnesses [11]. Patients who die of different diseases may go through different trajectories of terminal decline [17], which could lead to multiple transitions between different care settings near the end of life. However, little is known about the use of advance directives and care planning at the end of life between veteran and non-veteran older adults in the United States.

For male Americans who were born before the 1940s, veteran status is an important mediator of their aging experiences, because many of them had been drafted into the military and a large proportion of these veterans had served in World War II, the Korean War, or the Vietnam War. A theoretical perspective in social gerontology, the life course perspective, highlights the link between early experiences and later developments in human lives. In a similar vein, the lifespan view of military influences on aging US veterans also asserts that the effects of military service are lifelong [18]. Veterans usually form strong network ties through their military experiences and people's social networks provide a structure where potential resources are embedded [19,20]. The literature of healthcare utilization and the social process of help-seeking behavior have suggested that an individual's network is important in channeling their entrance into care [21].

Furthermore, as the largest healthcare delivery system in the country, the Veterans Health Administration (VHA) is charged with the provision of healthcare to qualified US veterans. The increasing number of aging veterans has been an important driving force for the VHA to take the lead in developing end-of-life care programs and initiatives (e.g., hospice and palliative care) [22,23]. There have been reports on the VHA's investment in improving the access and quality of end-of-life care since the 1990s [5,24,25]. Several policy evaluation studies also found that these programs have improved the quality, availability, and accessibility of end-of-life care in the VHA system [23,26]. However, most of these studies analyzed data from the medical records kept within the VHA system, so that their samples consisted mainly of the veterans covered by the VHA. In this study, we used data from a nationally representative survey, in which both veterans and non-veteran older adults were sampled. We compared the difference in the use of advance directives (either a living will or DPAHC) between the deceased veterans and non-veterans from a longitudinal survey over two decades.

2. Methods

2.1. Data and Samples

Launched in 1992, the Health and Retirement Study (HRS) is a panel-designed longitudinal survey of those over the age of 50 in the United States [27]. The survey draws a multistage probability sample that is nationally representative of the U.S. population. Using both face-to-face and telephone interviews, the survey collects information addressing many important questions related to the aging experiences in America. Core interviews were conducted every two years and, for the deceased HRS participants, exit interviews were arranged with their proxies to seek information about the decedents, including the diseases and causes of deaths, healthcare utilization, and end-of-life planning.

Data for the current study were taken from the Harmonized HRS End of Life data files, a streamlined collection of variables derived from the first HRS Exit Interviews from 1994 to 2014 [28]. A total of 12,952 HRS participants had died between 1992 and 2014. However, 2623 of the decedents whose proxies did not provide information on advance directives. Plus, for these cohorts of older Americans, military service was predominantly a male role, we further excluded all of the 5471 female decedents from the analyzed sample. After excluding another 30 cases with missing values on other variables, a total of 4828 male decedents were available for the current analysis.

2.2. Measures

For the dependent variable, the provision of advance directives was measured by two questions: "whether the deceased respondent ever provided written instructions about the treatment or care he/she wanted to receive during the final days of his/her life?" and "whether the deceased respondent had a Durable Power of Attorney for health care?" If the answers to either of the two items were "yes", the dependent variable was coded 1 (having an established advance directive). It was coded 0 if both answers were "no", indicating that the decedent had neither of the two types of advance directive.

For the independent variables, age at death was treated as a continuous measure. Over 96 percent of the male decedents were either white or Black, so race was dichotomized into Black (=1) and all others (=0). Educational attainment was measured as years of schooling and this measure was treated as a continuous variable. Marital status at death was also a dichotomous measure. The proxy was asked if the respondent was married (or partnered) at the time of death (yes = 1; otherwise = 0).

Caring for dying patients can be both physically and emotionally challenging for their family caregivers. Two indicators of care burden were also included to predict the dependent variable, the likelihood of having an established advance directive before death. In the survey, proxies were asked whether a spouse, child/grandchild, or other relatives had helped with Activity of Daily Living (ADLs) in the three months prior to death. A "yes" to any of the six ADLs (eating, bathing, dressing, walking, toileting, and getting in and out of bed) was coded as 1 and 0 for otherwise. Bedridden status was coded as 1 and 0 for otherwise if the respondent spent more than half the day in bed over 85 days during the last three months before death. These measures could be indications of an expected death and a prompt for end-of-life care planning activities. Since the deaths in our sample occurred over a long period, the social norms regarding the use of advance directives and the availability of care-planning tools could change considerably over time. Thus, a dichotomous variable indicating whether the death occurred during the earlier half (from 1992 and 2003) or the latter half (from 2004 to 2014) of the study period was also included. Finally, the prognosis of patients dying of cancer is more predictable and consistent when compared to other common causes of mortality [29]. Decedents whose main cause of death was cancer were singled out as a predictor for the use of advance directives. The main cause of death in the survey was determined by asking the proxies the following open-ended question, "What was the major illness that led to (her/his) death?". The reported illnesses were then recoded according to the Health Conditions Master Code developed by the HRS [28]. If the main cause of death was cancer, it was coded 1. For all other causes of death, it was coded 0.

2.3. Analysis

Binary logistic regression models, where the dependent variable was constructed as the probability of having an advance directive in place versus not having an advance directive. The main independent variable, veteran status, was used to predict the likelihood of having an advance directive, while controlling for other covariates. Odds ratios (and their 95 percent of confidence intervals) were used to evaluate the significance of the included predictors. Separated analyses were performed for decedents whose death occurred during the earlier half (from 1992 to 2003) and those who died during the latter half of the study period (from 2004 to 2014).

3. Results

Among the 4828 male decedents, about 58 percent of them (2783 out of 4828) were identified as veterans. The high percentage of veterans in our sample is because over 90 percent of the male decedents in our sample were born before 1941. For this cohort of male Americans, a military conscription was in place until 1973. From the descriptive statistics presented in Table 1, we know that, on average, veterans died older and had more years of schooling than those of the non-veteran decedents. The percentage of African Americans was significantly lower among the veteran group when compared to the non-veterans. The percentages of having a living will or a durable power of attorney for healthcare were also significantly higher among the veterans, when compared to their non-veteran counterparts.

Table 1. Selected characteristics of the male decedents of Health and Retirement Study participants by veteran status, 1992 to 2014.

Predictors	Veteran (N = 2783)	Non-Veteran (N = 2045)
Mean Age at death	78.2 (9.3)	77.4 (11.8)
Years in schools	12.3 (3.1)	10.0 (4.2)
African Americans (yes)	296 (10.6)	430 (21.0)
Marital status at death (married)	1858 (66.8)	1214 (59.4)
Death occurred between 1992 and 2003 (yes)	1178 (42.3)	897 (43.9)
Cancer as the main cause of death (yes)	803 (28.9)	530 (25.9)
Needed help with any activities of daily living 3 months before death (yes)	1320 (47.4)	921 (45.0)
Bedridden 3 months before death (yes)	674 (24.2)	512 (25.0)
Had a living will (yes)	1276 (45.8)	687 (33.6)
Had a durable power of attorney (yes)	1531 (55.0)	916 (44.8)

Note: For categorical variables, the number of cases and percentage (in parentheses) are presented and for continuous variables (age and years of schooling), means and standard deviations (in parentheses) are presented. Numbers and percentages for the two types of advance directives, a living will and a durable power of attorney for healthcare (DPAHC) were presented separately here, but they were combined to form the dependent variable in the logistic regression analyses.

Table 2 presents the logistic regression results for the whole sample. Veterans were more likely to have an established advance directive (odds ratio, OR = 1.15, $p < 0.05$) than that of the non-veterans, after controlling for other covariates. Deceased HRS participants who died at an older age (OR = 1.04, $p < 0.001$) and who had more years of schooling (OR = 1.12, $p < 0.001$) were more likely to have an established advance directive. Decedents who needed ADL assistance three months before death, those who were bedridden three months before death, and those who died during the latter half of the study period, had a significantly higher chance of having an advance directive. On the other hand, African

Americans and those who were married at the time of death were less likely to have an advance directive in place.

Table 2. Odds ratios of having an established advance directive among the male decedents of the Health and Retirement Study, 1992 to 2014.

Predictors	Odds Ratio (95% Confidence Intervals)
Veteran status	
No	1.0
Yes	1.15 (1.01, 1.31) *
Age at death	1.04 (1.04, 1.05) ***
Years in schools	1.12 (1.10, 1.14) ***
African American	
No	1.0
Yes	0.36 (0.30, 0.43) ***
Marital status at death	
No	1.0
Yes	0.74 (0.65, 0.85) ***
Cancer as the main cause of death	
No	1.0
Yes	1.35 (1.17, 1.56) ***
Needed help with any activities of daily living 3 months before death	
No	1.0
Yes	2.26 (1.94, 2.62) ***
Bedridden 3 months before death	
No	1.0
Yes	2.27 (1.91, 2.69) ***
Death occurred	
Between 1992 and 2003	1.0
Between 2004 and 2014	1.45 (1.28, 1.65) ***
−2 Log Likelihood (degrees of freedom)	5743.98 (9)

Note: * $p < 0.05$, *** $p < 0.001$.

Table 3 presents separated logistic regression models in predicting the use of advance directives for decedents who died earlier (from 19992 to 2003) and whose deaths occurred later in time (from 2004 to 2014). We found that there was no significant difference in having an established advance directive between male veteran and non-veteran decedents whose death occurred during the earlier-half study period. The significant difference between veterans and non-veterans happened to concentrate on decedents who died during the latter half of the study period (OR = 1.24, $p = 0.02$). For other covariates, the association patterns stayed the same.

Table 3. Odds ratios of having an established advance directive among male decedents of the Health and Retirement Study, separated by death period.

Predictors	Decedents Whose Death Occurred between 1992 and 2003 (N = 2075)	Decedents Whose Death Occurred between 2004 and 2014 (N = 2753)
Veteran status		
No	1.0	1.0
Yes	1.04 (0.85, 1.27)	1.24 (1.03, 1.48) *
Age at death	1.04 (1.03, 1.05) ***	1.04 (1.03, 1.05) ***
Years of schooling	1.12 (1.09, 1.15) ***	1.11 (1.08, 1.14) ***
African American		
No	1.0	1.0
Yes	0.36 (0.27, 0.47) ***	0.37 (0.29, 0.46) ***
Married at death		
No	1.0	1.0
Yes	0.77 (0.63, 0.94) *	0.73 (0.60, 0.87) **
Cancer as the main cause of death		
No	1.0	1.0
Yes	1.37 (1.11, 1.70) **	1.34 (1.10, 1.63) **
Needed help with any activities of daily living or 3 months before death		
No	1.0	1.0
Yes	2.15 (1.72, 2.69) ***	2.34 (1.91, 2.87) ***
Bedridden 3 months before death		
No	1.0	1.0
Yes	2.13 (1.66, 2.72) ***	2.41 (1.90, 3.05) ***
−2 log likelihood (degrees of freedom)	2569.43 (8)	3171.99 (8)

Note: * $p < 0.05$, ** $p < 0.01$, *** $p < 0.001$.

4. Discussion

As a tool to facilitate decision-making and communication at the end of life, ACP is associated with better end-of-life care, such as dying in preferred place and healthcare cost savings [12]. Furthermore, having an advance directive and ACP at the end of life are also associated with a reduced decision-making burden and improved well-being for dying patients' family members [30]. In this study, we used data collected from both the proxies and the deceased participants of a longitudinal survey to compare the rates of having an established advance directive between male veterans and non-veterans. The results show that male veterans had a significantly higher use of advance directives, an indicator of quality end-of-life care, than their non-veteran counterparts during the latter half of the study period (from 2004 to 2014). We also found that, regardless of their veteran status, male decedents, who died at older ages and who had higher educational attainment, were more likely to have an established advance directive. African American decedents and those who were married at the time of death were less likely to have an advance directive in place. Decedents with a higher care burden (those who needed ADL assistance and were bedridden three months before death) were also more likely to have an established advance directive.

The percentage of older adults with a written advance directive has been rising since the Patient Self-determination Act was passed in 1990 [1]. When asked, a great majority of Americans believe that having a family conversation about their wishes regarding life-sustaining treatments at the end of life are important, but much lower percentages of people have done so [5]. Conducted on adults of various ages, surveys on ACP activities indicated that some 23 to 54 percent Americans had a written advance directive in place and the rates were as high as 70 percent among older adults who had a terminal illness [1,5,9]. In the current analysis, the percentages of having either a living will or a DPAHC among the decedents who died during the first half of the study period were 47.8 percent for non-veterans and 54.2 percent for veterans. By the latter half of the study period (from 2004 to 2014), the rate difference had increased to 54.8 percent for non-veterans and 69.2 percent for veterans.

We are not completely clear about all the factors contributing to the observed difference in the use of advance directives between veteran and non-veteran HRS decedents. However, our findings indicate that the difference was significant only in the latter half of the study period (from 2004 to 2014). This time frame overlaps with a period when several end-of-life care programs and initiatives were launched and implemented by the VHA system. For example, the VHA was the first to require hospice consultation teams to be established in all its care facilities in 1992 and the Hospice–Veteran Partnership Program (launched in 2001) made hospice and palliative care widely available to veterans and their caregivers [22,24,25]. The Bereaved Family Survey was also launched in 2008 by the VHA to evaluate performance and monitor family members' perceptions of veterans' end-of-life care [29,31].

Moreover, for non-veteran older Americans covered by Medicare (the federal health insurance program for older people aged 65 or older in the United States), they must waive aggressive treatments in order to be eligible for hospice care. In contrast to Medicare beneficiaries, the VHA allows for the provision of concurrent care while the patient is in hospice [32,33]. Thanks to veterans' sacrifice to the country, these generous care benefits often receive bipartisan support in Congress. It is reasonable to speculate that these programs and initiatives have significantly improved the quality of end-of-life care and access to care planning tools within the VHA system.

There might be another organizational advantage of the VHA system in carrying through its end-of-life care policies. The VHA is the largest integrated healthcare delivery system in the United States. Different from Medicare, which functions as a healthcare purchaser, the VHA provides healthcare directly to qualified veterans. Over the past decades, Medicare has also expanded its coverage for end-of-life counseling on advance directives and hospice use [1,34]. However, as a care purchaser, Medicare can only implement its policy initiatives through incentives in reimbursing contracted care providers and managed-care organizations. The centralized VHA system with a salaried medical staff makes coordination more likely to occur, so it would be easier to put established policies into place.

Finally, it should be noted that there are several limitations in our study. First, this study focusses mostly on the birth cohorts of male HRS participants who lived through a time when military conscription was instituted in the United States. Military drafting was ended when the All-Volunteer Force (AVF) policy was established in 1973. Additionally, the centralized VHA healthcare system is supervised by the Department of Veteran Affairs, a US cabinet-level agency under the executive branch. These cohort-historic factors are culture- and country-specific, so the findings and implications of this study may not be applicable internationally.

Second, many veterans are eligible for both VHA care and Medicare. It is possible that some veterans could seek care in a non-VHA facility, meaning they would not be exposed to the organizational advantages and end-of-life care benefits provided by the VHA system. A survey in 2010 found that 77 percent of the veterans enrolled in the VHA were eligible for additional healthcare coverage and VHA care users were more likely to be older [35]. However, over 90 percent of the male veterans in our sample were born before 1941 (the pre-Vietnam-era veteran) [36]. It is reasonable to believe that, when presented with multiple options for end-of-life care, most veterans would seek VHA care, where better end-of-life benefits were offered.

Third, the HRS exit surveys were conducted by interviewing the proxy informants, so information reported by the proxies is subject to recall biases. Plus, not all the proxies for the HRS decedents knew all the details of end-of-life care planning pertaining to the deceased participants. About 20.3 percent of the decedents in the Harmonized HRS End of Life data (out of the 12,952 deaths of HRS participants recorded between 1992 and 2014) had missing information on the details of advance directives. It is possible that potential biases could be introduced due to the missing observations. Fortunately, the variables included in this study were mostly restricted to observable behaviors and facts of the deceased respondents reported by their proxies. According to the data description documents, about 95 percent of the proxies interviewed in the Exit Interview Surveys were related to the deceased participants [28], so reporting errors should be minimal.

Lastly, it is still possible that some unmeasured confounders might explain the observed difference between veterans and non-veterans in the use of advance directives. More studies are needed to confirm whether the observed difference in the use of advance directives can be attributed to the improved access and quality end-of-life care provided by the VHA system.

Author Contributions: Conceptualization, H.-J.T.; methodology, H.-J.T.; writing—original draft, H.-J.T.; writing—review and editing, M.-C.Y. All authors have read and agreed to the published version of the manuscript.

Funding: This research received no external funding.

Institutional Review Board Statement: Not applicable.

Informed Consent Statement: Not applicable.

Data Availability Statement: Study data were downloaded from a publicly accessible website, the Health and Retirement Study.

Acknowledgments: This analysis uses data or information from the Harmonized HRS End of Life dataset and Codebook, Version A as of March 2019 developed by the Gateway to Global Aging Data. The development of the Harmonized HRS End of Life was funded by the National Institute on Aging. For more information, please refer to www.g2aging.org (Accessed on 16 May 2023).

Conflicts of Interest: The authors declare no conflict of interest.

References

1. Carr, D.; Luth, E. End-of-Life Planning and Health Care. In *Handbook of Aging and the Social Sciences*; Elsevier: Amsterdam, The Netherlands, 2016; pp. 375–394. [CrossRef]
2. Wilkinson, A.M.; Lynn, J. The end of life. In *Handbook of Aging and the Social Sciences*, 5th ed.; Academic Press: Cambridge, MA, USA, 2001; pp. 444–461.
3. Steinhauser, K.E. Factors Considered Important at the End of Life by Patients, Family, Physicians, and Other Care Providers. *JAMA* **2000**, *284*, 2476. [CrossRef] [PubMed]
4. Teno, J.M. Advance Directives for Nursing Home Residents. *JAMA* **2007**, *283*, 1481–1482. [CrossRef] [PubMed]
5. Institute of Medicine. *Dying in America: Improving Quality and Honoring Individual Preferences Near the End of Life*; The National Academies Press: Washington, DC, USA, 2015. [CrossRef]
6. Morrison, R.S.; Meier, D.E.; Arnold, R.M. What's Wrong with Advance Care Planning? *JAMA* **2021**, *326*, 1575. [CrossRef] [PubMed]
7. Molloy, D.W.; Guyatt, G.H.; Russo, R.; Goeree, R.; O'Brien, B.J.; Bédard, M. Systematic Implementation of an Advance Directive Program in Nursing Homes: A Randomized Controlled Trial. *JAMA* **2000**, *283*, 1437. [CrossRef] [PubMed]
8. Shrank, W.H.; Russell, K.; Emanuel, E.J. Hospice Carve-In—Aligning Benefits With Patient and Family Needs. *JAMA* **2020**, *324*, 35. [CrossRef]
9. Silveira, M.J.; Langa, K.M. Advance Directives and Outcomes of Surrogate Decision Making before Death. *N. Engl. J. Med.* **2010**, *362*, 1211–1218. [CrossRef]
10. Teno, J.M.; Gozalo, P.; Trivedi, A.N.; Bunker, J.; Lima, J.; Ogarek, J.; Mor, V. Site of Death, Place of Care, and Health Care Transitions among US Medicare Beneficiaries, 2000–2015. *JAMA* **2018**, *320*, 264. [CrossRef]
11. Christakis, N.A. Survival of Medicare Patients after Enrollment in Hospice Programs. *N. Engl. J. Med.* **1996**, *335*, 172–178. [CrossRef]
12. Jimenez, G.; Tan, W.S.; Virk, A.K.; Low, C.K.; Car, J.; Ho, A.H.Y. Overview of Systematic Reviews of Advance Care Planning: Summary of Evidence and Global Lessons. *J. Pain Symptom Manag.* **2018**, *56*, 436–459.e25. [CrossRef]
13. Detering, K.M.; Hancock, A.D.; Reade, M.C.; Silvester, W. The impact of advance care planning on end of life care in elderly patients: Randomised controlled trial. *BMJ* **2010**, *340*, c1345. [CrossRef]

14. Higel, T.; Alaoui, A.; Bouton, C.; Fournier, J.P. Effect of Living Wills on End-of-Life Care: A Systematic Review. *J. Am. Geriatr. Soc.* **2019**, *67*, 164–171. [CrossRef] [PubMed]
15. Carr, D. Racial and Ethnic Differences in Advance Care Planning: Identifying Subgroup Patterns and Obstacles. *J. Aging Health* **2012**, *24*, 923–947. [CrossRef] [PubMed]
16. Smith, A.K.; McCarthy, E.P.; Paulk, E.; Balboni, T.A.; Maciejewski, P.K.; Block, S.D.; Prigerson, H.G. Racial and Ethnic Differences in Advance Care Planning Among Patients with Cancer: Impact of Terminal Illness Acknowledgment, Religiousness, and Treatment Preferences. *JCO* **2008**, *26*, 4131–4137. [CrossRef]
17. Cohen-Mansfield, J.; Skornick-Bouchbinder, M.; Brill, S. Trajectories of End of Life: A Systematic Review. *J. Gerontol. Ser. B* **2018**, *73*, 564–572. [CrossRef]
18. Spiro, A.; Settersten, R.A.; Aldwin, C.M. Long-term Outcomes of Military Service in Aging and the Life Course: A Positive Re-envisioning. *Gerontologist* **2016**, *56*, 5–13. [CrossRef] [PubMed]
19. Tung, H.-J. *Ethnicity, Use of Chinese Medicine Physicians, and Health Status among the Elderly in Taiwan*; University of North Carolina at Chapel Hill: Chapel Hill, NC, USA, 2001.
20. Perry Brea, L.; Pescosolido Bernice, A. Social network activation: The role of health discussion partners in recovery from mental illness. *Soc Sci Med.* **2015**, *125*, 116–128. [CrossRef] [PubMed]
21. Freidson, E. *Profession of Medicine: A Study of the Sociology of Applied Knowledge*; The University of Chicago Press: Chicago, IL, USA, 1970.
22. Daratsos, L.; Howe, J.L. The Development of Palliative Care Programs in the Veterans Administration: Zelda Foster's Legacy. *J. Soc. Work End-Life Palliat. Care* **2007**, *3*, 29–39. [CrossRef]
23. Kutney-Lee, A.; Smith, D.; Griffin, H.; Kinder, D.; Carpenter, J.; Thorpe, J. Quality of end-of-life care for Vietnam-era Veterans: Implications for practice and policy. *Healthcare* **2021**, *9*, 100494. [CrossRef]
24. Edes, T.; Shreve, S.; Casarett, D. Increasing Access and Quality in Department of Veterans Affairs Care at the End of Life: A Lesson in Change: Transforming va Care at the End of Life. *J. Am. Geriatr. Soc.* **2007**, *55*, 1645–1649. [CrossRef]
25. Miller, S.C.; Intrator, O.; Scott, W.; Shreve, S.T.; Phibbs, C.S.; Kinosian, B. Increasing Veterans' Hospice Use: The Veterans Health Administration's Focus on Improving End-Of-Life Care. *Health Aff.* **2017**, *36*, 1274–1282. [CrossRef]
26. Casarett, D.; Pickard, A.; Bailey, F.A.; Ritchie, C.; Furman, C.; Rosenfeld, K. Do Palliative Consultations Improve Patient Outcomes?: Palliative Care Consultation. *J. Am. Geriatr. Soc.* **2008**, *56*, 593–599. [CrossRef] [PubMed]
27. Servais, M. Overview of HRS Public Data Files for Cross-Sectional and Longitudinal Analysis. Published Online 2010. Available online: https://hrs.isr.umich.edu/sites/default/files/biblio/OverviewofHRSPublicData.pdf (accessed on 16 May 2023).
28. Ailshire, J.; Chien, S.; Phyllip, D.; Wilkens, J.; Lee, J. Harmonized HRS End of Life Documentation. Published Online 2019. Available online: https://www.g2aging.org (accessed on 16 May 2023).
29. Gidwani-Marszowski, R.; Needleman, J.; Mor, V.; Faricy-Anderson, K.; Boothroyd, D.B.; Hsin, G. Quality Of End-Of-Life Care Is Higher in The VA Compared to Care Paid for by Traditional Medicare. *Health Aff.* **2018**, *37*, 95–103. [CrossRef] [PubMed]
30. Stein, R.A.; Sharpe, L.; Bell, M.L.; Boyle, F.M.; Dunn, S.M.; Clarke, S.J. Randomized Controlled Trial of a Structured Intervention to Facilitate End-of-Life Decision Making in Patients with Advanced Cancer. *JCO* **2013**, *31*, 3403–3410. [CrossRef] [PubMed]
31. Kutney-Lee, A.; Carpenter, J.; Smith, D.; Thorpe, J.; Tudose, A.; Ersek, M. Case-Mix Adjustment of the Bereaved Family Survey. *Am. J. Hosp. Palliat. Care* **2018**, *35*, 1015–1022. [CrossRef] [PubMed]
32. Mor, V.; Joyce, N.R.; Coté, D.L.; Gidwani, R.A.; Ersek, M.; Levy, C.R. The rise of concurrent care for veterans with advanced cancer at the end of life: EOL Care for Veterans with Advanced CA. *Cancer* **2016**, *122*, 782–790. [CrossRef] [PubMed]
33. Presley, C.J.; Kaur, K.; Han, L.; Soulos, P.R.; Zhu, W.; Corneau, E. Aggressive End-of-Life Care in the Veterans Health Administration versus Fee-for-Service Medicare among Patients with Advanced Lung Cancer. *J. Palliat. Med.* **2022**, *25*, 932–939. [CrossRef]
34. Gold, D.T. Late life death and dying in 21st century America. In *Hanbook of Aging and Social Sciences*, 7th ed.; Academic Press: Cambridge, MA, USA, 2011; pp. 235–247.
35. Radomski, T.R.; Zhao, X.; Thorpe, C.T.; Thorpe, J.M.; Good, C.B.; Mor, M.K. VA and Medicare Utilization Among Dually Enrolled Veterans with Type 2 Diabetes: A Latent Class Analysis. *J. Gen. Intern. Med.* **2016**, *31*, 524–531. [CrossRef]
36. Spiro, A., III; Wilmoth, J.M.; London, A.S. *Assessing the Impact of Military Service in the Health and Retirement Study: Current Status and Suggestions for the Future*; National Institute on Aging: Bethesda, MD, USA, 2016; pp. 1–25. Available online: https://hrs.isr.umich.edu/documentation/dmc-review-papers (accessed on 16 May 2023).

Disclaimer/Publisher's Note: The statements, opinions and data contained in all publications are solely those of the individual author(s) and contributor(s) and not of MDPI and/or the editor(s). MDPI and/or the editor(s) disclaim responsibility for any injury to people or property resulting from any ideas, methods, instructions or products referred to in the content.

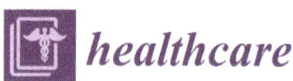

Review

School Health Services and Health Education Curricula in Greece: Scoping Review and Policy Plan

Pelagia Soultatou [1,*], Stamatis Vardaros [2] and Pantelis G. Bagos [3,*]

1. Department of Public and Community Health, University of West Attica, 11521 Athens, Greece
2. Department of Political Science, University of Crete, 74100 Rethymno, Greece; st.vardaros@gmail.com
3. Department of Computer Science and Biomedical Informatics, University of Thessaly, 35100 Lamia, Greece
* Correspondence: psoultatou@uniwa.gr (P.S.); pbagos@compgen.org (P.G.B.)

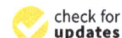

Citation: Soultatou, P.; Vardaros, S.; Bagos, P.G. School Health Services and Health Education Curricula in Greece: Scoping Review and Policy Plan. *Healthcare* **2023**, *11*, 1678. https://doi.org/10.3390/healthcare11121678

Academic Editors: Areti Stavropoulou and Sofia Koukouli

Received: 7 May 2023
Revised: 24 May 2023
Accepted: 5 June 2023
Published: 7 June 2023

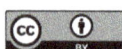

Copyright: © 2023 by the authors. Licensee MDPI, Basel, Switzerland. This article is an open access article distributed under the terms and conditions of the Creative Commons Attribution (CC BY) license (https://creativecommons.org/licenses/by/4.0/).

Abstract: The new generation's health and wellbeing is of paramount importance: it constitutes United Nations' priority, complies with Children's Rights and responds to the Sustainable Development Goals of the United Nations. In this perspective, school health and health education, as facets of the public health domain targeted at young people, deserve further attention after the unprecedented COVID-19 pandemic crisis in order to revise policies. The key objectives of this article are (a) to review the evidence generated over a span of two decades (2003–2023), identifying the main policy gaps by taking Greece as a case study, and (b) to provide a concrete and integrated policy plan. Following the qualitative research paradigm, a scoping review is used to identify policy gaps in school health services (SHS) and school health education curricula (SHEC). Data are extracted from four databases: Scopus, PubMed, Web of Science and Google Scholar, while the findings are categorized into the following themes following specific inclusion and exclusion criteria: school health services, school health education curricula, school nursing, all with reference to Greece. A corpus of 162 out 282 documents in English and Greek initially accumulated, is finally used. The 162 documents consisted of seven doctoral theses, four legislative texts, 27 conference proceedings, 117 publications in journals and seven syllabuses. Out of the 162 documents, only 17 correspond to the set of research questions. The findings suggest that school health services are not school-based but a function of the primary health care system, whereas health education retains a constantly changing position in school curricula, and several deficiencies in schoolteachers' training, coordination and leadership impede the implementation. Regarding the second objective of this article, a set of policy measures is provided in terms of a problem-solving perspective, towards the reform and integration of school health with health education.

Keywords: public health; policy plan; school health; health education; youth

1. Introduction

The unprecedented crisis of the COVID-19 pandemic provoked a discussion in respect to public health policies fueled by the need to respond to the wide spectrum of emerging challenges aligned to the plethora of exacerbated vulnerabilities and inequalities evidenced through the humanitarian crisis, as a growing corpus of literature shows [1–4]. The imperative to invent a new vision for public health which addresses the challenges, takes seriously into account the lessons emerging from the humanitarian crisis and reorganizes public health upon the ideal of a common good is also echoed in the literature [5–7]. However, little attention has been paid to school health services (SHS) and school health education curricula (SHEC), as two inter-linked dimensions of public health aiming at youth.

The new generation's health and wellbeing is of paramount importance, constitutes United Nations' priority and complies with Children's Rights [8]. Seventeen Sustainable Development Goals (SDG) have been adopted by governments at the UN General Assembly relating the SDG3 directly to health, prompting the states to ensure healthy lives and promote well-being for all at all ages. The SDG declaration emphasizes that to achieve the overall health goal, universal health coverage and access to quality health care will be encompassed in health policies. The UN Convention on the Rights of the Child entails that states need to ensure institutions, services and facilities responsible for the care and protection of children will conform with the standards established by competent authorities, in respect to health [9]. It is advocated to work towards "a revitalized global effort to fully protect, nurture, and support the health and development potential for every child everywhere, from before conception to adulthood" [10] (p. 1761).

Primary health care has the potential to fulfill the SDG in line with the Declaration of Astana, which defines three key areas of primary health care as: service provision, multi-sectoral actions and the empowerment of citizens. It also provides the framework to achieve the ideal of universal health coverage as it may prevent disease, promote health, reduce growth in costs and inequality, if the core primary health care principles (outlined as first contact, continuous, comprehensive and coordinated care) are translated into practice [11]. In terms of public health crises, it was found that countries that offer either universal medical care or universal health insurance systems ensured a better response to the disastrous effect of the pandemic on the most at-risk populations [12]. However, the provision of PCH and the achievement of the SDGs may be impeded by inadequate government spending on health, the shortage and maldistribution of the health workforce and an inadequate multi-sectoral health workforce [13,14].

School health services may be provided by health professionals and allied professionals either employed in local centers of the primary health care system or other public health units. SHS have the potential to address health inequalities for vulnerable children in deprived regions and lower socioeconomic strata and provide in situ health services and effective interventions fulfilling the goals of disease prevention and health promotion. However, as a recent large-scale study documented though a comparative study of 30 European countries, substantial disparities exist between countries as to the provision of services and most of the countries under consideration report a shortage in school health professionals, whilst training in school health is deficient [15].

School health education is aligned with SHS in that it constitutes the essentially pedagogical tenet of public health traced basically in school setting. SHE may adopt the values of neoliberal public health policies representing public health crises as unique and accidental, concurrently emphasizing individual responsibility, and adopting a victim-blaming perspective [16]. A new curriculum needs to be devised based on the ideals of democracy, social justice and solidarity and adopting a whole-school, bottom-up, pupil-centered and collaborative methodology. A paradigm shift from the individualistic and victim-blaming conception of health which is a product of the neoliberal ideas' dominance [17] will take seriously into account the lessons derived from this unprecedented health crisis which exacerbated social inequalities.

The pandemic health crisis is arguably not isolated from the wider crises of the capitalist system since the root causes of the pandemic include such things as "capitalist agriculture, its destruction of natural habitat, and the industrial production of meat" [18] (p. 55). School health education is founded on the principles of equality and equity, and incorporating also an ecological dimension will serve this purpose. For instance, it is suggested that the health promotion agenda should be reframed, based on three aspects: (a) planetary issues, (b) governance and (c) civil society and social change [19]. Similarly, the "5 Ps model" of global health education, which refers to parity, people, planet, priorities and practices, where parity stands for health equity, may be taken as an example of how the new health promotion agendas, imbued with humanitarian values, may expand to planetary issues, viewing individual and community health as inseparable from climate change [20].

It is evident from the above that in the post-pandemic world the new vision of public health services with emphasis on youth should not be viewed in isolation from the persistent and overlapping capitalist crises and the dismantling effects of neoliberal policies against state capabilities in favor of the markets. Quite the contrary, we argue that health inequalities, especially the exacerbated vulnerabilities of young people, may be alleviated if a radical and substantive change is planned and implemented in the post-pandemic world. This change needs to take the social determinants discourse seriously but also to include several aspects, such as the economy, the environment, social protection labor markets, education and skills formation as a public good, and an international obligation is proposed.

2. The Context of This Study

School health and health education constitute distinct responsibilities between two public executive bodies, the Hellenic Ministry of Health, and the Ministry of Education. This creates space for dichotomy, disintegration and lack of coordination, which therefore may lead to an expansion of unmet health needs, an indicator that signals social inequalities in health and in which Greece lags behind significantly [21]. Second, Greece has suffered the effects of a prolonged and severe economic crisis for nearly a decade (2009–2018) which was then succeeded by the multitude of capitalist crises provoked by the pandemic of COVID-19, which also impact on the supply of the health system and the educational system.

First, school health and health education, as interlinked fields of theory and practice, constitute a shared institutional responsibility between, respectively, the Ministry of Health (MoH) and the Ministry of Education (MoE). The MoH is responsible for delivering health services and health education programs in the school setting, whereas the MoE is accountable for educational policies that will encompass elements of health education. To date, there is no legislation or memorandum of understanding between the two executive bodies towards a common framework of policy planning. Within this framework, the health policy, represented by school health services, and the educational policy, represented by school health education, are deficient in respect of: (a) a common understanding of what children's and adolescents' health entails conceptually and how health needs may be met methodologically and (b) a concrete partnership and coordination mechanism between MoH and MoE to translate theory into practice [22].

Second, school health services are offered by Local Primary Care Units (TOMY) for urban regions units according to the legislative framework (law 4486/2017) that sought to reform and reinforce Primary Health Care (PHC). However, in practical terms, this is rarely the case due to TOMYs' limited capacity due to the prolonged period of austerity measures and neoliberal policies. Moreover, PHC services have been for long devalued as the health care system has been strongly hospital-oriented [10] and it has been characterized by lack of integration, fragmentation, shortcomings in efficiency and inequalities in access [23,24]. However, access to PHC through a multidisciplinary team was intended to ensure universal coverage [13]. The legal framework was enacted within months of the announcement. However, it encountered severe problems such as the significantly low availability of general practitioners and pediatricians, who resisted the idea of working exclusively for PHC [14], while it also met the undermining critique of organized economic interests and the neoliberal political party of New Democracy which was profoundly against the idea of expanding the social state. Under the circumstances, from 2017 to 2019 just over 100 TOMY have been initiated and become fully operational. From 2019, when the neoliberal government of New Democracy came to power, until now only six new TOMY were launched.

Third, although the significance of school nursing is recognized by school actors in Greece, the professionals are restricted to the daily, scheduled care of children and adolescents with special needs and emergency care, as a systematic review of relative legislative data through a span of three decades (1982–2011) reveals [25]. Although a decade has passed since the above review, little if any progress has been achieved and equally little evidence has been generated in the field. As confirmed in a recent work, school nurses are typically employed in special education schools at the request of parents of children with special healthcare needs after a relevant medical diagnosis has been issued by a public hospital doctor [26]. Given the above, two conclusions are extracted: (a) the duties of school nurses have not been expanded to cover the health needs of the total school population and (b) school nurse presence in schools remains sporadic and limited to the needs of children with special needs.

Fourth, school heath education as a subject is delivered within the context of the Greek educational system, basically in primary and secondary education, on a non-compulsory and voluntary basis. As a field of knowledge, within applied educational practice, it may adopt two distinct forms of curricula implementation: either as a cross-thematic subject within the compulsory timetable or as an extracurricular school activity, outside teaching hours. However, the constant modifications in its pedagogical methods and its place in the school curricula led to further marginalization of health education in schools [16,22].

Fifth, and in relation to the wider sociopolitical context, it is important to emphasize that health services and the public educational system, as facets of the social welfare state, suffered the effects a of a decade (2009–2018) of harsh austerity measures imposed by Greek governments in return loans from the International Monetary Fund, the European Union and the European Central Bank (widely acknowledged as the "Troika") following a debt crisis, which contributed to the deregulation and deterioration of labor, standards of living and the welfare system. The prolonged financial crisis and the imposition of austerity measures resulted in a reduction in health expenditures, the widening inequalities in access and downgrade of the quality of services [27].

Taking a critical public health and critical pedagogy point of view, we aim to produce a radical policy proposal informed by the principles of equality, equity, democracy, inclusion and grassroots participation decisions, following an ecological model framework which advocates embracing ecological approaches, political economic theory and critical pedagogy [28], and arguing against the de-politicization of public health [29]. At the heart of this theoretical model lies empowerment education which ensures community participation and dialogue at a personal level but also in social arenas to reinforce the individuals' and communities' ability to gain control over their own health.

3. Research Methods

This scoping review aimed to explore and systematically map the school health services and school health education curriculum in Greek primary, secondary and higher education, seeking to identify key problems, drawbacks and disadvantages in policy implementation. The objective, therefore, of this work was to locate certain gaps in the current literature and legislation as for the above-mentioned fields of action and then to highlight the gaps that need to be covered by policymaking, adopting a problem-solving perspective. This purpose is served by synthesizing the evidence thematically. The search strategy utilized the following categories: school health services, school health education curricula, school nursing, integration and critical pedagogy, all with reference exclusively to Greece, since this country is taken as a case study. The search followed two stages, one search with English and one with Greek key-terms. Irrespectively of the language employed, the terms remained identical, i.e., "health education & Greece" "school health & Greece", "school health services & Greece", "school health education & Greece", "health programs & school & Greece", "health interventions & school & Greece", etc.

3.1. Research Questions

The following research questions provided the framework of this scoping review:
1. To what extent and how school health services are offered in Greek primary and secondary education?
2. To what extent and how school education is included in the curricula of Greek primary and secondary education?
3. To what extent is health education included in the medical schools' curricula?
4. To what extent and how is school nursing included in schools?

3.2. Inclusion and Exclusion Criteria

A set of inclusion criteria was utilized from the outset of this work in order to exclude a multitude of irrelevant findings.

First, as this review aimed to trace evolution in policies, documents that focused merely on experiments, interventions and randomized-control trials were excluded.

Second, the time of the accumulated documents covered a period of two decades, i.e., from 2003 to 2023, thus allowing enough space to observe the evolution of the two fields of knowledge and action (i.e., school health services and school health curricula in primary and secondary education), whilst as for the syllabuses of the medical schools we scrutinized only the current ones (i.e., 2023). Hence, documents before 2003 have been excluded.

Third, the spectrum of the genres of the collected documents ranged from publications in journals (original research, reviews or editorials), syllabuses of medical schools, doctoral theses, conference proceedings and policy texts extracted from the official websites of the MoH and MoE, whilst publications in mass media or other sources were excluded.

Fourth, relevant data extracted from the corpus of documents by locating key terms in them were then classified into the above categories, thus building a narrative synthesis. For instance, the data had to be necessarily relevant to Greece, as this was the case studied.

3.3. Findings

During the first round of our scoping review, 282 documents were initially identified by searching the above-mentioned databases that fit the set of specific inclusion criteria. Subsequently, the duplicates were removed and the titles and abstracts of 202 have been scrutinized for further consideration. Out of 202 documents screened, six have not been accessible in full text and have consequently been excluded as well as 12 more documents due to the exclusion criteria above. During the second round, 184 full text records were assessed for eligibility, excluding 22 documents that did not meet all of the inclusion criteria. The third round ended up with 162 documents that have been finally included in this scoping review, consisting of seven doctoral theses, 14 legislative texts, 27 conference proceeding, 107 publications in peer reviewed journals and seven syllabuses of tertiary education. From the 162 documents, only 17 correspond to the set of research questions.

In what follows (Table 1) a detailed process of search in databases is depicted. All the following search terms included also "Greece" or "Greek" to limit the data to our case study.

Table 1. Scoping Review Selection Process.

Key Concepts	Search Terms	Time Span	Genres
School health	Health services primary school Health services secondary education Health services preschool education TOMY Health Centers Primary Healthcare Service	2003–2023	Academic publications Legislation
School health education	Health education primary school Health education secondary school School health education	2003–2023	Academic publications Legislation
Health Education	Health education Health literacy	2023	Syllabuses of Medical Schools

3.4. The CriSHEP Plan

This article attempts to fill in this gap by presenting an innovative radical integrated policy plan bringing together school health services with health education curricula embedded in critical public health and critical pedagogy. The fundamental axes of a Critical School Health and Education Policy (CriSHEP) is presented below (Figure 1).

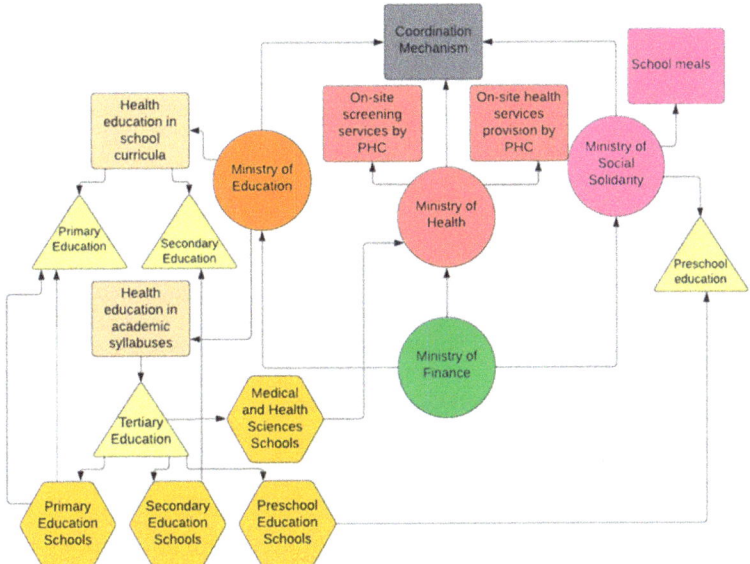

Figure 1. Critical School Health and Education Policy (CriSHEP).

- On-site provision of health services at school, adopting the settings approach of health promotion, will be organized and implemented by the PPH units in deprived urban areas, giving priority to pupils from lower social strata and disadvantaged regions;
- The on-site provision of health services includes early detection, treatment and monitoring of health problems of children and adolescents, covering almost the entire age range of the minor population. Organization of medical and school nursing services, which will provide on-site screening tests to check: (a) visual acuity and color blindness, (b) oral hygiene, (c) diseases of the spine (e.g., scoliosis), (d) vaccination coverage and infectious diseases, (e) development (body measurements—weight, height, head circumference), (f) checking vaccination coverage, (g) carrying out Mantoux tuberculosis reactions, (h) carrying out vaccinations;
- Design of school health education curricula based on the principles of critical pedagogy, oriented to equality, social justice and solidarity, and aiming to re-conceptualize health as a social good and not an individual responsibility. In this frame, the whole-school approach is adopted in order to engage the entire school community, i.e., students, parents, teachers at all levels of basic education (preschool education, primary education, secondary education), thus enhancing participation towards an ecological model;
- Ensuring provision of school meals to all primary schools of the country and including special school meals for pupils with special nutritional needs;
- Pre-service teachers' education: Rejuvenation of health education curricula in primary and preschool education departments of tertiary education based on critical pedagogy;
- Pre-service medical doctors' education: Rejuvenation of health education curricula in medical schools of tertiary education based on critical pedagogy.

4. Discussion

In summary, this article reviewed the evolution of school health services and health education curricula in Greece over a span of two decades, aiming to produce thereafter am integrated and radical policy plan, based on a vision of certain principles and theoretically underpinned by critical public health and critical pedagogy paradigms.

First, it is found that school health services are rarely based in a permanent and sustainable mode in a school setting, and they are rarely accessible for the whole school population. In contrast, SHS constitute a non-compulsory duty of PHC and as such operate in a sporadic and fragmented mode in primary and secondary education delivered basically by school nurses recruited for children with special condition.

Second, it is observed that the vast majority (reaching 75%) of the studies under consideration in terms of the scoping review focus on single interventions or health-related topics, disregarding the contextual factors that impede or promote the enactment of curricula. The political context of the policies implemented in practice is dismissed from studies exploring or surveying SHS and SHE, arguably because of the allegedly neutral public-health domain [29].

Third, SHE as a subject does not retain a permanent position in school curricula; it has operated as an extracurricular and cross-curricular activity [30,31]. Moreover, SHE operates under the medical hegemony retaining a bio-medical and individualistic character focusing on personal health and disease prevention [16], whereas schoolteachers lack training, experience and leadership from the health education officers [32]. In addition, the optional character of SHE in the school curricula is identified as a barrier to its implementation [31]. In respect to school nursing, it is restricted to the daily, scheduled care of children and adolescents with special needs and emergency care. Finally, it is noted that none of the seven medical schools in Greece have health education as an autonomous module, although several relevant subjects, such as public health and preventive medicine, include elements of health education and health literacy [25,26].

In line with a recent large observational study conducted in 30 EU countries, this review emphasizes the need to adapt to the contemporary and perplexed health priorities of pupils and extend SHS beyond traditional screening or vaccination procedures [15]. The two distinctive executive bodies of Ministry of Health and Ministry of Education need to establish a sustainable collaboration aiming to integrate SHS with SHE into a robust health and education policy which will protect and foster the real needs of the new generation in the post pandemic world.

The lack of school-based health services in conjunction with the absence of a primary healthcare system, at least recently, increases pupils' unmet health needs, especially for those from lower social strata. By contrast the development of a concrete and comprehensive integrated system of school health is expected to fill in the gaps. From this perspective, based upon the deficiencies identified in this review, we devised and propose the Critical School Health and Education Policy (CriSHEP).

The CriSHEP is embedded in critical public health and critical pedagogy paradigms, in that it interrogates the current status, it views public health as political endeavor and not a neutral field of science and it seeks to bring social justice and solidarity. Within this framework, it is anticipated that the universal health coverage, initiated in the major reform of PHC in 2018, will be expanded and deepened through the reform of school health services and unmet health needs, as exemplified in the OECD's (2021) "Health at a glance" edition [21], signaling that inequalities in access to health services due to structural and economic barriers will be reduced.

5. Conclusions

The imperative for the post-pandemic world and future generations is to revisit and reinvent public health policies that apply in the school setting. The two cardinal components of what constitutes school health, that is health services on the one hand and health education on the other, need to be integrated. However, the new vision of public health policies needs to address the disastrous effects of the humanitarian crisis and the lessons stemming from this. In this light, the problem-solving perspective that produces evidence towards a new egalitarian and integrated perspective in school health and health education is at stake at a time of crises.

Author Contributions: Conceptualization P.S. and S.V.; Methodology P.S. and P.G.B.; Original draft preparation P.S.; Writing, review and editing S.V. and P.G.B.; Supervision P.G.B. All authors have read and agreed to the published version of the manuscript.

Funding: This research received no external funding.

Institutional Review Board Statement: Not applicable.

Informed Consent Statement: Not applicable.

Data Availability Statement: Not applicable.

Acknowledgments: The authors would like to thank the anonymous reviewers and the associate editor whose valuable comments helped in improving the quality of the manuscript.

Conflicts of Interest: The authors declare no conflict of interest.

References

1. Marmot, M.; Allen, J. COVID-19: Exposing and amplifying inequalities. *J. Epidemiol. Community Health* **2020**, *74*, 681–682. [CrossRef] [PubMed]
2. Mishra, V.; Seyedzenouzi, G.; Almohtadi, A.; Chowdhury, T.; Khashkhusha, A.; Axiaq, A.; Wong, W.Y.E.; Harky, A. Health Inequalities During COVID-19 and Their Effects on Morbidity and Mortality. *J. Healthc. Leadersh.* **2021**, *13*, 19–26. [CrossRef]
3. Cheater, S. Health inequalities—COVID-19 will widen the gap. *Int. J. Health Promot. Educ.* **2020**, *58*, 223–225. [CrossRef]
4. McGowan, V.J.; Bambra, C. COVID-19 mortality and deprivation: Pandemic, syndemic, and endemic health inequalities. *Lancet Public Health* **2022**, *7*, e966–e975. [CrossRef]
5. Sacco, P.L.; De Domenico, M. Public health challenges and opportunities after COVID-19. *Bull. World Health Organ.* **2021**, *99*, 529–535. [CrossRef] [PubMed]
6. Bashier, H.; Ikram, A.; Khan, M.A.; Baig, M.; Al Gunaid, M.; Al Nsour, M.; Khader, Y. The Anticipated Future of Public Health Services Post COVID-19: Viewpoint. *JMIR Public Health Surveill.* **2021**, *7*, e26267. [CrossRef]
7. Brownson, R.C.; Burke, T.A.; Colditz, G.A.; Samet, J.M. Reimagining Public Health in the Aftermath of a Pandemic. *Am. J. Public Health* **2020**, *110*, 1605–1610. [CrossRef]
8. United Nations. Convention on the Rights of the Child. In *United Nations Treaty Series*; United Nations: New York, NY, USA, 1989.
9. United Nations. *The 2030 Agenda for Sustainable Development*; United Nations: New York, NY, USA, 2015.
10. Bhutta, Z.A.; Boerma, T.; Black, M.M.; Victora, C.G.; Kruk, M.E.; Black, R.E. Optimising child and adolescent health and development in the post-pandemic world. *Lancet* **2022**, *399*, 1759–1761. [CrossRef]
11. Pettigrew, L.M.; De Maeseneer, J.; Anderson, M.I.P.; Essuman, A.; Kidd, M.R.; Haines, A. Primary health care and the Sustainable Development Goals. *Lancet* **2015**, *386*, 2119–2121. [CrossRef]
12. Navarro, V. The Consequences of Neoliberalism in the Current Pandemic. *Int. J. Health Serv.* **2020**, *50*, 271–275. [CrossRef]
13. Myloneros, T.; Sakellariou, D. The effectiveness of primary health care reforms in Greece towards achieving universal health coverage: A scoping review. *BMC Health Ser. Res.* **2021**, *21*, 628–632. [CrossRef] [PubMed]
14. Lionis, C.; Symvoulakis, E.K.; Markaki, A.; Petelos, E.; Papadakis, S.; Sifaki-Pistolla, D.; Papadakakis, M.; Souliotis, K.; Tziraki, C. Integrated people-centred primary health care in Greece: Unravelling Ariadne's thread. *Prim. Health Care Res. Dev.* **2019**, *20*, e113. [CrossRef] [PubMed]
15. Michaud, P.A.; Vervoort, J.P.M.; Visser, A.; Baltag, V.; Reijneveld, S.A.; Kocken, P.L.; Jansen, D. Organization and activities of school health services among EU countries. *Eur. J. Public Health* **2021**, *31*, 502–508. [CrossRef]
16. Soultatou, P.; Duncan, P.; Athanasiou, K.; Papadopoulos, I. Health needs: Policy plan and school practice in Greece. *Health Edu.* **2011**, *111*, 266–282. [CrossRef]
17. Cardona, B. The pitfalls of personalization rhetoric in time of health crisis: COVID-19 pandemic and cracks on neoliberal ideologies. *Health Prom. Int.* **2020**, *36*, 714–721. [CrossRef]
18. Waitzkin, H. Confronting the Upstream Causes of COVID-19 and Other Epidemics to Follow. *Int. J. Health Serv.* **2020**, *51*, 55–58. [CrossRef]
19. Baum, F. How can health promotion contribute to pulling humans back from the brink of disaster? *Global Health Prom.* **2021**, *28*, 4. [CrossRef]
20. Jacobsen, K.H.; Waggett, C.E. Global health education for the post-pandemic years: Parity, people, planet, priorities, and practices. *Global Health Res. Policy* **2022**, *7*, 1. [CrossRef]
21. OECD. *Health at a Glance 2021: OECD Indicators*; OECD Publishing: Paris, France, 2021. [CrossRef]

22. Soultatou, P.; Duncan, P. Exploring the reality of applied partnerships: The case of the Greek school health education curriculum. *Health Educ. J.* **2009**, *68*, 34–43. [CrossRef]
23. Economou, C.; Kaitelidou, D.; Karanikolos, M.; Maresso, A. *Greece: Health System Review, Health Systems in Transition*; World Health Organization Regional Office for Europe: Copenhagen, Denmark, 2017. Available online: https://apps.who.int/iris/handle/10665/330204 (accessed on 12 January 2023).
24. Papakosta-Gaki, E.; Zissi, A.; Smyrnakis, E. Evaluation of primary health care and improvement of the services provided. *Arch. Hell. Med.* **2022**, *39*, 439–451.
25. Siamaga, E.; Koutsouki, N.; Koulouri, A.; Lianou, I.; Karasavvidis, S. School Nurses and Their Role in Emergency Health Care at Schools in the Last Thirty Years (1982–2011) in Greece: A Systematic Review Based on Greek Legislation Data. *Int. J. Caring Sci.* **2012**, *5*, 3–12.
26. Drakopoulou, M.; Begni, P.; Mantoudi, A.; Mantzorou, M.; Gerogianni, G.; Adamakidou, T.; Alikari, V.; Kalemikerakis, I.; Kavga, A.; Plakas, S.; et al. Care and Safety of Schoolchildren with Type 1 Diabetes Mellitus: Parental Perceptions of the School Nurse Role. *Healthcare* **2022**, *10*, 1228. [CrossRef]
27. Koukiadaki, A.; Kretsos, L. Opening Pandora's Box: The Sovereign Debt Crisis and Labour Market Regulation in Greece. *Ind. Law J.* **2012**, *41*, 276–304. [CrossRef]
28. Martinson, M.; Elia, J.P. Ecological and political economy lenses for school health education: A critical pedagogy shift. *Health Educ.* **2018**, *118*, 131–143. [CrossRef]
29. Daher-Nashif, S. In sickness and in health: The politics of public health and their implications during the COVID-19 pandemic. *Sociol. Compass* **2021**, *16*, e12949. [CrossRef]
30. Soultatou, P. School Health Education in Greek secondary schools: Searching for a place in the National Curriculum. *Educ. Health* **2007**, *25*, 63–67.
31. Psarouli, S.; Mavrikaki, E.; Alexopoulos, C.; Gavriil, D.; Vantarakis, A. Implementation of Health Promotion Programmes in Schools: An Approach to Understand Knowledge, Perceptions and Barriers. *J. Community Med. Public Health* **2022**, *6*, 233. [CrossRef]
32. Cholevas, N.K.; Loucaides, C.A. Factors that facilitate and barriers towards the implementation of health educational programmes in primary education schools of the prefecture of Achaia, Greece. *Health Educ. J.* **2012**, *71*, 365–375. [CrossRef]

Disclaimer/Publisher's Note: The statements, opinions and data contained in all publications are solely those of the individual author(s) and contributor(s) and not of MDPI and/or the editor(s). MDPI and/or the editor(s) disclaim responsibility for any injury to people or property resulting from any ideas, methods, instructions or products referred to in the content.

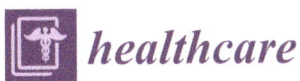

Article

Understanding the Experience of Long COVID Symptoms in Hospitalized and Non-Hospitalized Individuals: A Random, Cross-Sectional Survey Study

Jacqueline A. Krysa [1,2], Mikayla Buell [1,3], Kiran Pohar Manhas [1,3], Katharina Kovacs Burns [4,5], Maria J. Santana [3], Sidney Horlick [1,6], Kristine Russell [1], Elizabeth Papathanassoglou [1,6] and Chester Ho [1,2,*]

1. Neurosciences, Rehabilitation and Vision, Strategic Clinical Network, Alberta Health Services, Edmonton, AB T5J 3E4, Canada
2. Division of Physical Medicine and Rehabilitation, University of Alberta, Edmonton, AB T6G 2E1, Canada
3. Community Health Sciences, Cumming School of Medicine, University of Calgary, Calgary, AB T2N 1N4, Canada
4. School of Public Health, University of Alberta, Edmonton, AB T6G 1C9, Canada
5. Department of Clinical Quality Metrics, Alberta Health Services, Edmonton, AB T5J 3E4, Canada
6. Faculty of Nursing, University of Alberta, Edmonton AB T6G 1C9, Canada
* Correspondence: chester.ho@albertahealthservices.ca; Tel.: +1-780-735-8870

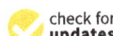

Abstract: The relationship between initial COVID-19 infection and the development of long COVID remains unclear. The purpose of this study was to compare the experience of long COVID in previously hospitalized and non-hospitalized adults in a community-based, cross-sectional telephone survey. Participants included persons with positive COVID-19 test results between 21 March 2021 and 21 October 2021 in Alberta, Canada. The survey included 330 respondents (29.1% response rate), which included 165 previously hospitalized and 165 non-hospitalized individuals. Significantly more previously hospitalized respondents self-reported long COVID symptoms (81 (49.1%)) compared to non-hospitalized respondents (42 (25.5%), $p < 0.0001$). Most respondents in both groups experienced these symptoms for more than 6 months (hospitalized: 66 (81.5%); non-hospitalized: 25 (59.5), $p = 0.06$). Hospitalized respondents with long COVID symptoms reported greater limitations on everyday activities from their symptoms compared to non-hospitalized respondents ($p < 0.0001$) and tended to experience a greater impact on returning to work (unable to return to work—hospitalized: 20 (19.1%); non-hospitalized: 6 (4.5%), $p < 0.0001$). No significant differences in self-reported long COVID symptoms were found between male and female respondents in both groups ($p > 0.05$). This study provides novel data to further support that individuals who were hospitalized for COVID-19 appear more likely to experience long COVID symptoms.

Keywords: long COVID; hospitalization; patient experience; COVID-19 recovery; COVID-19 severity and impact

Citation: Krysa, J.A.; Buell, M.; Pohar Manhas, K.; Kovacs Burns, K.; Santana, M.J.; Horlick, S.; Russell, K.; Papathanassoglou, E.; Ho, C. Understanding the Experience of Long COVID Symptoms in Hospitalized and Non-Hospitalized Individuals: A Random, Cross-Sectional Survey Study. *Healthcare* 2023, *11*, 1309. https://doi.org/10.3390/healthcare11091309

Academic Editors: Sofia Koukouli and Areti Stavropoulou

Received: 21 March 2023
Revised: 21 April 2023
Accepted: 28 April 2023
Published: 3 May 2023

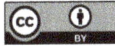

Copyright: © 2023 by the authors. Licensee MDPI, Basel, Switzerland. This article is an open access article distributed under the terms and conditions of the Creative Commons Attribution (CC BY) license (https://creativecommons.org/licenses/by/4.0/).

1. Introduction

In Canada, 4.42 million individuals have recovered from COVID-19, of which over 100,000 were hospitalized [1]. The World Health Organization defines post-COVID conditions as any new, recurring, or lingering symptoms that persist for at least 12 weeks following acute COVID-19 infection and cannot be explained by an alternative diagnosis [2]. Long COVID is a more general term used to describe new or ongoing signs and symptoms that develop after recovery from acute COVID-19 and includes ongoing symptomatic COVID-19 (4–12 weeks since initial recovery) and post-COVID conditions (12 weeks or more since initial recovery) [3]. Current estimates of long COVID prevalence vary regionally and between COVID-19 variants [4,5]. The Canadian COVID-19 Antibody and Health Survey (CCAHS-2) described the experience of long-term symptoms after a COVID-19 infection between January 2020 and August 2022 [6]. Prior to December 2021 (pre-Omicron variant), one in four persons with confirmed or suspected COVID-19 infection reported long COVID symptoms [6]. Conversely, of those that experienced COVID-19 after December 2021, about one in ten persons reported long COVID symptoms [6]. This highlights the changing severity and experience of long COVID over time.

Long COVID includes common, diverse, and varying symptomology that affect multiple organ systems, as well as functional, cognitive, and mental health outcomes [7–12]. Common long COVID symptoms include anosmia, anxiety, cognitive problems, exercise intolerance, fatigue, headaches, impaired sleep, and shortness of breath [2,12–15]. These lasting health consequences, manifesting as chronic symptoms, have been found to significantly impact physical and cognitive function, participation in daily activities, and overall quality of life [16]. The underlying pathophysiology and long-term impact of these symptoms remain largely unknown [4,5].

Considering the recency and burden of long COVID on persons recovering from COVID-19, there is increasing interest in understanding the relationship between initial COVID-19 recovery and the development of long COVID [17]. Although long COVID is frequently observed in those that experienced milder forms of acute COVID, recent evidence indicates some association between hospitalization for COVID-19 and an increased likelihood of developing long COVID [17–23]. A retrospective cohort study of 133 inpatients that tested positive for COVID-19 found that 64.7% self-reported long COVID symptoms four months after the index date (the date on which hospitalization for COVID-19 occurred) [24]. Conversely, individuals who were not hospitalized for COVID-19 appeared less likely to develop long COVID [25]. One study reviewed over 400,000 recorded COVID-19 cases in non-hospitalized adults between January 2020 and April 2021 and found that 5.4% of patients reported at least one long COVID symptom 12 weeks after the index date [25]. This evidence suggests a role for early hospitalization in the development of long COVID and has Implications for those more at risk and requiring hospitalization, including older age groups and those with underlying conditions [24,26].

Evidence on the impact of previous hospitalization for acute COVID-19 on the development of long COVID is emerging [27–29]. A 2022 systematic review and meta-analysis found that independent of hospitalization status, 45% of COVID-19 survivors experienced a diversity of unresolved symptoms after 4 months [27]. Moreover, a 2022 prospective cohort study reported that long COVID symptoms were more common in hospitalized patients compared to outpatients after 6 months (52.3% vs. 38.2%, respectively) [28]. Due to the limited availability of validated tools and lack of a unified definition of long COVID during the pandemic, most studies rely on the self-reporting of symptoms to understand the impact of long COVID [30]. Given the current limitations to identifying long COVID with lower self-selection bias and the challenges of monitoring recovery outcomes following COVID-19, more evidence is required to determine the relationship between previous hospitalization and the development and severity of long COVID. To better understand the relationship between previous hospitalization and long COVID, this study aimed to compare the patient experience of long COVID following a positive COVID-19 test in a random sample of previously hospitalized and non-hospitalized adults.

2. Materials and Methods

2.1. Study Design

In this cross-sectional, provincial, observational study, a telephone survey was administered to a random sample of persons recovering from COVID-19 to understand their experience with long COVID and navigating health services. This study was approved by the University of Alberta Research Ethics Board (Pro00113182) and complied with all relevant guidelines and regulations. All respondents consented to participate in this study. Reporting was guided by the Checklist for Reporting of Survey Studies (CROSS) (Supplemental Table S1) [31].

2.2. Study Population

Persons recovering from acute COVID-19 infection in Alberta, Canada, were recruited. Inclusion criteria were individuals aged >18 years with a laboratory-confirmed COVID-19 polymerase chain reaction (PCR) test between 21 March 2021 and 21 October 2021 and able to read and understand English (with or without the assistance of an available family member/friend). There were no explicit exclusion criteria for study respondents.

2.3. Sampling

This study aimed to recruit 300 respondents. This number was estimated to ensure representation within each stratum, the feasibility of recruitment, and to account for limited numbers of previously hospitalized, COVID-19 positive individuals. This estimated target was also selected to reduce the burden of survey fatigue and to account for the sensitivity and emotional context of COVID-19, as these factors can impact the survey response rate [29]. Professional and experienced telephone surveyors developed a proportional stratified random sampling frame based on pre-specified inclusion criteria and applied this to existing administrative databases for hospitalized and non-hospitalized individuals with a positive COVID-19 test. The sampling frame was based on hospitalization status during the study window (50% hospitalized and 50% non-hospitalized) and geographical location (60% metropolitan-urban residence and 40% regional-urban/rural residence). Alberta is a province in western Canada with five geographical zones with an overall population of 4.54 million [32]. The 2021 Census profile of Alberta reported that approximately 50% of residents were female, and the most commonly reported ethnic backgrounds included English (18.0%), German (15.0%), Scottish (14.8%), and Irish (13.2%) [33]. In Alberta, two zones, Calgary and Edmonton, represent metropolitan-urban regions, with densely populated areas exceeding 100,000 individuals. The other three zones, North, Central, and South, represent regional-urban/rural areas, with generally between 10,000 and 100,000 individuals in densely populated regions [33].

Telephone surveyors randomly selected and called eligible individuals from relevant administrative databases and would call back those that agreed or continued to call those that did not respond to the initial call for up to three-call backs, as needed. This process ensured that all randomly selected individuals had the opportunity to respond to or decline the survey. Telephone surveyors would continue to draw random samples until targeted numbers of cases and strata were achieved. Recruitment continued past the target of 300 respondents to further minimize response and non-response bias and ensure saturation of data responses.

2.4. Survey Content Development

The survey was co-designed with input from provincial stakeholders, including patient and family advisors with lived experience of long COVID, clinicians, and administrative, operational, and health system leadership. Figure 1 summarizes the process involved in the survey design. To inform the co-design process, a one-time virtual focus group was held with provincial stakeholders and patient and family advisors to determine priority concepts regarding the patient experience of navigating long COVID care to inform health service planning. Five core concepts emerged from the focus group: patient and provider knowledge, appropriateness of the information, peer and family support, accessibility of care, and appropriateness of care. These core concepts informed the development of the draft survey. Five cognitive interviews were conducted with persons with lived experience of long COVID to reduce the likelihood of item non-response error and measurement error [34,35]. Verbal probing was used throughout the cognitive interviews to explore how respondents understood and answered survey questions. The probes were used to assess concern about the content of the survey questions, survey construction, overall comprehension, and possible reactions from respondents for each question. Textual analysis of interview notes allowed for comparison of responses across respondents for each item. These interviews led to changes in survey content, formatting, and layout to determine the final version of the survey. An additional literacy/language correction to grade 5/6 level was completed. The final survey and results of the survey were shared with participating patient and family advisors by email and presentation. The final survey was designed for online or phone delivery, consisting of 33 questions (including 6 demographic questions) (see Supplemental File S2). Survey items included closed, multiple-response, and open-ended questions. Survey questions probed to better understand the experience or lack of experience of prolonged symptoms after COVID-19 recovery, as well as the impact of long COVID symptoms on daily activities and return to work. In order to identify those with long COVID symptoms, respondents were asked whether they were experiencing 'any new or lasting/ongoing symptoms after recovery from COVID-19'. This wording was recommended to avoid confusion about the definition of long COVID by respondents. Prior to the start of the survey, telephone surveyors overviewed the definition of long COVID to ensure participants could differentiate between the experience of COVID-19 recovery and long COVID. Additional questions (not discussed in the present manuscript) included general and specific experiences regarding health system navigation, as well as open-ended questions on perceived challenges, positive experiences, and improvement suggestions.

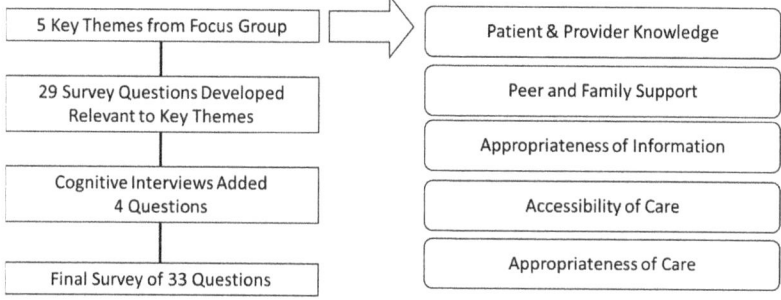

Figure 1. Item Selection in the Development of a Long COVID Patient Experience Survey.

2.5. Recruitment and Data Collection

Eligible hospitalized and non-hospitalized COVID-19 respondents were identified through Alberta Health Services' administrative COVID-19 databases between April and June 2022. Potential respondents within the hospitalized and non-hospitalized databases were randomized and recruited by health system-employed, professionally trained telephone surveyors [36]. Surveyors provided a brief study introduction and outlined participation requirements over the telephone. Those that agreed to participate provided verbal consent. Survey questions were read to the study respondents by the telephone surveyors, who then recorded their responses. Survey responses were recorded and stored in VOXCO, a secured and private survey software (VOXCO Survey Software, Montréal, QC, Canada, 2022). Only select telephone surveyors had access to VOXCO to prevent unauthorized access. Recruitment continued until stratification and a minimum sample size of at least 150 hospitalized and 150 non-hospitalized individuals was reached.

2.6. Data Analysis

Survey data were de-identified and cleaned for analysis by telephone surveyors before analysis by the research team. SPSS (IBM SPSS Statistics 25, New York, NY, United States) was used to analyze data. Descriptive statistics were used to describe and summarize the results. Comparisons of proportions between groups (including hospitalization status, gender, and geographical location) were examined using Pearson's Chi-square test of independence. Independent comparisons were conducted between self-identified ethnicity as respondents were invited to select multiple options. Missing data (either due to omitted answers or 'not applicable' answers) is reported for all variables and was adjusted for in the analysis. Statistical significance was set at $p < 0.05$.

3. Results

3.1. Response Rate and Respondent Demographics

A total of 1131 persons were invited to participate in the survey. Telephone surveyors contacted 514 previously hospitalized individuals that were randomly selected from a larger pool of 4728 eligible participants. Of these, 222 were disqualified, 112 refused to participate, 15 had indeterminant responses, and 165 completed the survey (59.6% response rate). Out of 112,449 eligible non-hospitalized participants, 617 were randomly selected. Of these, 305 were disqualified, 6 had indeterminant responses, 141 refused to participate, and 165 completed the telephone survey (53.92%). In total, the survey had 330 respondents (Figure 2). The telephone survey took between 7 and 64 min (median 10 min) to complete. Table 1 reports the demographics of the 330 survey respondents. Per pre-defined sampling strata, 50% of the COVID-19 positive respondents experienced hospitalization due to COVID-19 and 60% of respondents in both groups lived in a metropolitan-urban residence. Hospitalized respondents reported significantly different age groups than non-hospitalized respondents, with more respondents being in older age groups ($p < 0.0001$). 72 (43.6%) previously hospitalized respondents and 73 (44.2%) non-hospitalized) identified as female ($p = 0.99$). Significantly more non-hospitalized respondents self-identified as Caucasian (106 (63.5%) compared to previously hospitalized respondents (124 (75.9%), $p = 0.03$). Employment status prior to a positive diagnosis of COVID-19 was significantly different between groups ($p < 0.0001$), with more than 74 (44.8%) of the previously hospitalized and 100 (60.6%) of the non-hospitalized respondents self-reported full-time employment status.

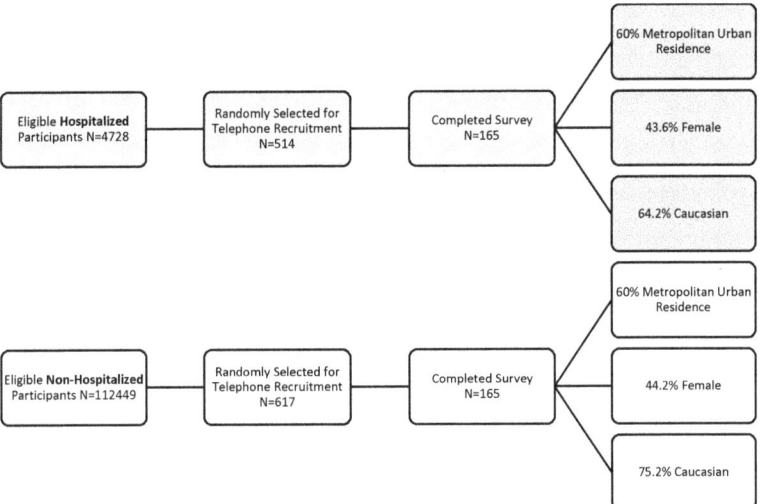

Figure 2. Survey Response Rate.

Table 1. Survey Respondent Demographics by Hospitalization Status.

Item	Hospitalized (n = 165)	Non-Hospitalized (n = 165)	p Value χ^2
Age Group (Years)			
18–24	0 (0.0%)	16 (9.7%)	
25–40	23 (13.9%)	61 (37.0%)	
41–55	43 (26.1%)	53 (32.1%)	<0.0001
56–65	45 (27.3%)	19 (11.5%)	
66–75	42 (25.5%)	9 (5.5%)	
>75	12 (7.3%)	6 (3.6%)	
Refused	-	1 (0.6%)	

Table 1. Cont.

Item	Hospitalized (n = 165)	Non-Hospitalized (n = 165)	p Value χ^2
Female Gender	72 (43.6%)	73 (44.2%)	0.99
Metropolitan-Urban Residence.	99 (60%)	99 (60%)	1.00
Racial/Ethnic Groups *			
Arab	5 (3.0%)	1 (0.6%)	0.10
Black	4 (2.4%)	5 (3.0%)	0.74
Caucasian	106 (63.5%)	124 (75.9%)	0.03
Chinese	2 (1.2%)	3 (1.8%)	0.65
Filipino	11 (6.6%)	8 (4.8%)	0.48
Indigenous	8 (4.8%)	6 (3.5%)	0.56
Latin American	4 (2.4%)	4 (2.4%)	1.00
South Asian	7 (4.2%)	9 (5.3%)	0.61
Southeast Asian	3 (1.8%)	2 (1.2%)	0.65
West Asian	1 (0.6%)	0 (0.0%)	0.32
Other	16 (9.6%)	8 (4.7%)	0.09
Hospital Length of Stay (Days (mean, SD))	9.4 (12.6)	N/A	N/A
What was your employment status before you were infected by COVID-19?			
Full-Time	74 (44.8%)	100 (60.6%)	
Part-Time	7 (4.2%)	13 (7.9%)	
Casual	3 (1.8%)	4 (2.4%)	<0.0001
Student	2 (1.2%)	7 (4.2%)	
Not Employed	16 (9.7%)	15 (9.1%)	
Retired	44 (26.7%)	16 (9.7%)	
Other	19 (11.5%)	10 (6.1%)	

* Participants were invited to select multiple options as appropriate to their racial/ethnic identity.

3.2. Self-Reported Post-COVID Symptoms by Hospitalization Status

Almost half of the previously hospitalized respondents self-reported long COVID symptoms following a positive diagnosis of COVID-19 (81 (49.1%)). This was significantly greater compared to self-reported symptoms by non-hospitalized respondents (42 (25.5%), $p < 0.0001$) (Table 2). Most respondents in both groups self-reported long COVID symptoms lasting for longer than 6 months (hospitalized 66 (81.5%); non-hospitalized 25 (59.5%), $p = 0.06$)). Previously hospitalized respondents reported significant impairment from their long COVID symptoms on their everyday activities (24 (29.6%)) compared to non-hospitalized respondents (1 (2.4%), $p < 0.0001$). Of the individuals that reported full-time working status prior to COVID-19, significantly more non-hospitalized respondents (115 (85.8%)) were able to return to this work after recovery compared to previously hospitalized respondents (65 (61.9%, $p < 0.0001$) (Table 2).

Table 2. Self-Reported Long COVID Symptoms by Hospitalization Status.

Item	Hospitalized (n = 165)	Non-Hospitalized (n = 165)	p Value χ^2
Are you having new or lasting/ongoing symptoms (e.g., physical, cognitive, emotional, etc.) since you first tested positive for COVID-19?			
Yes	81 (49.1%)	42 (25.5%)	<0.0001
No	78 (47.3%)	118 (71.5%)	
Do Not Know	6 (3.6%)	5 (3.0%)	

Table 2. Cont.

Item	Hospitalized (n = 165)	Non-Hospitalized (n = 165)	p Value χ²
How long have you been experiencing these symptoms?			
<1 Month	4 (4.9%)	3 (7.1%)	
1–3 Months	2 (2.5%)	2 (4.8%)	0.06
3–6 Months	8 (9.9%)	12 (28.6%)	
>6 Months	66 (81.5%)	25 (59.5%)	
Do Not Know	1 (0.6%)	-	
Since your experience of long-COVID, have you been able to return to your previous employment status?			
Yes	65 (61.9%)	115 (85.8%)	
Partially	15 (14.3%)	6 (4.5%)	<0.0001
No	20 (19.1%)	6 (4.5%)	
Other	3 (2.9%)	5 (3.7%)	
Please select the choice that best describes how your symptoms could have had an impact on your usual, everyday activities.			
My Usual, Everyday Activities are Not Impacted by My Symptoms.	10 (12.3%)	17 (41.5%)	
I Can Perform Most of my Usual Activities.	8 (9.9%)	8 (19.5%)	
I Sometimes Need to Stop or Cut Down on My Usual Activities.	23 (12.3%)	12 (29.3%)	<0.0001
I Often Need to Stop or Cut Down My Usual Activities.	10 (12.3%)	3 (7.3%)	
I Suffer from Limitations in My Everyday Life and Am Not Able to Perform My Usual Activities.	24 (29.6%)	1 (2.4%)	
Do Not Know	6 (3.6%)	1 (0.6%)	

3.3. Self-Reported Long COVID by Gender

Table 3 reports a comparison of self-reported long COVID symptoms by gender and hospitalization status. No significant differences were observed in self-reported long COVID symptoms between male and female respondents in hospitalized (males 42 (45.6%); females: 39 (52.2%), $p = 0.34$)) and non-hospitalized groups (males 18 (19.7%); females 23 (31.0%), $p = 0.10$). Significantly fewer female respondents were able to return to their previous level of employment since their experience of long COVID (males 43 (46.7%), females 21 (29.1%)). No significant differences in returning to work were observed between males and females in the non-hospitalized groups (males 66 (72.5%), females 48 (65.7%), $p = 0.91$). Comparable duration of symptoms and impact of symptoms on daily activities were reported between genders in both groups ($p > 0.05$).

Table 3. Self-Reported Long COVID Symptoms by Gender and Hospitalization Status.

Item	Hospitalized (n = 164)		p Value χ²	Non-Hospitalized (n = 164)		p Value χ²
	Male (n = 92)	Female (n = 72)		Male (n = 91)	Female (n = 73)	
Age Group (Years)						
18–55	40 (43.4%)	26 (36.1%)	0.42	72 (79.1%)	58 (79.5%)	0.85
56–Greater than 75	52 (56.5%)	46 (63.9%)		19 (20.9%)	15 (20.5%)	
Are you having new or lasting/ongoing symptoms (e.g., physical, cognitive, emotional, etc.) since you first tested positive for COVID-19?						
Yes	42 (45.6%)	39 (54.2%)	0.25	18 (19.7%)	23 (31.0%)	0.10
No	50 (54.4%)	33 (45.8%)		73 (80.3%)	50 (69.0%)	

Table 3. Cont.

Item	Hospitalized (n = 164)		p Value χ^2	Non-Hospitalized (n = 164)		p Value χ^2
	Male (n = 92)	Female (n = 72)		Male (n = 91)	Female (n = 73)	
How long have you been experiencing these symptoms?						
<6 Months	8 (19.0%)	6 (15.5%)	0.25	8 (44.5%)	9 (39.1%)	0.24
>6 Months	33 (78.6%)	33 (84.6%)		10 (55.6%)	14 (60.9%)	
Do Not Know	1 (2.4%)	-		-	-	
Since your experience of post-COVID, have you been able to return to your previous employment status?						
Yes	43 (46.7%)	21 (29.1%)		66 (72.5%)	48 (65.7%)	
Partially	10 (10.9%)	5 (6.9%)	0.02	0 (0.0%)	6 (8.2%)	0.91
No	11 (12.0%)	9 (12.5%)		5 (5.5%)	1 (1.4%)	
Other	3 (3.3%)	1 (1.4%)		1 (1.0%)	4 (5.4%)	
Missing	25 (27.2%)	36 (50.0%)		19 (20.9%)	14 (19.2%)	
Please select the choice that best describes how your symptoms could have had an impact on your usual, everyday activities.						
My Usual, Everyday Activities are Not Impacted by My Symptoms.	5 (11.9%)	5 (12.8%)		12 (66.7%)	4 (17.4%)	
I Can Perform Most of my Usual Activities.	3 (7.1%)	5 (12.8%)		2 (11.1%)	6 (26.1%)	
I Sometimes Need to Stop or Cut Down on My Usual Activities.	9 (21.4%)	14 (35.9%)	0.13	2 (11.1%)	10 (43.4%)	0.49
I Often Need to Stop or Cut Down My Usual Activities.	7 (16.7%)	3 (7.7%)		2 (11.1%)	1 (4.3%)	
I Suffer from Limitations in My Everyday Life and Am Not Able to Perform My Usual Activities.	13 (31.0%)			0 (0%)	1 (4.3%)	
Do Not Know	5 (11.9%)			-	1 (4.3%)	

2 participants refused to identify a gender.

3.4. Comparison of Self-Reported Long COVID by Geographical Region

Table 4 reports on respondents from metropolitan-urban residences compared to those from regional-urban/rural residences that were or were not hospitalized for COVID-19. Comparable self-reported long COVID symptoms and the impact of symptoms on daily activities were reported between metropolitan-urban and regional-urban respondents amongst previously hospitalized and non-hospitalized groups ($p > 0.05$).

Table 4. Self-Reported Long COVID Symptoms by Geographical Region.

Item	Hospitalized (n = 165)		p Value χ²	Non-Hospitalized (n = 165)		p Value χ²
	Metropolitan-Urban (n = 99)	Regional-Urban/Rural (n = 66)		Metropolitan-Urban (n = 99)	Regional-Urban/Rural (n = 66)	
Age Group (Years)						
18–55	39 (39.4%)	26 (39.4%)	0.90	83 (83.8%)	46 (69.7%)	0.04
56 –>75	60 (60.6%)	40 (60.6%)		16 (16.2%)	19 (28.8%)	
Refused	-	-		-	1 (1.5%)	
Gender (% Female)	40 (40.4%)	30 (45.5%)	0.48	46 (46.5%)	27 (40.9%)	0.34
Are you having new or lasting/ongoing symptoms (e.g., physical, cognitive, emotional, etc.) since you first tested positive for COVID-19?			0.25			0.23
Yes	45 (45.4%)	36 (54.5%)		25 (25.2%)	18 (27.3%)	
No	54 (54.5%)	30 (45.4%)		74 (74.7%)	48 (72.7%)	

4. Discussion

The COVID-19 recovery trajectory and experience of long COVID symptoms remain unclear [37]. In this present study, we investigated the experience of COVID-19 recovery in a random sample of individuals that tested positive for COVID-19 between the 21 March 2021 and the 21 October 2021. Our results found that individuals previously hospitalized for COVID-19 were more likely to self-report long COVID symptoms and experienced a greater duration and severity of symptoms compared to those that had not been hospitalized. Due to the recency and emerging evidence on underlying risks and outcomes of long COVID, this study contributes to rigorous, generalizable knowledge to advance our understanding of long COVID in the general population.

Our findings align with the recent Canadian CCAHS-2 survey, which found that respondents with more mild, initial COVID-19 symptoms reported fewer longer-term symptoms than those that reported moderate symptoms (6.3% versus 15%, respectively) [6]. More severe acute COVID-19 infection has been identified as a significant risk factor for developing long COVID [6,23,38,39]. A 2021 systematic review of ten international cohort studies revealed that individuals with milder acute COVID-19 experienced a faster estimated recovery (median duration of symptoms: 3.99 months (interquartile range (IQR) 3.84–4.20)) compared to those admitted for hospitalization for acute infection (median duration of symptoms: 8.84 months (IQR 8.10–9.78)) [38]. Additional findings from this systematic review found that 15.1% (IQR 10.3–21.1) of respondents continue to experience long COVID symptoms after one year [38]. The present study adds and strengthens these findings by directly comparing the experience of long COVID in previously hospitalized and non-hospitalized respondents and further emphasizes the relationship between the severity of acute COVID-19 symptoms and the development of long COVID symptoms.

Further analysis of our survey findings revealed comparable self-reported long COVID, duration of symptoms, and impact of symptoms on daily activities between male and female respondents. This contrasts with recent findings from the Canadian CCAHS-2 survey, which demonstrated a higher percentage of women experiencing long COVID symptoms compared with men (18.0% versus 11.6%, respectively) [6]. A recent study explored risk factors associated with long COVID in over 480,000 COVID positive adults, finding that the female sex was a significant risk factor for developing long COVID (adjusted Hazard Ratio 1.52 95% CI 1.48–1.56) [25]. The lack of significant difference in long COVID symptoms between males and females in this study may be due to the approach for self-reporting long COVID symptoms.

Common long COVID symptoms, such as fatigue, dyspnea, muscle weakness, and mood disturbances, can significantly impact an individual's ability to perform activities of daily living (ADLs) [40]. ADLs describe the collective, fundamental skills necessary to independently care for oneself (e.g., mobility, eating, and bathing) [41,42]. The Canadian CCAHS-2 survey revealed that 21.3% of adults with self-reported PCC symptoms experienced limits in their daily activities [6]. In a systematic review (n = 9 articles), ADL performance significantly declined following COVID-19 infection [40]. Similarly, 7.9% of respondents from a longitudinal prospective cohort of adults with laboratory-confirmed COVID-19 reported negative impacts to at least one ADL up to 9 months after their acute infection [43]. In this present study, a survey item modified from the post-COVID functional scale (PCFS) was used to assess the impact of long COVID symptoms on function and ADLs [44]. The PCFS is an ordinal tool designed to measure and track functional outcomes, focusing on changes in ADLs following COVID-19 [44]. PCFS scoring ranges from grade 0–4, where grade 0 reflects the absence of functional limitations and grade 4 reflects severe functional limitations requiring assistance with ADLs [44]. Our survey revealed that almost one-third of previously hospitalized respondents with self-reported PCC symptoms reported severe limitations to their everyday activities (comparable to PCFS grade 4), compared to very few (2%) of non-hospitalized respondents with self-reported long COVID. A cross-sectional study of over 100 patients recovering from COVID-19 identified that more than half (56.6%) of respondents reported no functional limitations (PCFS grade 0), while 43.4% of respondents indicated some degree of functional limitations (grade 1 to 4) [45]. By designing a survey item based on the PCFS, our survey was able to clarify that previous hospitalization was associated with greater severity of long COVID symptoms and impact on ADLs.

The persistence and impact of long COVID symptoms on ADLs have significant implications for returning to work [46]. Our survey results indicated that over 30% of previously hospitalized respondents and 10% of non-hospitalized respondents were unable to maintain their previous level of employment following recovery from COVID-19. Results from the Wuhan follow-up cohort study revealed that 12 months after hospitalization for COVID-19, 12% of respondents had not returned to work, and 24% of respondents were unable to return to their pre-COVID level of work [47]. Likewise, a patient-led survey of over 3700 individuals with suspected or confirmed COVID-19 reported that 45.2% had a reduced work schedule compared to pre-COVID, and 22.3% were not working at the time of the survey because of their current health condition [15]. Our study was able to report changes in employment status up to 13 months following initial infection and adds to the growing evidence of the impact of long COVID on productivity and the global workforce.

The strengths of this study include the process followed by professional, experienced telephone surveyors to support study recruitment. The random sampling approach resulted in respondent demographics that aligned closely with the population characteristics of the province of Alberta and, therefore, is a representative sample [29,30]. The survey was conducted between April 2022 and June 2022, allowing between 6 and 13 months of follow-up, which allows for a better understanding of the longer-term COVID-19 recovery trajectory. Another strength of the survey was the co-design of a novel survey tool by a multidisciplinary group of stakeholders, including patient and family advisors, refined using cognitive interviews. This allowed for an investigation of experience regarding a novel condition based on the experiences and needs of professionals caring for and persons living with long COVID. The novelty of this tool is also a limitation, as this tool has not been validated to assess long COVID symptoms and, therefore, limits comparability between subjects or studies. Additional limitations of this study included an estimated sample size and self-reporting of long COVID symptoms, which may misrepresent the true prevalence of long COVID in this sample. This study also focused on individuals that experienced COVID-19 in Waves 3 and 4 of the pandemic in Canada (between March 2021 and October 2021). Therefore, the experiences of respondents may not reflect the experiences of those who had COVID-19 prior to March 2021 or after October 2021. Recent studies have indicated that the Omicron COVID-19 variant and vaccination may have contributed to a decrease in the likelihood of developing long COVID compared to earlier variants [6,48,49]. In the present study, we did not retrieve the vaccination status of our respondents, which limited inferences about the impact of vaccination status and COVID-19 recovery. Although we were able to stratify sampling by metropolitan-urban and regional-urban/rural areas of the province, we did not have adequate numbers of COVID positive individuals, either hospitalized or non-hospitalized, to directly compare rural and urban living status. Therefore, we were not able to accurately describe all the differences we observed between groups. The present survey was also not designed to include questions regarding socioeconomic status, anthropometrics, lifestyle habits (i.e., smoking, alcohol use), or pre-existing conditions. Additional risk factors identified for long COVID include belonging to an ethnic minority group, a gradient of decreasing age, socioeconomic deprivation, smoking status, high body mass index, and presence of comorbidities [25]. Respondents in the survey were English-speaking and primarily identified as Caucasian (64% hospitalized and 75% non-hospitalized), and, therefore, the results may not be generalizable to other ethnic/racial groups. Future studies should investigate the prevalence, incidence, and experience of long COVID in other diverse populations to better understand the types of recovery services required.

5. Conclusions

The underlying pathophysiology recovery trajectory of long COVID remains unclear [38]. This study provides novel insights into the recovery from COVID-19 and the experience of long COVID by directly comparing self-reported long COVID symptoms as well as the perceived impact of symptoms on everyday activities and returning to work in previously hospitalized and non-hospitalized individuals. It also supports that individuals at greater risk of hospitalization from COVID-19 may have an increased likelihood of developing long COVID and require additional follow-up care and supports after discharge. Collectively, these findings add to the growing evidence on the existence and impact of long COVID and have implications for the development of novel care pathways and post-hospitalization follow-up to support patient recovery, returning to work, and overall quality of life.

Supplementary Materials: The following supporting information can be downloaded at: https://www.mdpi.com/article/10.3390/healthcare11091309/s1, Table S1: Checklist for Reporting of Survey Studies; File S2: Accessing Care and Services After COVID-19: A Patient Experience Survey.

Author Contributions: All authors have contributed to the manuscript in accordance with the criteria for authorship. Conceptualization, J.A.K., C.H., K.P.M., E.P., K.K.B. and S.H.; methodology, J.A.K., C.H., K.P.M., K.K.B., M.B., K.R. and M.J.S.; software, K.K.B.; validation, J.A.K., K.R., K.K.B. and K.P.M.; formal analysis, J.A.K. and M.B.; investigation, J.A.K. and M.B.; resources, C.H., E.P. and K.P.M.; data curation, J.A.K. and K.K.B.; writing—original draft preparation, J.A.K.; writing—review and editing, J.A.K., C.H., K.P.M., E.P., K.K.B., K.R., M.J.S. and S.H.; visualization, J.A.K. and M.B.; supervision, C.H., E.P. and K.P.M.; project administration, C.H.; funding acquisition, C.H. All authors have read and agreed to the published version of the manuscript.

Funding: J.A.K. was funded by the Canadian Institutes for Health Research Operating Grant, 'Emerging COVID-19 Research Gaps and Priorities Emerging COVID-19 Research Gaps and Priorities'. M.B. was funded by the Program from Undergraduate Research Experience Award. C.H. is a Canadian Institutes of Health Research Principal Investigator.

Institutional Review Board Statement: The study was conducted in accordance with the Declaration of Helsinki and approved by the University of Alberta Research Ethics Board (Pro00113182, 3 September 2021).

Informed Consent Statement: Informed consent was obtained from all subjects involved in the study.

Data Availability Statement: Data available on request due to restrictions, e.g., privacy or ethical. The data presented in this study are available on request from the corresponding author. The data are not publicly available due to participant confidentiality.

Acknowledgments: The authors would like to thank all respondents that volunteered their time to participate in this study. We further acknowledge the participation of the persons with lived experience that volunteered their time to support the co-design of the survey. We would also like to acknowledge Alberta Health Services Primary Data Support team for leading the recruitment and administration of the survey.

Conflicts of Interest: The authors declare no conflict of interest.

References

1. Canadian Institute for Health Information. COVID-19 Hospitalization and Emergency Department Statistics. Available online: https://www.cihi.ca/en/covid-19-hospitalization-and-emergency-department-statistics (accessed on 22 November 2022).
2. World Health Organization. Coronavirus disease (COVID-19): Post COVID-19 Condition. Available online: https://www.who.int/news-room/questions-and-answers/item/coronavirus-disease-(covid-19)-post-covid-19-condition (accessed on 9 March 2022).
3. National Institute for Health and Care Excellence (NICE). COVID-19 Rapid Guideline: Managing the Long Term Effects of COVID-19. Available online: https://www.nice.org.uk/guidance/ng188/resources/covid19-rapid-guideline-managing-the-longterm-effects-of-covid19-pdf-51035515742 (accessed on 22 November 2022).
4. Pavli, A.; Theodoridou, M.; Maltezou, H.C. Post-COVID Syndrome: Incidence, Clinical Spectrum, and Challenges for Primary Healthcare Professionals. *Arch. Med. Res.* **2021**, *52*, 575–581. [CrossRef] [PubMed]
5. Wiersinga, W.J.; Rhodes, A.; Cheng, A.C.; Peacock, S.J.; Prescott, H.C. Pathophysiology, Transmission, Diagnosis, and Treatment of Coronavirus Disease 2019 (COVID-19): A Review. *JAMA* **2020**, *324*, 782–793. [CrossRef] [PubMed]
6. Statistics Canada. Long-Term Symptoms in Canadian Adults Who Tested Positive for COVID-19 or Suspected an Infection, January 2020 to August 2022. Available online: https://www150.statcan.gc.ca/n1/daily-quotidien/221017/dq221017b-eng.htm (accessed on 18 October 2022).
7. Alberta Health Services Scientific Advisory Group. *Rapid Review: Rehabilitation Needs for COVID-19 Patients*; Alberta Health Services Scientific Advisory Group: Edmonton, AB, Canada, 2020. Available online: https://www.albertahealthservices.ca/assets/info/ppih/if-ppih-covid-19-sag-rehabilitation-needs-rapid-review.pdf (accessed on 13 October 2020).
8. Turner-Stokes, P.L. Rehabilitation in the wake of COVID-19—A phoenix from the ashes. *Br. Soc. Rehabil. Med.* **2020**, *1*, 1–19.
9. Demeco, A.; Marotta, N.; Barletta, M.; Pino, I.; Marinaro, C.; Petraoli, A.; Moggio, L.; Ammendolia, A. Rehabilitation of patients post-COVID-19 infection: A literature review. *J. Int. Med. Res.* **2020**, *48*, 0300060520948382. [CrossRef] [PubMed]
10. Barker-Davies, R.M.; O'Sullivan, O.; Senaratne, K.P.P.; Baker, P.; Cranley, M.; Dharm-Datta, S.; Ellis, H.; Goodall, D.; Gough, M.; Lewis, S.; et al. The Stanford Hall consensus statement for post-COVID-19 rehabilitation. *Br. J. Sports Med.* **2020**, *54*, 949–959. [CrossRef]
11. Tenforde, M.W.; Kim, S.S.; Lindsell, C.J.; Rose, E.B.; Shapiro, N.I.; Files, C.D.; Gibbs, K.W.; Erickson, H.L.; Steingrub, J.S.; Smithline, H.A.; et al. Symptom Duration and Risk Factors for Delayed Return to Usual Health Among Outpatients with COVID-19 in a Multistate Health Care Systems Network—United States, March–June 2020. *MMWR Morb. Mortal. Wkly. Rep.* **2020**, *69*, 993–998. [CrossRef]
12. Scientific Advisory Group. *COVID-19 Scientific Advisory Group Rapid Evidence Report on Chronic COVID-19 Symptoms*; Scientific Advisory Group: Calgary, AB, Canada, 2020; p. 45.
13. López-León, S.; Wegman-Ostrosky, T.; Perelman, C.; Sepulveda, R.; Rebolledo, P.A.; Cupaio, A.; Villapol, S. More than 50 Long-Term Effects of COVID-19, A Systematic Review and Meta-Analysis. *Sci. Rep.* **2021**, *11*, 16144. [CrossRef]
14. Razak, F.; Katz, G.M.; Cheung, A.M.; Herridge, M.S.; Atzema, C.L.; Born, K.B.; Chan, K.; Chien, V.; Kaplan, D.M.; Kwong, J.; et al. Understanding the Post COVID-19 Condition (Long COVID) and the Expected Burden for Ontario. Available online: https://covid19-sciencetable.ca/sciencebrief/understanding-the-post-covid-19-condition-long-covid-and-the-expected-burden-for-ontario (accessed on 14 November 2020).
15. Davis, H.E.; Assaf, G.S.; McCorkell, L.; Wei, H.; Low, R.J.; Re'em, Y.; Redfield, S.; Austin, J.P.; Akrami, A. Characterizing long COVID in an international cohort: 7 months of symptoms and their impact. *eClinicalMedicine* **2021**, *38*, 101019. [CrossRef]
16. Tabacof, L.; Tosto-Mancuso, J.; Wood, J.; Cortes, M.; Kontorovich, A.; McCarthy, D.; Rizk, D.; Rozanski, G.; Breyman, E.; Nasr, L.; et al. Post-acute COVID-19 Syndrome Negatively Impacts Physical Function, Cognitive Function, Health-Related Quality of Life, and Participation. *Am. J. Phys. Med. Rehabil.* **2021**, *101*, 48. [CrossRef]
17. National Institute for Health and Care Excellence, Practitioners RC of G, Scotland HI. *COVID-19 Rapid Guideline: Managing the Long-Term Effects of COVID-19*; NICE Guidance: London, UK, 2020; pp. 1–35.
18. Sudre, C.H.; Murray, B.; Varsavsky, T.; Graham, M.S.; Penfold, R.S.; Bowyer, R.C.; Pujol, J.C.; Klaser, K.; Antonelli, M.; Canas, L.S.; et al. Attributes and predictors of long COVID. *Nat. Med.* **2021**, *27*, 626–631. [CrossRef]

19. Carvalho-Schneider, C.; Laurent, E.; Lemaignen, A.; Neaufils, E.; Tournois-Bourbao, C.; Laribi, S.; Flament, T.; Ferreia-Maldent, N.; Bruyère, F.; Stefic, K.; et al. Follow-up of adults with noncritical COVID-19 two months after symptom onset. *Clin. Microbiol. Infect.* **2021**, *27*, 258–263. [CrossRef]
20. Galal, I.; Hussein, A.A.R.M.; Amin, M.T.; Saad, M.M.; Zayan, H.E.E.; Abdelsayed, M.Z.; Moustafa, M.M.; Ezzat, A.R.; Helmy, R.E.D.; Abd-Elaal, H.K.; et al. Determinants of persistent post-COVID-19 symptoms: Value of a novel COVID-19 symptom score. *Egypt. J. Bronchol.* **2021**, *15*, 1–8. [CrossRef]
21. Tung, Y.-J.; Huang, C.-T.; Lin, W.-C.; Cheng, H.H.; Chow, J.C.; Ho, C.H.; Chou, W. Longer length of post-acute care stay causes greater functional improvements in poststroke patients. *Medicine* **2021**. Epub ahead of print. [CrossRef]
22. Al-Aly, Z.; Xie, Y.; Bowe, B. High-dimensional characterization of post-acute sequelae of COVID-19. *Nature* **2021**, *594*, 259–264. [CrossRef]
23. Huang, C.; Huang, L.; Wang, Y.; Li, X.; Ren, L.; Gu, X.; Kang, L.; Guo, L.; Liu, M.; Zhou, X.; et al. 6-month consequences of COVID-19 in patients discharged from hospital: A cohort study. *Lancet* **2021**, *397*, 220–232. [CrossRef]
24. Yaksi, N.; Teker, A.G.; Imre, A. Long COVID in Hospitalized COVID-19 Patients: A Retrospective Cohort Study. *Iran. J. Public. Health* **2022**, *51*, 88. [CrossRef]
25. Subramanian, A.; Nirantharakumar, K.; Hughes, S.; Myles, P.; Williams, T.; Gokhale, K.M.; Taverner, T.; Chandan, J.S.; Brown, K.; Simms-Williams, N.; et al. Symptoms and risk factors for long COVID in non-hospitalized adults. *Nat. Med.* **2022**, *28*, 1706–1714. [CrossRef]
26. Carfì, A.; Bernabei, R.; Landi, F. Persistent Symptoms in Patients After Acute COVID-19. *JAMA* **2020**, *324*, 603. [CrossRef]
27. O'Mahoney, L.L.; Routen, A.; Gillies, C.; Ekezie, W.; Wilford, A.; Zhang, A.; Karamchandani, U.; Simms-Williams, N.; Cassambai, S.; Ardavani, A.; et al. The prevalence and long-term health effects of Long Covid among hospitalized and non-hospitalized populations: A systematic review and meta-analysis. *EClinicalMedicine* **2022**, *55*, 101762. [CrossRef]
28. Pérez-González, A.; Araújo-Ameijeiras, A.; Fernández-Villar, A.; Crespo, M.; Poveda, E.; Cohort COVID-19 of the Galcia Sur Health Research Institute. Long COVID in hospitalized and non-hospitalized patients in a large cohort in Northwest Spain, a prospective cohort study. *Sci. Rep.* **2022**, *12*, 3369. [CrossRef]
29. Katsarou, M.S.; Iasonidou, E.; Osarogue, A.; Kalafatis, E.; Stefanatou, M.; Pappa, S.; Gatzonis, S.; Verentzioti, A.; Gounopoulous, P.; Demponeras, C.; et al. The Greek Collaborative Long COVID Study: Non-Hospitalized and Hospitalized Patients Share Similar Symptom Patterns. *J. Pers. Med.* **2022**, *12*, 987. [CrossRef] [PubMed]
30. Groff, D.; Sun, A.; Ssentongo, A.E.; Djibril, M.; Parsons, N.; Poudel, G.R.; Lekoubou, A.; Oh, J.S.; Ericson, J.E.; Ssentongo, P.; et al. Short-term and Long-term Rates of Postacute Sequelae of SARS-CoV-2 Infection: A Systematic Review. *JAMA Netw. Open* **2021**, *4*, e212856. [CrossRef] [PubMed]
31. Sharma, A.; Minh Duc, N.T.; Luu Lam Thang, T.; Nam, N.H.; Ng, S.J.; Abbas, K.S.; Huy, N.T.; Marušić, A.; Paul, C.L.; Kowk, J.; et al. A Consensus-Based Checklist for Reporting of Survey Studies (CROSS). *J. Gen. Intern. Med.* **2021**, *36*, 3179–3187. [CrossRef] [PubMed]
32. Government of Alberta. Alberta Population Statistics. Available online: https://www.alberta.ca/population-statistics.aspx (accessed on 20 December 2022).
33. Statistics Canada. 2021 Census of Population—Alberta. Available online: https://www12.statcan.gc.ca/census-recensement/2021/dp-pd/prof/details/page.cfm?Lang=E&SearchText=Alberta&DGUIDlist=2021A000248&GENDERlist=1,2,3&STATISTIClist=1&HEADERlist=0 (accessed on 3 January 2023).
34. Nápoles-Springer, A.M.; Santoyo-Olsson, J.; O'Brien, H.; Stewart, A.L. Using cognitive interviews to develop surveys in diverse populations. *Med. Care* **2006**, *44*, S21–S30. [CrossRef]
35. Tourangeau, R.; Rips, L.J.; Rasinski, K. *The Psychology of Survey Response*; Cambridge University Press: Cambridge, UK, 2000. [CrossRef]
36. Alberta Health Services. AHS Public Surveys. Available online: https://www.albertahealthservices.ca/about/page13181.aspx (accessed on 23 August 2022).
37. Perlis, R.H.; Santillana, M.; Ognyanova, K.; Safarpour, A.; Trujillo, K.L.; Simonson, M.D.; Green, J.D.; Quintana, A.; Druckman, J.; Baum, M.A.; et al. Prevalence and Correlates of Long COVID Symptoms Among US Adults. *JAMA Netw. Open.* **2022**, *5*, e2238804. [CrossRef]
38. Hanson, S.W.; Abbafati, C.; Aerts, P.J.G.; Al-Aly, Z.; Ashbaugh, C.; Ballouz, T.; Blyuss, O.; Bobkova, P.; Bonsel, G.; Borzakova, S.; et al. A global systematic analysis of the occurrence, severity, and recovery pattern of long COVID in 2020 and 2021. *medRxiv* **2022**. Epub ahead of print. [CrossRef]
39. Ayoubkhani, D.; Khunti, K.; Nafilyan, V.; Maadox, T.; Humberstone, B.; Diamond, I.; Banerjee, A. Post-covid syndrome in individuals admitted to hospital with COVID-19, Retrospective cohort study. *BMJ* **2021**, *372*, n693. [CrossRef]
40. Pizarro-Pennarolli, C.; Sánchez-Rojas, C.; Torres-Castro, R.; Vera-Uribe, R.; Sanchez-Ramirez, D.C.; Vasconcello-Castillo, L.; Solís-Naravarro, L.; Rivera-Lillo, G. Assessment of activities of daily living in patients post COVID-19, A systematic review. *PeerJ* **2021**, *9*, e11026. [CrossRef]
41. Edemekong, P.F.; Bomgaars, D.L.; Sukumaran, S.; Schoo, C. Activities of Daily Living. *Encycl. Neurol. Sci.* **2022**. Available online: https://pubmed.ncbi.nlm.nih.gov/29261878 (accessed on 20 February 2023).
42. Katz, S. Assessing self-maintenance: Activities of daily living, mobility, and instrumental activities of daily living. *J. Am. Geriatr. Soc.* **1983**, *31*, 721–727. [CrossRef]

43. Logue, J.K.; Franko, N.M.; McCulloch, D.J.; McDonald, D.; Magedson, A.; Wolf, C.R.; Chu, H.Y. Sequelae in Adults at 6 Months After COVID-19 Infection. *JAMA Netw. Open.* **2021**, *4*, e210830. [CrossRef]
44. Klok, F.A.; Boon, G.J.A.M.; Barco, S.; Endres, M.; Geelhoed, M.J.J.; Knauss, S.; Rezek, S.A.; Spruit, M.A.; Veherschild, V.; Siegerink, B. The post-COVID-19 functional status scale: A tool to measure functional status over time after COVID-19. *Eur. Respir. J.* **2020**, *56*, 2001494. [CrossRef]
45. Pant, P.; Joshi, A.; Basnet, B.; Shrestha, B.M.; Bista, N.R.; Bam, N.; Das, S.K. Prevalence of Functional Limitation in COVID-19 Recovered Patients Using the Post COVID-19 Functional Status Scale. *JNMA J. Nepal. Med. Assoc.* **2021**, *59*, 7. [CrossRef]
46. Gaber, T.; Ashish, A.; Unsworth, A. Persistent post-covid symptoms in healthcare workers. *Occup. Med.* **2021**, *71*, 144–146. [CrossRef]
47. Huang, L.; Yao, Q.; Gu, X.; Wang, Q.; Ren, L.; Wang, Y.; Hu, P.; Guo, L.; Liu, M.; Xu, J.; et al. 1-year outcomes in hospital survivors with COVID-19, A longitudinal cohort study. *Lancet* **2021**, *398*, 747–758. [CrossRef]
48. Antonelli, M.; Pujol, J.C.; Spector, T.D.; Ourselin, S.; Steves, C.J. Risk of long COVID associated with delta versus omicron variants of SARS-CoV-2. *Lancet* **2022**, *399*, 2263–2264. [CrossRef]
49. UK Health Security Agency. The Effectiveness of Vaccination against Long COVID: A Rapid Evidence Briefing. Available online: https://www.icpcovid.com/sites/default/files/2022-02/Ep 241-9 UK Health Security Agency The effectiveness of vaccination against long COVID Feb 2022.pdf (accessed on 7 November 2022).

Disclaimer/Publisher's Note: The statements, opinions and data contained in all publications are solely those of the individual author(s) and contributor(s) and not of MDPI and/or the editor(s). MDPI and/or the editor(s) disclaim responsibility for any injury to people or property resulting from any ideas, methods, instructions or products referred to in the content.

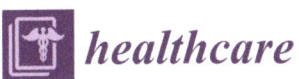

Article

Clinical and Social Features of Patients with Eye Injuries Admitted to a Tertiary Hospital: A Five-Year Retrospective Study from Crete, Greece

Elli D. O. Kyriakaki [1,*], Efstathios T. Detorakis [2], Antonios K. Bertsias [3], Nikolaos G. Tsakalis [4], Ioannis Karageorgiou [5], Gregory Chlouverakis [6] and Emmanouil K. Symvoulakis [1]

[1] Clinic of Social and Family Medicine, School of Medicine, University of Crete, 71003 Heraklion, Greece
[2] Department of Ophthalmology, University Hospital of Heraklion, Crete, 71500 Heraklion, Greece
[3] Clinic of Social and Family Medicine, Faculty of Medicine, University of Crete, 71003 Heraklion, Greece
[4] Department of Ophthalmology, General Hospital of Ierapetra, 72200 Ierapetra, Greece
[5] School of Medicine, University of Crete, 71003 Heraklion, Greece
[6] Department of Social Medicine, Biostatistics Lab, School of Medicine, University of Crete, 71003 Heraklion, Greece
* Correspondence: ellkiriakaki@yahoo.com or medp2011940@med.uoc.gr; Tel.: +30-6945832472

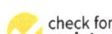

Citation: Kyriakaki, E.D.O.; Detorakis, E.T.; Bertsias, A.K.; Tsakalis, N.G.; Karageorgiou, I.; Chlouverakis, G.; Symvoulakis, E.K. Clinical and Social Features of Patients with Eye Injuries Admitted to a Tertiary Hospital: A Five-Year Retrospective Study from Crete, Greece. *Healthcare* 2023, 11, 885. https://doi.org/10.3390/healthcare11060885

Academic Editors: Sofia Koukouli and Areti Stavropoulou

Received: 13 January 2023
Revised: 6 March 2023
Accepted: 17 March 2023
Published: 18 March 2023

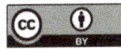

Copyright: © 2023 by the authors. Licensee MDPI, Basel, Switzerland. This article is an open access article distributed under the terms and conditions of the Creative Commons Attribution (CC BY) license (https://creativecommons.org/licenses/by/4.0/).

Abstract: Eye injuries are a major cause of visual disability worldwide and may present a burden to both quality of life of the sufferers and healthcare services. The aim of this study was to extract and triangulate information on the demographic, clinical, and social features of eye-injured adult patients admitted to a tertiary hospital in Greece. The design was a five-year retrospective study of eye-injured adult patients, admitted to the General University Hospital of Heraklion, Crete (GUHH), the single tertiary referral hospital on the island. Drawing the profile of eye-injured patients may add to future health planning. Data collected from 1 January 2015 to 31 December 2019, such as sociodemographic features and clinical information, were extracted. One hundred twenty-eight patients were included. Of those, there was no available information on activity during injury for 6 patients, 78 (60.9%) had work-related ocular injuries, and 44 (34.4%) had non-work-related ocular injuries. Patients with no current formal employment, those who were retired, and formally unemployed and manual force workers had the higher rates of work-related injuries. The most common work-related injuries were closed globe injuries, specifically contusions, while ruptures and penetrating wounds were the most frequent of the open globe injuries. Within the univariate analyses, work-related eye injuries were significantly associated with male gender, middle age, and the place related to daily work activity. Determinants of poor final visual acuity (VA) were the initial VA, the type of injury ($p < 0.0001$), the distance of the place of residence from the hospital, and the time to hospital admission ($p < 0.013$). In a multivariate analysis, referred patients and those with open globe injuries arrived at hospital after a two-hour interval compared with those who were not referred and those with closed globe injuries ($p \leq 0.05$). A reduction in the time to hospital admission deserves further attention. The interconnection of community and health system services through a capacity increase and networking needs further research in order to obtain targeted and viable access for eye-injured patients.

Keywords: eye injury; occupation; retrospective; visual outcomes; prevention

1. Introduction

Ophthalmic traumas include injuries of the eyelids, corneal and conjunctival abrasion, contusion of the globe, rupture, intraocular hemorrhage, optic nerve and orbital trauma, and retinal or chorio-retinal trauma [1]. According to Birmingham Eye Trauma Terminology (BETT), ophthalmic trauma can be classified into Open and Closed globe injuries [2]. Open globe injuries are full thickness wounds that are grouped into ruptures and lacerations, while lacerations are further classified as penetrating and perforating wounds and intraocular foreign bodies [2]. Closed globe injuries are sub-grouped into lamellar lacerations and contusions of the eye globe [2]. Eye injuries are a major cause of avoidable visual disability worldwide. They can be caused by falls, car accidents, chemical burns, or assaults, or during agricultural, sport, or occupational activities, among other methods [3]. They represent a significant burden to healthcare systems [4] and can reduce the quality of life of sufferers [5]. Of the 55 million estimated ocular injuries occurring yearly, approximately 750,000 require hospital admission, with 250,000 being open-globe injuries [1].

Ophthalmic trauma is associated with various factors, such as the geographic location, culture, and socioeconomic status of the population [1,6]. Many studies show that most eye wound injuries are work-related [7,8] and mainly occur among men as they are usually exposed to more higher-risk activities than women are [9]. A 15-year retrospective study from Portugal revealed that, apart from gender and the location of the injury, the economic situation may be included as a high-risk determinant [10]. The study showed that ocular eye injury incidents were related to Portugal's economic recession period, and the authors stated that job uncertainty and work-related pressure may be associated with this rise [10]. Additionally, the same study showed that 7.3% of the ocular injuries were related to substance or alcohol use [10]. Both elements link social and economic determinants with eye injuries.

Moreover, ocular injuries have psychological and economic impacts on individuals, because they lead to loss of work capacity and productivity limitations [11]. They also present an economic burden to the insurance system of a country, because of the constantly increasing hospitalization costs [12,13]. General practitioners and occupational health providers may be able to play a role in the prevention of these injuries and limit complications by providing a care network for mild eye injuries and by giving prompt referrals for severe cases [14]. Regarding the prevention of occupational eye injuries, employers and occupational health and safety professionals should develop personalized messages for the proper use of protective eye equipment and other measures in workplaces.

This study aims to extract and triangulate information regarding the demographic, clinical, and social features of eye-injured adult patients admitted to the General University Hospital of Heraklion (GUHH), Crete, Greece. Drawing the profiles of eye-injured patients can offer some baseline input for future service adjustments.

2. Materials and Methods

2.1. Study Design, Population, and Ethics Approval

Crete is relatively isolated from mainland Greece and has a fully supported healthcare system with primary healthcare centers and secondary and tertiary hospital units. The single tertiary hospital in the geographical region of Crete provides medical services to a population of over 632,674 permanent inhabitants living in all four prefectures of Crete in a catchment area of 8336 km^2. In the summer the population grows significantly due to tourism. We conducted a retrospective study of patients admitted to the GUHH, with ocular injuries from 1 January 2015 to 31 December 2019, prior to the COVID-19 pandemic. Therefore, COVID-19 did not affect the hospitalization length, doctor availability, or overall capacity of the hospital. The medical records of patients who presented to the Ophthalmology emergency department were screened and reviewed by the first author to determine their eligibility. Participants included in the study were adults with ocular injuries severe enough to require hospitalization at the ophthalmology department. The total sample included 128 patients. The gender, age, occupation, family status, nationality, and insurance status of the patients as well as several clinical variables were analyzed. Missing information was added, when possible, via telephone interviews.

The GUHH is the only reference center on Crete and is on duty every second day. All departments are active to deal with emergencies, thus, there is no process or management variation between weekdays and weekends. Most participants included in the study were insured. However, in Greece, all patients, whether they are insured, uninsured, or foreigners/tourists, benefit equally from emergency care. Due to the available on-call system, most emergency cases that need surgical treatment undergo interventions without a prolonged delay. For instance, in the case of vitreoretinal surgery, patients are hospitalized for posturing, and the surgeon is called to perform the surgery in due time. All procedures associated with serious eye injuries are performed under general anesthesia.

Age was classified into three categories: 18–40, 41–66, and over 67 years. Work activity was defined as any paid formal professional activity with a job contract agreement with an employer. Secondary occupational activities were defined as any working activities without a job contract but conducted for indirect profit. These were mainly related to agriculture, which is a socio-cultural commonality for the inhabitants of Crete, even after retirement.

The source of injury was coded into four categories: solid object injury, chemical burns, livestock–agricultural activity, fall and sport leading injuries. The classification of open and closed globe injuries was based on the BETT criteria [2] and the Ocular Trauma Classification Group [15,16]. The Initial and Final Visual Acuity (VA) were used to define the visual outcomes. Additionally, a conversion of all VAs from the Snellen chart to the Logarithm of the Minimum Angle of Resolution (LogMAR) was applied. The geometric mean of the LogMAR values was used for the statistical analysis and comparisons of different datasets and variables [17]. Moreover, the LogMAR measurement was used for research purposes, because it has the potential to accurately calibrate low VA and to practically facilitate its analysis [18,19]. VA was assessed on presentation at the clinic and upon recovery. The final VA was the last value recorded in a patient's record file following hospitalization in the ophthalmology department or after outpatient follow-up. Eleven patients with initial and final VA scores of 10/10 on the Snellen scale (LogMAR = 0.00) were not included. VA was arbitrarily coded into poor ($\leq$0.5/10 or $\leq$20/400 on the Snellen scale, $\geq$1.3 on the LogMAR scale) and not poor (>0.5/10 or >20/400 on the Snellen scale, <1.3 in LogMAR scale) [20]. Time to admission was coded as $\leq$2 or >2 h. The residence distance from the hospital (in kilometers) was categorized as 0–20 km, 21–60 km, or over 61 km. Given the variance in the road network and island geography, a linear relation between time and distance could not be estimated.

The patients' insurance statuses were coded into four main categories: public, social, agricultural, and self-employment insurance, according to the Greek insurance system, whilst data were also recorded for uninsured patients. Data on the cost of care included the cost of all days for hospitalized patients. These were provided by the pertinent administrative authorities. The cost was classified into categories of less than EUR 500; EUR 501–1000; EUR 1001–1500; and over EUR 1501.

Children and adolescents aged under 18 years were not included. Patient data were collected according to the guidelines of the Declaration of Helsinki, assuring confidentiality, and the study was approved by the Scientific Council of the 7th Health District of Crete (Prot. Number:17/30-10-2019) and the Scientific Ethics and Deontology Committee of the University of Crete (Prot. Number:28/07-02-2020).

2.2. Statistical Analysis

Descriptive statistics were used to summarize all variables. An analysis between work-related injuries and selected variables was performed using Pearson's chi-square test. A comparison between the initial and final LogMAR performance (poor vs. not poor) was performed using the McNemar test. An analysis of the initial LogMAR values, the delay time, and the risk category was performed using the nonparametric Mann–Whitney test. An analysis of the number of days of hospitalization (0–7 days vs. 8+ days) and certain parameters was performed using Pearson's chi-square test and a simple logistic regression. An analysis of the delay time ($\leq$2 h vs. >2 h) and selected factors was performed using Pearson's Chi-Square test. Finally, an analysis of the final LogMAR (poor vs. not poor) and selected variables was performed using Pearson's Chi-square test and a simple logistic regression. All continuous variables were checked for normality using both histograms and the Kolmogorov–Smirnov Test. A multiple logistic regression model was performed with the dependent variable being the time of admittance ($\leq$2 h vs. >2 h). Independent variables used in the model were the initial visual acuity (not poor vs. poor), the final visual acuity (not poor vs. poor), the type of injury (open globe injury vs. closed globe injury), and referral to hospital by any doctor (yes/no). The adopted level of significance was $p = 0.05$, and data were analyzed with the statistical software IBM SPSS, version 24.3.

3. Results

Among the 128 ocular injury patients, 113 (88.3%) were males and 15 (11.7%) were females. The mean age was 52.39 ± 17.64 years. The majority of patients did not have an active employment status (39.4%), but most of them (30.7%) had retired and were involved in secondary non-formal agricultural work, while 8.7% were formally unemployed. Fifty percent of patients had social insurance/self-employment insurance (Table 1). The BETT system classifications [2] of the ocular injuries reported in our study analysis are shown in Table 2.

Table 1. Socio-demographic characteristics of eye injuries (N = 128).

		n * (%)
Gender		
	Male	113 (88.3%)
	Female	15 (11.7%)
Age group		
	18–40	37 (28.9%)
	41–66	59 (46.1%)
	66+	32 (25.0%)
Family status		
	Married	107 (88.4%)
	Unmarried, divorced, widow	14 (11.6%)
Nationality		
	Greeks	101 (79%)
	Foreigners	27 (21%)
Occupation		
	Manual force workers	28 (22%)
	Farmers/livestock workers	18 (14.2%)
	Self-employed/private-public sector employees	31 (24.4%)
	With no currently formal employment	50 (39.4%)
Insurance status		
	Public insurance	19 (14.8%)
	Private insurance	3 (2.3%)
	Agricultural insurance	34 (26.6%)
	Social insurance/self-employment insurance	64 (50%)
	Uninsured	8 (6.3%)

* Total counts may differ due to missing values.

Univariate comparisons were conducted between work-related/non-work-related injuries and several variables. Most injuries (78, 60.9%) were work-related, while 44 (34.4%) were non-work-related, and 6 patients (4.7%) had injuries with an unknown reason and were thus removed from this analysis. A higher proportion of men (98.7%) than women (1.3%) had work-related eye trauma ($p < 0.0001$) (Table 3). Statistically significant differences in work-related eye injuries among different age groups were observed, with a higher proportion of injuries occurring in those aged 41–66 years (56.4%), compared with those aged 18–40 years and those older than 67 years ($p = 0.014$). The higher rates of work-related eye injuries, approximately 30%, were observed among manual force workers and in those with no currently formal employment. Significant differences between work- and non-work-related eye injuries in terms of the source and the place of injury were also observed ($p < 0.0001$). Solid-object injuries, livestock and agricultural injuries, and chemical burns were more common in the work-related injury subgroup (48.1%, 31.2%, and 18.2%, respectively). Solid-object injuries were more common in the non-work-related group (38.6%), followed by falls and sports injuries (34.1%). As for the place of injury, work-related ocular injuries occurred during formal or non-formal work activities, as previously defined, whereas most non-work-related injuries occurred at home ($p < 0.0001$, Table 3). Most patients with work-related eye injuries did not wear protective eye devices (PED) while performing their duties ($n = 57$, 90.5%).

Table 2. Work-related and non-work-related ocular trauma cases stratified from our data collection, according to the Birmingham Eye Trauma Terminology (BETT) [2].

	Work-Related	Non-Work-Related
	n *	n *
PATIENTS WITH OCULAR INJURIES	78	44
PATIENTS WITH CLOSED GLOBE INJURIES	48	23
Chemical burn lesions	14	6
Contusion lesions	22	12
Partial thickness wound lesions	15	7
PATIENTS WITH OPEN GLOBE INJURIES	30	21
Rupture lesions	29	19
Full thickness wound lesions		
Perforating wound lesions	28	19
Penetrating wound lesions	29	19
Intraocular foreign body lesions	7	5

* Number of lesions may differ from the number of patients because they may be more than one lesion per patient.

Within the current patient study group, there were registered 31 lesions of vitreous hemorrhage, 30 lesions of traumatic cataract, 22 lesions of partial iris loss, and one lesion of total iris loss. Seven lesions of retinal detachment were recorded. No case of endopthalmitis was reported.

There was no significant association of the duration of hospitalization with gender, age, or occupation. On the contrary, patients with closed globe injuries had increased rates of hospitalization over 8 days (33, 73.3%) compared with those with open globe injury (12, 26.7%) ($p < 0.0001$). Moreover, the season was associated with the duration of hospitalization. In terms of the hospitalization length, eye injuries that occurred in autumn differed when compared to those occurring in spring (<8 days of hospitalization: 17.8% in autumn vs. 37.8% in spring); ($p = 0.041$). The hospitalization length did not show a statistically significant correlation with the distance from the hospital (Table 4).

Univariate comparisons between the time to hospital admission and specific variables are presented in Table 5. There was a statistically significant correlation between the initial and final VA and the time to admission. Patients who arrived at the hospital after more than two hours were more frequently assessed as having "poor" initial and final VA than those admitted within two hours (Table 5). Moreover, patients admitted after two hours had a higher likelihood of undergoing surgical intervention compared to those admitted in less than two hours (63.4% vs. 24.1%, $p < 0.0001$). There were significantly more patients with a poor final VA following delayed admission compared with those admitted in less than two hours (23.9% vs. 7.3%, $p = 0.013$). In addition, the cost of hospitalization was increased for patients who took over two hours to be admitted ($p = 0.010$), and the same was true for the median personal expenses ($p = 0.010$). Patients referred from private practitioners or public units were admitted significantly later than those who were not referred ($p < 0.0001$, Table 5).

Comparisons between the final VA (not poor/poor) and selected factors are presented in Table 6. The final VA was significantly associated with the initial VA. Patients who did not have a poor initial VA also did not have a poor final VA (74.8%, $p < 0.0001$). Closed globe injuries had more "not poor" final visual outcomes compared with open globe injuries (65.4% vs. 34.6%; $p < 0.0001$). Additionally, patients who lived at a distance of greater than 61 km away from the hospital, and were thus likely admitted late, had a higher percentage of poor outcomes compared with those who lived closer (65.0%, $p = 0.005$).

Participants with no currently formal employment had a greater rate of poor final visual outcomes (71.4%) compared with the rest of the occupational categories (manual force workers, farmers/locksmiths and private/public sector employees, and self-employed) ($p = 0.031$).

Table 3. Demographic and injury characteristics of work- and non-work-related eye injuries (N = 122 *).

		Work-Related	Non-Work-Related	p-Value
		N ** (%)	N ** (%)	
Gender				<0.0001
	Male	77 (98.7%)	31 (70.5%)	
	Female	1 (1.3%)	13 (29.5%)	
Age groups				0.014
	18–40	19 (24.4%)	15 (34.1%)	
	41–66	44 (56.4%)	13 (29.5%)	
	67+	15 (19.2%)	16 (36.4%)	
Occupation				0.016
	Manual force workers	23 (29.5%)	4 (9.1%)	
	Farmers/livestock workers	12 (15.4%)	6 (13.6%)	
	Self-employed/private-public sector employees	19 (24.4%)	9 (20.5%)	
	With no currently formal employment	24 (30.8%)	25 (56.8%)	
Days of hospitalization		5 (1, 26; 6)	6 (1, 22; 7)	0.323
Surgery				0.448
	Yes	33 (42.9%)	22 (50.0%)	
	No	44 (57.1%)	22 (50.0%)	
Cost of care		701 (60, 2615; 551)	799 (188, 2203; 548)	
Type of injury				0.319
	Closed globe injuries	48 (61.5%)	23 (52.3%)	
	Open globe injuries	30 (38.5%)	21 (47.7%)	
Source of injury				<0.0001
	Solid object injury	37 (48.1%)	17 (38.6%)	
	Chemical burns	14 (18.2%)	8 (18.2%)	
	Livestock and agricultural injuries	24 (31.2%)	4 (9.1%)	
	Falls and sport injuries	2 (2.6%)	15 (34.1%)	
Place of injury				<0.0001
	Daily work activity (formal or non-formal)	69 (89.6%)	0 (0.0%)	
	Road and traffic accidents	0 (0.0%)	5 (11.9%)	
	Assaults	0 (0.0%)	1 (2.4%)	
	Sport activities	0 (0.0%)	2 (4.8%)	
	Domestic and other	8 (10.4%)	34 (81.0%)	
Use of protective eye devices				0.823
	Yes	6 (9.5%)	2 (8.0%)	
	No	57 (90.5%)	23 (92.0%)	

* 6 patients were excluded due to having a non-specified reported activity during injury. ** Total counts may differ due to missing values.

Table 4. Variables associated with hospitalization (N = 128).

	Hospital Stay (0–7 Days)	Hospital Stay (8+ Days)	p-Value
	n * (%)	n * (%)	
Gender			0.117
Male	76 (91.6%)	37 (82.2%)	
Female	7 (8.4%)	8 (17.8%)	
Age groups			0.268
18–40	26 (31.3%)	11 (24.4%)	
41–66	40 (48.2%)	19 (42.2%)	0.799

Table 4. Cont.

	Hospital Stay (0–7 Days)	Hospital Stay (8+ Days)	p-Value
	n * (%)	n * (%)	
67+	17 (20.5%)	15 (33.3%)	0.145
Occupation			0.189
Manual force workers	21 (25.6%)	7 (15.6%)	
Farmers/livestock workers	23 (28.0%)	8 (17.8%)	0.943
Self-employed/private-public sector employees	10 (12.2%)	8 (17.8%)	0.174
With no currently formal employment	28 (34.1%)	22 (48.9%)	0.100
Type of injury			<0.0001
Closed globe	21 (25.3%)	33 (73.3%)	
Open globe	62 (74.7%)	12 (26.7%)	
Season			0.041
Spring	14 (16.9%)	17 (37.8%)	
Summer	20 (24.1%)	11 (24.4%)	0.128
Autumn	28 (33.7%)	8 (17.8%)	0.007
Winter	21 (25.3%)	9 (20.0%)	0.053
Time of admittance			0.082
≤2 h	40 (49.4%)	15 (33.3%)	
>2 h	41 (50.6%)	30 (66.7%)	
Residence distance from hospital (km)			0.144
0–20	34 (41.5%)	14 (32.6%)	
21–60	26 (31.7%)	10 (23.3%)	0.889
61+	22 (26.8%)	19 (44.2%)	0.097

* Total counts may differ due to missing values.

Table 5. Injury and cost outcomes related to the time of access (N = 126 *).

	Time of Admittance to Hospital (≤2 h)	Time of Admittance to Hospital (>2 h)	p-Value
	N ** (%)	N ** (%)	
Initial visual acuity (LogMAR scale)			0.010
Not poor	41 (74.5%)	37 (52.1%)	
Poor	14 (25.5%)	34 (47.9%)	
Final visual acuity (LogMAR scale)			0.013
Not poor	51 (92.7%)	54 (76.1%)	
Poor	4 (7.3%)	17 (23.9%)	
Days of hospitalization			0.082
0–7	40 (72.7%)	41 (57.7%)	
8+	15 (27.3%)	30 (42.3%)	
Surgical intervention			<0.0001
Yes	13 (24.1%)	45 (63.4%)	
No	41 (75.9%)	26 (36.6%)	
Cost of care			0.010
≤500 €	31 (57.4%)	20 (28.2%)	
501–1000 €	17 (31.5%)	33 (46.5%)	
1001–1500 €	3 (5.6%)	9 (12.7%)	
1501+	3 (5.6%)	9 (12.7%)	
Pocket payments			
Median(min, max; IQP)	80 (0, 10.000; 150)	150 (0, 15.000; 600)	0.010
Referral by			<0.0001
Private practice	0 (0.0%)	16 (23.2%)	
Public practice	3 (5.5%)	28 (40.6%)	
None	52 (94.5%)	25 (36.2%)	

* 2 patients were excluded due to having a non-specified time of admittance. ** Total counts may differ due to missing values.

The results from a multiple logistic regression analysis indicated that the initial and final visual acuity were not significant predictors of the time to hospital admittance (≤2 h vs. >2 h; $p > 0.05$ for both). On the other hand, patients with an open globe injury had

2.78 times higher odds of hospital admittance in >2 h compared to patients with a closed globe injury (OR 2.718; 95% CI from 1.001 to 7.740; $p = 0.050$). Finally, patients who were referred to the hospital from other health-care settings had 23.9 times higher odds of hospital admittance in >2 h compared to patients without a referral (OR 23.94; 95% CI from 6.534 to 87.76; $p < 0.0001$).

Table 6. Factors associated with visual outcomes (N = 128).

	Final Visual Acuity (LogMAR Scale)	Final Visual Acuity (LogMAR Scale)	p-Value
	Not Poor	Poor	
	n * (%)	n * (%)	
Initial visual acuity (LogMAR scale)			<0.0001
Not poor	80 (74.8%)	0 (0.0%)	
Poor	27 (25.2%)	21 (100.0%)	
Type of injury			<0.0001
Closed globe injury	70 (65.4%)	4 (19.0%)	
Opened globe injury	37 (34.6%)	17 (81.0%)	
Occupation			0.022
Manual force workers	26 (24.5%)	2 (9.5%)	
Farmers/livestock workers	16 (15.1%)	2 (9.5%)	0.644
Self-employed/private-public sector employees	29 (27.4%)	2 (9.5%)	0.916
With no currently formal employment	35 (33.0%)	15 (71.4%)	0.031
Residence distance from hospital (km)			0.003
0–20	45 (42.9%)	3 (15.0%)	
21–60	32 (30.5%)	4 (20.0%)	0.431
61+	28 (26.7%)	13 (65.0%)	0.005
Time of admittance to hospital			0.013
≤2 h	51 (48.6%)	4 (19.0%)	
>2 h	54 (51.4%)	17 (81.0%)	
Surgical intervention			<0.0001
No	68 (64.2%)	1 (4.8%)	
Yes	38 (35.8%)	20 (95.2%)	

* Total counts may differ due to missing values.

4. Discussion

This study provides the first analysis of work-related ophthalmic trauma on the Mediterranean island of Crete. Closed globe injuries were the most common type of work-related ocular injury, whilst 4 out of 10 were open globe cases. This is similar to the results reported by another Greek study in 2005 [21]. Closed globe injuries were also associated with increased rates of hospitalization for ≥8 days compared with open globe injuries (73.3% vs. 26.7%, $p < 0.0001$). This finding is in contrast with that of another study, where the most common duration of hospital stay was 3 to 5 days for all types of globe injury [22]. Because closed injuries are managed conservatively, the hospitalization duration may be prolonged. Additionally, as many patients were older than 50 years of age, their health status or overall pharmacotherapy profile might have influenced the duration of hospital stay.

A final not poor VA was found to be strongly correlated with a not poor initial VA, as shown in other studies [23,24]. Comparable results have emerged from a prospective data collection branch study that has been recently published [25]. Open globe injuries were more frequently related to a poor final VA compared to closed globe injuries, showing that visual outcomes depend on the clinical characteristics and the nature of eye damage [23,24]. Within the present study, patients with vitreous hemorrhage received a two-month eye drop medication prescription. Follow-up monitoring, to assess vitreous hemorrhage absorption, was scheduled for these patients. Those with persistent vitreous hemorrhage, after the two-month period, underwent vitrectomy. Patients with traumatic cataract underwent lensectomy. Patients with iris loss underwent iridoplasty. Finally, patients with retinal detachment underwent surgical restoration.

Most of the eye injuries were work-related (60.9%), as observed by other authors [21,26,27]. Manual force workers (construction, welding, electric work, plumbing, farming) formed one of the most commonly affected groups among the admitted patients (29.5%), indicating that these patients have a higher risk of sustaining an eye injury, as highlighted by other studies [21,28–30]. A large proportion of patients were retired and spent their spare time in agricultural labor, which also involves high-risk activities [29,30]. Occupation was also strongly correlated with poor final VA, as shown in another study [24].

Most sufferers with work-related injuries had not used protective measures (90.5%), as reported in other studies [21,27]. It is therefore possible that a significant number of eye injuries could be prevented or avoided. However, any effort geared towards increasing PED use compliance should take into consideration the specific social and occupational features of the residents of that region [31], as the occupational characteristics of each region's population are very important in determining the major sources of ocular injury in that area [1,9,30].

The mean age of the patients was 52.39 ± 17.64 years, which is older than what has been reported in other studies [21,27]. This could be attributed to the fact that, in Crete, many people own properties with crops and work there unofficially after retirement. Injuries that occurred during spring and summer were associated with increased rates of hospitalization over 8 days. In rural Crete, many agricultural activities are carried out during those seasons, thus, more serious eye injuries tend to occur then.

In the univariate analysis, patients admitted to the hospital more than two hours after the occurrence of the injury had poorer initial and final VA compared to those admitted in less than two hours ($p = 0.010$ and $p = 0.013$, respectively). Thus, the final VA depends, among the other factors highlighted in our study, on early hospital admission. This is in line with the results of other studies [23,32]. The multivariate analysis did not confirm this finding. The use of larger sample size groups and different time cut-offs may offer answers in future research efforts. A study conducted in Bosnia did not find an association between the final VA and the time to hospital admission [33]. A recently published study showed that a delay of almost 4 h caused by interhospital transfer led to a lower final VA [34].

Patients with a delayed admission had increased rates of surgical interventions and an increased cost of care and personal cost. To the authors' current knowledge, few studies have investigated the relationship between time to admission and economic parameters. As shown in Table 5, both the overall cost of care and the out-of-pocket payment of patients were significantly lower when the time to admission was less than 2 h ($p = 0.010$). It could, therefore, be assumed that late eye injury management is likely to lead to poorer outcomes [32], and this may be reflected in the cost of care and personal expenses for the sufferers and the healthcare system. A study from the United States found that the cost of care was higher for patients from high-income households, probably, as discussed by the authors, because health providers were more willing to order tests and because the patients themselves demanded a higher care level [12].

The multiple regression analysis showed that patients with open globe injuries had significantly higher odds of being admitted to the hospital in >2 h from the incident compared to those with closed globe injuries, while another study showed that the median time to hospital admittance was 4 h for patients with an open globe injury [35]. A possible explanation for this is that open globe injuries are likely to occur in the context of more complex trauma, which may lead to a process involving service prioritization, and this may influence the time to arrival at the hospital. The GUHH is on duty every second day, so we cannot exclude the fact that visit timing may have been influenced by this parameter in some cases. For closed globe eye care, access may directly emerge, and time of arrival may be anticipated. It also appears that referred patients are more likely to arrive at the hospital more than two hours after the injury than those who are not referred. Both findings show that the initial assessment and management of ocular injuries deserve an evidence-based design in terms of the roles, flows, and care network, as this might increase the viability of moving patients from community and primary settings to tertiary care.

4.1. Implications

Primary care physicians can assist with early hospital admission by assessing and promptly referring patients with severe ocular injuries to the hospital while managing mild cases. This can lead to earlier recognition, and therefore better visual outcomes of serious ocular injuries as well as appropriate management of mild ocular injuries without burdening large referral centers.

PED use compliance was minimal in our study. To increase compliance, the special geographical, occupational, and cultural characteristics of a region should be taken into consideration when designing prevention and protective measures [36]. Occupational health and safety professionals could contribute to the prevention of ocular injuries by educating and counseling workers regarding the importance of using PED in the workplace. A focus on rural areas should be given to inform low-educated, elderly, and residents about the risk of not wearing PED, while local municipalities could provide suitable and well-fitted protective equipment, as a public health measure initiative.

4.2. Limitations

This was a retrospective observational study conducted in Crete; thus, the study results are not representative of the whole country. The study included hospitalized patients, therefore, patients with less severe injuries that were managed in local first aid health units or secondary hospitals were not recorded. Considering that the study's data reflect a pre-COVID-19 period, there were no irregularities regarding the hospitalization length, doctor availability, or overall capacity of the hospital. Additionally, up to the study's end date, COVID-19 did not affect access or greatly influence possible follow-up consultation, as mentioned in other studies [37,38]. However, it was difficult to collect data retrospectively due to a ban on physical hospital access and the strict measures undertaken for COVID-19, because the data record search and collection were performed during the pandemic. Recall biases cannot be excluded for missing information that was retrieved via phone calls.

5. Conclusions

This study concluded that most cases of ocular injury requiring hospitalization in Crete were work-related. Those with no current formal employment, those who were retired or formally unemployed, and manual force workers had higher rates of work-related injuries. Patients with open globe injuries were more likely to attend hospital in >2 h compared to patients with closed globe injuries. Finally, patients who were referred from other health-care settings had an increased likelihood of accessing the hospital in >2 h compared to patients without a referral. Major efforts to improve the initial management of ocular injuries should include an evidence-based design of the roles, flows, and care network to increase the interconnectivity of services.

Author Contributions: Conceptualization, E.D.O.K., E.K.S. and E.T.D.; methodology, E.D.O.K., E.K.S., E.T.D. and G.C.; formal analysis, A.K.B.; resources, N.G.T.; data curation, E.D.O.K. and N.G.T.; writing—original draft preparation, E.D.O.K. and I.K.; writing—review and editing, E.T.D., E.K.S. and E.D.O.K.; supervision, E.K.S., E.T.D. and E.D.O.K.; project administration, E.D.O.K. All authors have read and agreed to the published version of the manuscript.

Funding: This research received no external funding.

Institutional Review Board Statement: Patient data were collected according to the guidelines of the Declaration of Helsinki, assuring confidentiality, and the study was approved by the Scientific

Council of the 7th Health District of Crete (Prot. Number: 17/30-10-2019) and the Scientific Ethics and Deontology Committee of the University of Crete (Prot. Number: 28/07-02-2020).

Informed Consent Statement: Not applicable.

Data Availability Statement: The data that support the findings of this study are available on request from the corresponding author. The data are not publicly available due to privacy or ethical restrictions.

Conflicts of Interest: The authors declare no conflict of interest.

References

1. Umarane, S.; Kale, T.; Tenagi, A.; Manavadaria, Y.; Motimath, A.S. A Clinical Study of the Evaluation and Assessment of the Etiology and Patterns of Ocular Injuries in Midfacial Trauma in a Tertiary Care Hospital. *Cureus* **2020**, *12*, e10216. [CrossRef]
2. Kuhn, F.; Morris, R.; Witherspoon, C.D. Birmingham Eye Trauma Terminology (BETT): Terminology and Classification of Mechanical Eye Injuries. *Ophthalmol. Clin. N. Am.* **2002**, *15*, 139–143. [CrossRef] [PubMed]
3. Ahn, J.Y.; Ryoo, H.W.; Park, J.B.; Moon, S.; Cho, J.W.; Park, D.H.; Lee, W.K.; Kim, J.H.; Jin, S.C.; Lee, K.W.; et al. Epidemiologic Characteristics of Work-Related Eye Injuries and Risk Factors Associated with Severe Eye Injuries: A Registry-Based Multicentre Study. *Ophthalmic Epidemiol.* **2020**, *27*, 105–114. [CrossRef]
4. Négrel, A.D.; Thylefors, B. The Global Impact of Eye Injuries. *Ophthalmic Epidemiol.* **1998**, *5*, 143–169. [CrossRef]
5. Yüksel, H.; Türkcü, F.M.; Şahin, M.; Çinar, Y.; Cingü, A.K.; Özkurt, Z.; Bez, Y.; Çaça, I. Vision-Related Quality of Life in Patients after Ocular Penetrating Injuries. *Arq. Bras. Oftalmol.* **2014**, *77*, 95–98. [CrossRef] [PubMed]
6. Ngo, C.; Leo, S. Industrial Accident-Related Ocular Emergencies in a Tertiary Hospital in Singapore. *Singap. Med. J.* **2008**, *49*, 280–285.
7. Shepherd, M.; Barker, J.; Scott, D.; Hockey, R.; Spinks, D.; Pitt, R. Occupational Eye Injuries. *Queensl. Inj. Surveill. Unit* **2006**. Available online: https://www.researchgate.net/publication/260909071_Occupational_Eye_Injuries (accessed on 17 March 2023).
8. Ye, C.; Wang, X.; Zhang, Y.; Ni, L.; Jiang, R.; Liu, L.; Han, C. Ten-Year Epidemiology of Chemical Burns in Western Zhejiang Province, China. *Burns* **2016**, *42*, 668–674. [CrossRef] [PubMed]
9. Tök, O.Y.; Tok, L.; Eraslan, E.; Ozkaya, D.; Ornek, F.; Bardak, Y. Prognostic Factors Influencing Final Visual Acuity in Open Globe Injuries. *J. Trauma* **2011**, *71*, 1794–1800. [CrossRef]
10. Marta, A.; Silva, N.; Correia, N.; Pessoa, B.; Ferreira, N.; Beirão, M.; Meireles, A. A 15-Year Retrospective Epidemiologic Study of Ocular Trauma in the North of Portugal. *Eur. J. Ophthalmol.* **2021**, *31*, 1079–1084. [CrossRef]
11. Chowdhury, S. Injuries in Marginal Workers and Social Trauma in Female: Important Cause of the Paradigm Shift in Eye Injury over a Decade. *Indian J. Occup. Environ. Med.* **2015**, *19*, 36–43. [CrossRef] [PubMed]
12. Iftikhar, M.; Latif, A.; Usmani, B.; Canner, J.K.; Shah, S.M.A. Trends and Disparities in Inpatient Costs for Eye Trauma in the United States (2001–2014). *Am. J. Ophthalmol.* **2019**, *207*, 1–9. [CrossRef] [PubMed]
13. American Academy of Ophthalmology. Falls and Brawls Top List of Causes for Eye Injuries in United States. Available online: https://www.aao.org/newsroom/news-releases/detail/falls-brawls-top-list-of-causes-eye-injuries-in-un (accessed on 13 January 2023).
14. Wallace, H.B.; Ferguson, R.A.; Sung, J.; McKelvie, J. New Zealand Adult Ocular Trauma Study: A 10-Year National Review of 332,418 Cases of Ocular Injury in Adults Aged 18 to 99 Years. *Clin. Experiment. Ophthalmol.* **2020**, *48*, 158–168. [CrossRef] [PubMed]
15. Kuhn, F.; Morris, R.; Witherspoon, C.D.; Heimann, K.; Jeffers, J.B.; Treister, G. A Standardized Classification of Ocular Trauma. *Ophthalmology* **1996**, *103*, 240–243. [CrossRef]
16. Pieramici, D.J.; Sternberg, P.J.; Aaberg, S.; Bridges, J.; Capone, A.J.; Cardillo, J.A.; De Juan, E.J.; Kuhn, F.; Meredith, T.A.; Mieler, W.F.; et al. A System for Classifying Mechanical Injuries of the Eye (Globe). The Ocular Trauma Classification Group. *Am. J. Ophthalmol.* **1997**, *123*, 820–831. [CrossRef]
17. Holladay, J.T. Visual Acuity Measurements. *J. Cataract Refract. Surg.* **2004**, *30*, 287–290. [CrossRef]
18. Oduntan, O.A.; Mashige, K.P.; Raliavhegwa-Makhado, M. A Comparison of Two Methods of LogMAR Visual Acuity Data Scoring for Statistical Analysis. *Afr. Vis. Eye Health* **2009**, *68*, 155–163. [CrossRef]
19. Lovie-Kitchin, J.E. Validity and Reliability of Visual Acuity Measurements. *Ophthalmic Physiol. Opt.* **1988**, *8*, 363–370. [CrossRef]
20. Upaphong, P.; Supreeyathitikul, P.; Choovuthayakorn, J. Open Globe Injuries Related to Traffic Accidents: A Retrospective Study. *J. Ophthalmol.* **2021**, *2021*, 6629589. [CrossRef]
21. Mela, E.K.; Mantzouranis, G.A.; Giakoumis, A.P.; Blatsios, G.; Andrikopoulos, G.K.; Gartaganis, S.P. Ocular Trauma in a Greek Population: Review of 899 Cases Resulting in Hospitalization. *Ophthalmic Epidemiol.* **2009**, *12*, 185–190. [CrossRef]
22. Chang, C.H.; Chen, C.L.; Ho, C.K.; Lai, Y.H.; Hu, R.C.; Yen, Y.L. Hospitalized Eye Injury in a Large Industrial City of South-Eastern Asia. *Graefes Arch. Clin. Exp. Ophthalmol.* **2008**, *246*, 223–228. [CrossRef] [PubMed]
23. Abu, E.K.; Ocansey, S.; Gyamfi, J.A.; Ntodie, M.; Morny, E.K.A. Epidemiology and Visual Outcomes of Ocular Injuries in a Low Resource Country. *Afr. Health Sci.* **2020**, *20*, 779–788. [CrossRef] [PubMed]

24. Atik, S.S.; Ugurlu, S.; Egrilmez, E.D. Open Globe Injury: Demographic and Clinical Features. *J. Craniofac. Surg.* **2018**, *29*, 628–631. [CrossRef] [PubMed]
25. Kyriakaki, E.D.O.; Detorakis, E.T.; Bertsias, A.K.; Markakis, G.; Tsakalis, N.G.; Volkos, P.; Spandidos, D.A.; Symvoulakis, E.K. Ocular Trauma, Visual Acuity Related to Time of Referral and Psychosocial Determinants, during COVID-19 Pandemic: A Prospective Study. *Exp. Ther. Med.* **2023**, *25*, 130. [CrossRef] [PubMed]
26. Northey, L.C.; Bhardwaj, G.; Curran, S.; Mcgirr, J. Eye Trauma Epidemiology in Regional Australia. *Ophthalmic Epidemiol.* **2014**, *21*, 237–246. [CrossRef] [PubMed]
27. Hui, R.N.; Shew, F.C.; Khai-Siang, C.; Mei, F.C.; Mushawiahti, M. The Epidemiological Profile of Open Globe Injuries and Prognostic Factors in a Tertiary Care Centre. *Cureus* **2021**, *13*, e15846. [CrossRef]
28. Sukati, V.N. Workplace Eye Injuries: A Literature Review. *Occup. Health South. Africa* **2014**, *20*, 18–22.
29. Mansouri, M.R.; Hosseini, M.; Mohebi, M.; Alipour, F.; Mehrdad, R. Work-Related Eye Injury: The Main Cause of Ocular Trauma in Iran. *Eur. J. Ophthalmol.* **2018**, *20*, 770–775. [CrossRef]
30. Al-Mahrouqi, H.; Al-Harthi, N.; Al-Wahaibi, M.; Hanumantharayappa, K. Ocular Trauma: A Tertiary Hospital Experience from Oman. *Oman J. Ophthalmol.* **2017**, *10*, 63–69.
31. Forrest, K.Y.Z.; Cali, J.M. Epidemiology of Lifetime Work-Related Eye Injuries in the U.S. Population Associated with One or More Lost Days of Work. *Ophthalmic Epidemiol.* **2009**, *16*, 156–162. [CrossRef]
32. Omotoye, O.J.; Ajayi, I.A.; Ajite, K.O.; Bodunde, O.F. Factors Responsible for Poor Visual Outcome Following Emergency Eye Surgery in a Tertiary Eye Centre. *Ethiop. J. Health Sci.* **2019**, *29*, 631. [CrossRef] [PubMed]
33. Jovanovic, N.; Peek-Asa, C.; Swanton, A.; Young, T.; Alajbegovic-Halimic, J.; Cavaljuga, S.; Nisic, F. Prevalence and Risk Factors Associated with Work-Related Eye Injuries in Bosnia and Herzegovina. *Int. J. Occup. Environ. Health* **2016**, *22*, 325–332. [CrossRef] [PubMed]
34. Fernandez, E.O.; Miller, H.M.; Pham, V.Q.; Fleischman, D. Comparison of Time-to-Surgery and Outcomes in Transferred Vs. Non-Transferred Open Globe Injuries. *Clin. Ophthalmol.* **2022**, *16*, 2733–2742. [CrossRef] [PubMed]
35. Amro, M.Y. Visual Outcomes Associated with Delay from Trauma to Surgery for Open Globe Eye Injury in Palestine: A Retrospective Chart Review Study. *Lancet* **2021**, *398*, S14. [CrossRef] [PubMed]
36. Kyriakaki, E.D.O.; Symvoulakis, E.K.; Chlouverakis, G.; Detorakis, E.T. Causes, Occupational Risk and Socio-Economic Determinants of Eye Injuries: A Literature Review. *Med. Pharm. Rep.* **2021**, *94*, 131–144. [CrossRef]
37. Lik Au, S.C. Anti-Vascular Endothelial Growth Factor Treatment Regimens Preference by Choroidal Neovascularization Patients under COVID-19. *Indian J. Ophthalmol.* **2020**, *68*, 2314. [CrossRef]
38. Au, S.C.L.; Ko, C.K.L. Delayed Hospital Presentation of Acute Central Retinal Artery Occlusion during the COVID-19 Crisis: The HORA Study Brief Report No. 4. *Indian J. Ophthalmol.* **2021**, *69*, 2904. [CrossRef]

Disclaimer/Publisher's Note: The statements, opinions and data contained in all publications are solely those of the individual author(s) and contributor(s) and not of MDPI and/or the editor(s). MDPI and/or the editor(s) disclaim responsibility for any injury to people or property resulting from any ideas, methods, instructions or products referred to in the content.

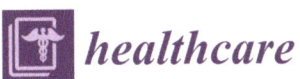

Article

Cultural Adaptation of a Health Literacy Toolkit for Healthcare Professionals Working in the Primary Care Setting with Older Adults

Areti Efthymiou [1,2,*], Argyroula Kalaitzaki [1,2,3] and Michael Rovithis [2,3,4]

1. Department of Social Work, Hellenic Mediterranean University (HMU), 71410 Heraklion, Crete, Greece
2. Laboratory of Interdisciplinary Approaches to the Enhancement of Quality of Life (Quality of Life Lab), Hellenic Mediterranean University (HMU), 71410 Heraklion, Crete, Greece
3. University Centre of Research and Innovation 'Institute of AgriFood and Life Sciences, Hellenic Mediterranean University (HMU), 71410 Heraklion, Crete, Greece
4. Department of Business Administration and Tourism, Hellenic Mediterranean University (HMU), 71410 Heraklion, Crete, Greece
* Correspondence: aefthymiou@hmu.gr

Abstract: Healthcare professionals' health literacy (HL) knowledge and skills influence their interaction with older adults. Healthcare professionals, when effectively communicating with older adults, can empower and enhance patients' skills to make informed decisions about their health. The study aimed to adapt and pilot test a HL toolkit to enhance the HL skills of health professionals working with older adults. A mixed methodology of three phases was used. Initially, the healthcare professionals' and older adults' needs were identified. Following a literature review of existing tools, a HL toolkit was selected, translated, and adapted into Greek. The HL toolkit was introduced to 128 healthcare professionals as part of 4 h webinars; 82 healthcare professionals completed baseline and post assessments, and 24 healthcare professionals implemented it in their clinical practice. The questionnaires used included an interview on HL knowledge, communication strategies, and self-efficacy using a communication scale. HL and communication strategies knowledge (13 items) and self-efficacy in communication ($t = -11.127$, $df = 81$, $p < 0.001$) improved after the end of the HL webinars, and improvement was retained during the follow-up after 2 months ($H = 8.99$, $df = 2$, $p < 0.05$). A culturally adapted HL toolkit was developed to support the needs of healthcare professionals working with older adults, taking into consideration their feedback in all phases of the development.

Keywords: communication; health literacy; healthcare professionals; older adults; self-efficacy; toolkit

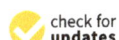

Citation: Efthymiou, A.; Kalaitzaki, A.; Rovithis, M. Cultural Adaptation of a Health Literacy Toolkit for Healthcare Professionals Working in the Primary Care Setting with Older Adults. *Healthcare* 2023, 11, 776. https://doi.org/10.3390/healthcare11050776

Academic Editor: Federico Longhini

Received: 29 December 2022
Revised: 26 February 2023
Accepted: 2 March 2023
Published: 6 March 2023

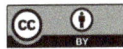

Copyright: © 2023 by the authors. Licensee MDPI, Basel, Switzerland. This article is an open access article distributed under the terms and conditions of the Creative Commons Attribution (CC BY) license (https://creativecommons.org/licenses/by/4.0/).

1. Introduction

According to WHO, strengthening the health literacy (HL) skills of the general population is a multicomponent process involving the participation of healthcare organizations, healthcare professionals, healthcare users, and the environment [1]. An improvement in healthcare organizations' and healthcare professionals' HL skills could be beneficial for national healthcare systems, considering that studies have associated patients' low HL with higher medical costs [2,3].

Older adults are considered a vulnerable population with low HL [4], who may face cognitive, sensory, and other physical challenges that prevent them from communicating effectively with healthcare professionals [5]. Older adults' low HL is associated with negative health outcomes, such as deteriorated physical and cognitive functioning, worse mental health, low medication adherence, worse disease management, fewer health-related preventive actions, longer hospital stays, frequent emergency admissions, and overall higher mortality rates [3,4].

Among the objectives of "Healthy People" for 2030, an initiative running for almost thirty years by the US Department of Health and Human Services, are access to healthcare services and an improvement in communication among healthcare providers and patients (i.e., involve patients in decision-making, assure understanding, increase clear communication) [6]. Older adults are coping with barriers in accessing and utilizing healthcare services [7]. Factors influencing access to healthcare services in primary care include individual (literacy and education, health beliefs, limited mobility, limited digital skills), socioeconomic, cultural/linguistic, environmental (geographical location, transportation, visit modality), and organizational (staff shortage) factors [8–10]. Healthcare professionals play a crucial role in assisting healthcare users to overcome the aforementioned barriers, as it was stated in Ottawa Chart [11], through the redistribution of power, participation, and healthcare users becoming experts.

The knowledge and comprehension of HL among healthcare professionals influence the communication between healthcare professionals and older individuals with chronic diseases and their families [5]. Communication and empowerment of the high-risk population are considered one of the ten attributes of HL organizations [12]. Organizational HL is gaining prominence within health organizations. The ten attributes of HL organizations include [12] leadership to promote HL; integration of HL in planning; evaluation measures; training of the workforce on HL issues; participation of healthcare users in the design, implementation, and evaluation of the health services; combating stigma; use of HL strategies in communication; accessible services and health resources provided by the organization; clear communication; and empowered users in high-risk situations (medication adherence) [12].

The use of clear language without medical jargon, the use of a person-centered approach, and the implementation of communication strategies according to healthcare professionals working with older adults improved communication with them [13]. According to the HL Universal Precautions, healthcare professionals should not assume the HL level of their patients based on their appearance [14]. The Agency of Healthcare and Research Quality developed a universal precautions toolkit for physicians including 20 tools [15], which was later updated to 21 tools [16]. The main categories included were raising awareness, improving spoken and written communication, and improving supportive systems [16]. To the authors' knowledge, there is no HL toolkit adapted to the needs of healthcare professionals working with older adults [17]. The study aimed to adapt and pilot a health literacy toolkit to enhance the HL skills of healthcare professionals working with older people to validly detect and empower patients' HL levels.

2. Materials and Methods

2.1. Study Design

The current study followed a mixed method design with three phases lasting 24 months (November 2020 to October 2022) and following the cultural adaptation process model (CAP): (1) examining the target groups' needs, (2) developing the adaptation methodology, and (3) adapting the selected tools and pilot testing them [18]. Target groups of the adaptation process were healthcare professionals working with older adults (Figure 1).

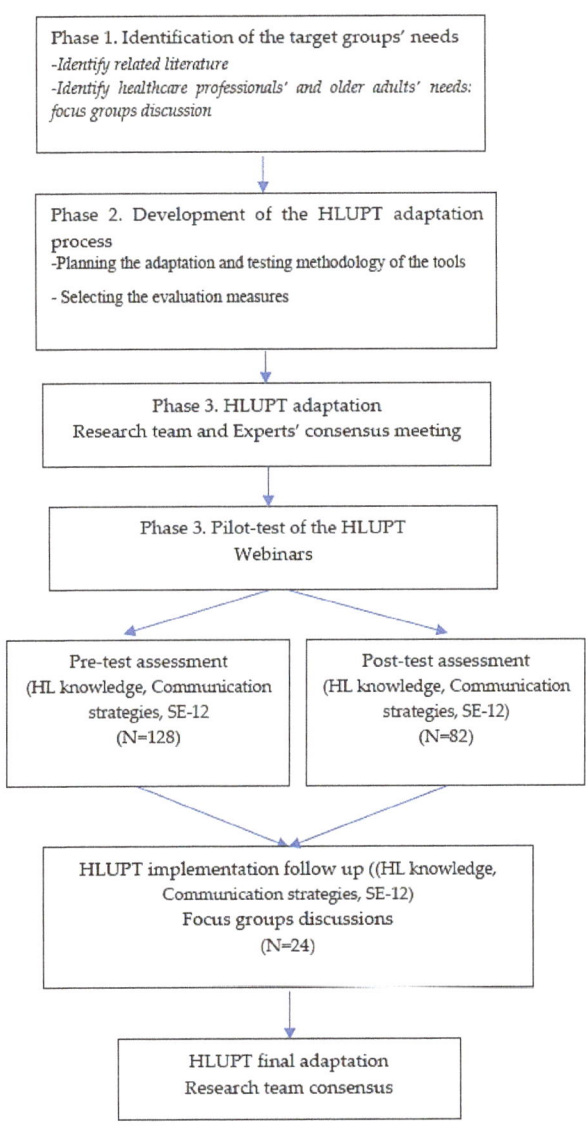

Figure 1. HLUPT cultural adaptation process.

2.1.1. Examining the Target Groups' Needs

Identify related literature. A scoping review was conducted by the research group for the period 2000 to 2020 to identify tools for translation and adaptation, HL training courses, and evaluation measures. The literature search of five electronic databases (PubMed, MEDLINE, CINAHL, PsychInfo, and Opengrey) resulted in 27 papers, and it was concluded that there is a lack of HL tools tailored for healthcare professionals working with older healthcare users [17]. The most used HL toolkit was the HLUPT. Information is available in the published scoping review [17].

Identify healthcare professionals' and older healthcare users' needs. Two focus groups were conducted to assess the HL knowledge and communication needs of healthcare professionals ($n = 7$) and older healthcare users ($n = 5$). Questions included topics on HL knowledge, perspectives on barriers and facilitators in patient–healthcare professional interaction, and healthcare professionals' training needs [13]. Healthcare professionals reported that trust, collaboration, patients' education, psychological resilience, carers' participation, use of plain language, and compassion facilitated their interaction with older healthcare users. On the other hand, the rigid lifestyle of older adults and any cognitive, emotional, sensory, and physical health issues comprised barriers. Older healthcare users considered as important elements in their interaction with healthcare professionals the appropriate preparation before their visit, the assessment of the severity of their health problems, their carers' participation, nonuse of medical jargon, patients' involvement in decision-making, equality, respect, compassion, and healthcare professionals' encouraging discussion [13].

2.1.2. Developing the HLUPT Adaptation Methodology

Permission to adapt the health literacy toolkit was granted by Advancing Excellence in Health Care. A certified translator from English to Greek and a group of HL experts were identified to evaluate the terminology, and cultural appropriacy of the selected tools, supplementary material, and inclusion criteria for the tools were agreed upon. The inclusion criterion set was that the tool to be in accordance with national health system processes in Greece.

This pilot test method has already been used in the adaptation of HLUPT for cardiology and rheumatology [19]. Healthcare professionals were initially informed about the HLUPT tools during a 4 h webinar and were then asked to use the toolkit for a two-month period. The webinars were delivered online for two main reasons: to facilitate participation from different regions of Greece and to ensure safety due to pandemic restrictions. Overall, six webinars of 12–20 participants each were delivered from October 2021 to June 2022.

The content of the webinars derived from the work by Kripalani et al. [14] with permission to use and adapt the workshop material, "Strategies to improve communication between pharmacy staff and patients: A training program for pharmacy staff curriculum guide". The webinar included a theoretical section in the form of a presentation on the definition of HL, red flags for identifying older patients with low HL, and an introduction to the HL toolkit. The second section outlined the most important communication strategies (plain language, teach-back, summarizing the main message, and searching for online information). The third section consisted of role-playing exercises. Evaluation of the knowledge and communication skills was designed at baseline, after the end of the webinar, and for the small sample that implemented the adapted HLUPT after the end of a two-month period.

2.1.3. HLUPT Adaptation

In collaboration with the research team, a group of four HL experts evaluated the terminology and cultural appropriacy of the selected tools and supplementary material. The research team tailored the language to be culturally sensitive to Greek content and values and ensured the content was applicable to healthcare professionals working with older adults according to the ecological validity model (16).

In the pre-piloting phase, the research team excluded information regarding private insurance forms, nonmedical support and medical resources, referrals, and literacy and math resources (Table 1).

Table 1. Health Literacy Universal Precautions Toolkit (HLUPT) selected tools before piloting.

	Selected HLUPT to Be Adapted for Healthcare Professionals Working with Older Adults	Tools Selected for Piloting	Content Modifications Focusing on Healthcare Professionals Working with Older Adults
1	Tool 1. Form a team		Partially included in Tool 3
2	Tool 2. Create a health literacy improvement plan		Not included

Table 1. Cont.

	Selected HLUPT to Be Adapted for Healthcare Professionals Working with Older Adults	Tools Selected for Piloting	Content Modifications Focusing on Healthcare Professionals Working with Older Adults
3	Tool 3. Raise awareness (path of improvement)	Tool 1. Raise awareness (path of improvement) + annexes	• Use of simple language focusing on healthcare professionals working with older adults • Presentation adapted to Greek context • Role-playing adapted to Greek context • Links updated for Greek context, including training resources for healthcare professionals • HL quiz adapted to Greek context
4	Tool 4. Communicate clearly (spoken communication)	Tool 2. Communicate clearly (spoken communication) + annexes	• Use of simple language focusing on healthcare professionals working with older adults • Person-centered communication strategies and tailored communication tips for older adults focusing on older adults were added • Links to videos for person-centered care were added • Adaptation of annexes in Greek
5	Tool 5. Teach-back (spoken communication)	Tool 3. Teach-back (spoken communication)	• Use of simple language focusing on healthcare professionals working with older adults • Links subtitled in Greek • Links to teach-back training.org • Modifying the person experience targeting older patients • Evidence added in relation to the implementation of the technique for older adults
6	Tool 6. Follow-up with patients		Not included
7	Tool 7. Improve telephone access		Not included
8	Tool 8. Brown bag medicine reviews (spoken communication)	Tool 4. Brown bag medicine reviews (spoken communication)	• Use of simple language focusing on healthcare professionals working with older adults • Including tips for polypharmacy, older adults' rigid attitudes in the use of medication, naming of medication. Exclusion of terms irrelevant to Greek context (medicine reconciliation), American Institute manual, Ohio toolkit
9	Tool 9. Address language differences		• (Partially included in tool of cultural customs and beliefs)
10	Tool 10. Consider culture, customs, and beliefs, incl. points for language differences (spoken communication)	Tool 5. Consider culture, customs, and beliefs, incl. points for language differences (spoken communication)	• Use of simple language focusing on healthcare professionals working with older adults • Points from the tool of language differences were added • Associations working with refugees and migrants and associations working with older adults in Greece were added • Links to eLearning courses for cultural skills in Greek language
11	Tool 11. Assess, select, and create easy-to-understand materials (written communication)	Tool 6. Assess, select, and create easy-to-understand materials (written communication)	• Use of simple language focusing on healthcare professionals working with older adults • Use of HLS-EU evidence on health literacy and of OECD for literacy in Greece • Link of a Greek readability online tool developed by the Centre of Greek language • Links to eLearning courses and manuals to enhance digital skills of older adults (in Greek) and to use applications

Table 1. *Cont.*

	Selected HLUPT to Be Adapted for Healthcare Professionals Working with Older Adults	Tools Selected for Piloting	Content Modifications Focusing on Healthcare Professionals Working with Older Adults
12	Tool 12. Use health education material effectively (written communication)	Tool 7. Use health education material effectively (written communication)	• Updating terminology focusing on Web 2.0 • Links for the eLearning course eLILY1 focusing on ehealth literacy skills of carers working with older adults • Exclusion of nonrelevant examples
13	Tool 13. Welcome patients: helpful attitude, signs, and more		Not included
14	Tool 14. Encourage questions (self-management and empowerment)	Tool 8. Encourage questions (self-management and empowerment) + annexes	• Use of simple language focusing on healthcare professionals working with older adults • Type of questions that older adults should ask when visiting a clinical practice
15	Tool 15. Make action plans		Not included
16	Tool 16. Help patients remember how and when to take their medicine (self-management and empowerment)	Tool 9. Help patients remember how and when to take their medicine (self-management and empowerment) + annexes	• Use of simple language focusing on healthcare professionals working with older adults • Tips to help older people to take their medication (memory game, naming game) • Links to medication reminder applications
17	Tool 17. Get patient feedback (self-management and empowerment)	Tool 10. Get patient feedback (self-management and empowerment) + annexes	Use of simple language focusing on healthcare professionals working with older adults
18	Link patient to nonmedical support		Not included
19	Direct patients to medicine resources		Not included
20	Connect patients with literacy and math resources		Not included
21	Make referrals easy		Not included

2.2. Sample and Recruitment Process of the HLUPT Pilot Phase

Over 250 professionals were invited to participate in the pilot phase of the HLUPT. Recruitment followed a convenience and snowball sampling procedure, according to which professionals invited colleagues via social media, online groups, healthcare services, and university departments. The eligibility criteria for the healthcare professionals included: being a physician, nurse, psychologist, or other healthcare professional, speaking and writing in Greek, and working in a primary healthcare setting (e.g., hospital, day center, day clinic). Initially, 128 healthcare professionals registered to attend the webinar, and 82 completed the post-training assessment. The most common explanations for drop-out were time constraints and an abundance of responsibilities. Other reasons concerned organization barriers and the inability to comprehend the task of this phase. After the webinar, a small sample of healthcare professionals ($n = 24$) implemented the adapted HLUPT in their clinical practice for a two-month period. The healthcare professionals used up to three tools in their daily clinical practice for two months under the supervision of the research team. Short calls were scheduled with the researchers for questions or clarification. At the end of this two-month period, healthcare professionals evaluated their communication skills and knowledge of HL and participated in three focus groups.

Three focus groups were organized with 15 participants. The discussion was facilitated with the use of a guide that included questions regarding the HL toolkit and the way they used the selected HL tools (i.e., how they implemented the tools, barriers to implementation, evaluation of the practicality of the tools, suggestions of HL tools from the toolkit, written language of the toolkit, organization and staff attitudes toward the toolkit, and future training needs). The focus group sessions lasted between 40 and 60 min. The principal author (A.E.) served as a moderator and the second author (A.K.) as an observer.

2.3. Questionnaires Used in the HLUPT Pilot Phase

Demographic information (e.g., gender, age, education, profession, professional experience, and type of healthcare service) was obtained from healthcare professionals at baseline. To assess HL knowledge and communication skills, 13 Likert-type questions were adapted based on the research conducted by Mackert [20], including HL perceived knowledge, perceived ability to identify low-HL patients, communication skills, and one open question on the definition of HL.

Self-Efficacy-12 questionnaire was validated in Greek for the purpose of pilot test phase [21]. The questionnaire consists of 12 items measuring healthcare professionals' self-efficacy of skills used during the patient–clinician encounter, rated on a 10-point Likert scale ranging from 1 = very uncertain to 10 = very certain. The sum of scores ranges from 12–120, and higher scores indicate higher levels of self-efficacy in skills [22]. The first 10 items measure "self-efficacy in communication skills and strategies", and the last two items measure "self-efficacy of successful interaction". Both factors of the Greek version have shown high internal consistency (factor 1: $\alpha = 0.95$ and factor 2: $\alpha = 0.93$), similar to the total scale ($\alpha = 0.96$).

2.4. Statistical Analysis

Descriptive statistics and dependent sample t-tests were computed to compare the pre- and post-assessments. The Kruskal–Wallis test was used to compare baseline, post-, and follow-up scores for the sample of 24 healthcare professionals. Three focus group discussions evaluated the usefulness of the HL toolkit after implementing the selected tools for a two-month period. Transcribed scripts, derived from the focus group discussions, were content analyzed.

2.5. Ethics and Informed Consent

Permission to conduct the study was granted by the bioethics committee of the Hellenic Mediterranean University (63/EMΠ 95). All participants were fully informed of the study aims and the requirements for their participation in the study. Consent forms were signed before the pilot testing, and all participants were informed that they could withdraw their participation and that their data could be excluded by contacting the main investigator. Researchers in all phases of the study promoted the wellbeing of the participants. The researcher/trainer tried to make participants feel comfortable and resolve any kind of conflict. To safeguard sensitive personal data, a database protected by password was developed and stored on the research team's university computers; only members of the research team had access to the database.

3. Results

3.1. Descriptive Characteristics

Most of the participants who attended the webinars were women ($n = 120$, 93.8%) with tertiary and postgraduate education (N = 105, 82%), a mean age of 44 years old, and worked in public healthcare services ($n = 103$, 83%). Nurses ($n = 36$, 28.1%), health visitors ($n = 30$, 23.4%), and social workers ($n = 22$, 17.2%) were the professions with the highest representation in the sample. Physicians, physiotherapists, and occupational therapists had the lowest participation. Almost half of the sample had over 10 years of experience with older healthcare users (Table 2).

Table 2. Descriptive characteristics of the participants.

	Variable	N (%) Pretraining (n = 128)	N (%) Post-Training (n = 82)	N (%) Follow-Up (n = 24)	N (%) Focus Group (n = 15)
Sex	Women	120 (93.8)	77 (93.9)	23 (95.8)	14 (93.3)
	Men	8 (6.3)	5 (6.1)	1 (4.2)	1 (6.7)
Education	Secondary/upper secondary	17 (13.3)	9 (11)	3 (12.5)	1 (6.7)
	Tertiary	52 (40.6)	35 (42.7)	11 (45.8)	8 (53.3)
	Postgraduate	53 (41.4)	35 (42.7)	10 (41.7)	6 (40)
	Doctoral	6 (4.7)	3 (3.7)	0	0
Age		43.16 (SD = 8.76)	44.63 (SD = 7.07)	46.21 (SD = 7.25)	46 (SD = 7.25)
Profession	Physician	3 (2.3)	1 (1.2)	0	0
	Nurse	36 (28.1)	25 (30.5)	5 (20.8)	4 (26.7)
	Social worker	22 (17.2)	15 (18.3)	5 (20.8)	5 (33.3)
	Physiotherapist	1 (.8)	0	0	0
	Nurse assistant	7 (5.5)	2 (2.4)	1 (4.2)	0
	Psychologist	14 (10.9)	11 (13.4)	2 (8.3)	2 (13.3)
	Health visitor	30 (23.4)	16 (19.5)	5 (20.8)	0
	Other (occupational therapist, linguist, sociologist)	15 (23.4)	12 (14.6)	6 (25)	4 (26.7)
Type of service	Private	21 (16.9)	13 (15.9)	4 (16.7)	2 (13.3)
	Public	103 (83.1)	69 (84.1)	20 (83.3)	13 (86.7)
Professional experience	<1 year	9 (7.1)	3 (3.7)	1 (4.2)	0
	1—less than 2 years	16 (12.5)	7 (8.5)	1 (4.2)	1 (6.7)
	2—less than 5 years	20 (15.6)	11 (13.4)	2 (8.3)	1 (6.7)
	5—less than 10 years	12 (9.4)	9 (11)	1 (4.2)	1 (6.7)
	>10	69 (53.9)	51 (62.2)	18 (75)	12 (80)

3.2. HL Definition, Knowledge, and Communication Self-Efficacy

More than two-thirds of the healthcare professionals (n = 83, 64%) provided at baseline the HL definitions, whereas the remaining gave vague definitions of health, skills, knowledge, clinical diagnosis, and communication skills of healthcare professionals. Most of the respondents identified the ability to comprehend medical recommendations and treatment plans in order to make health decisions as the central aspect of the HL definition, while others identified the ability to comprehend medical jargon. Examples of the HL definitions follow:

"the skill to understand medical jargon and to use the internet to support your health";

"the skill to understand the therapeutic plan";

"the skill to understand and process health information to make health decisions".

In the post-test assessment (after the end of the webinar), 82 participants had statistically significantly improved their HL knowledge in all 13 of Mackert's interview items (Table 3).

Table 3. Mackert's interview items (n = 82).

	Pre-Assessment M	Pre-Assessment SD	Post Assessment M	Post Assessment SD	t-Test (df)
Q1. I understand what it means for patients to have low health literacy	5.74	1.3	6.63	0.59	−6.532 *** (80)
Q2. I know the prevalence of low health literacy in Greece	4.24	1.65	6.01	1.04	−8.709 *** (80)
Q3. I know the groups that are more likely to be low health literate	5.8	1.15	6.43	0.72	−8.579 *** (80)
Q4. I understand the health outcomes associated with low health literacy	5.19	1.28	6.59	0.58	−6.726 *** (80)
Q5. Identifying low health literate patients	5.19	1.28	6.21	0.77	−6.963 *** (80)

Table 3. Cont.

	Pre-Assessment		Post Assessment		
	M	SD	M	SD	t-Test (df)
Q6. Paying attention to whether or not my patients understand what I'm telling them	5.77	0.98	6.45	0.63	−6.457 *** (80)
Q7. Maintaining a culturally sensitive healthcare experience	5.8	0.89	6.51	0.69	−6.077 *** (80)
Q8. Speaking slowly	5.79	1.2	6.62	0.58	−6.141 *** (80)
Q9. Using plain nonmedical language	6.28	0.85	6.66	0.57	−3.592 ** (80)
Q10. Show or draw pictures	5	1.69	6.29	0.97	−6.754 *** (80)
Q11. Limit the amount of information provided and repeat it	5.64	1.22	6.46	0.81	−6.192 *** (80)
Q12. Use the teach-back or show me techniques	4.58	1.61	6.51 ()	0.74	−10.511 *** (80)
Q13. Create a shame-free environment	6.16	0.94	6.61	0.6	−4.698 *** (80)

*** $p < 0.001$, ** $p = 0.01$.

There was a significant difference in SE-12-Gr between the baseline scores (M = 92.1, SD = 13.62) and the post-assessment scores for the 82 participants (M = 104.24, SD = 10.82) (t = −11.127, df = 81, $p < 0.001$) (Table 4).

Table 4. Self-Efficacy-12-Gr (SE-12-Gr) in pre- and post-assessments ($n = 82$).

Variable	Pre-Assessment		Post-Assessment		t
	Mean Score	SD	Mean Score	SD	
SE-12-Gr total	92.1	13.62	104.24	10.82	−11.13 ***
SE-1	77.4	11.22	78	8.2	ns
SE-2	14.69	2.65	17.3	1.99	−10.41 ***

*** $p < 0.001$.

3.3. Implementation of HLUPT Tools in Clinical Practice

The sample that continued to the implementation of the three tools from the HLUPT for healthcare professionals working with older adults retained a higher rank mean (39.17) in the SE-12-Gr at the follow-up assessment compared with baseline (26.42) (Table 5).

Table 5. Self-Efficacy-12-Gr (SE-12-Gr) in pre-, post-, and follow-up assessments ($n = 24$).

Variable	Group	Rank Mean	Kruskal–Wallis
SE 12-GR SUM	Pre	26.42	
	Post	43.92	8.990 *
	Follow-up	39.17	
SE_1	Pre	32.33	
	Post	31.92	6.313
	Follow-up	45.25	
SE_2	Pre	24.08	
	Post	46.15	14.313
	Follow-up	39.27	

* $p < 0.05$.

3.4. Focus Group Discussions

Of the 15 participants in the three groups, 29% ($n = 7$) used the HL toolkit for less than a week, 25% ($n = 6$) for 1 to 2 weeks, and the remaining participants (46%; $n = 11$) from 1 to 2 months. Half of the participants in the focus groups reported using the HL toolkit frequently during the aforementioned periods.

Three themes were discussed: (1) the preferred tools, (2) ways to improve the toolkit, and (3) HL toolkit usefulness and health organization acceptance.

1. *Preferred tools.* The most preferred tool was "Tool 3. Teach-back method" (n = 9, 60%). Participants reported that they informed their coworkers, and they planned meetings

to do so whenever possible using available material and instructions from "Tool 1. Raise awareness" of the HLUPT. Healthcare professionals working at home preferred "Tool 4. Brown bag medication review" and "Tool 10. Assisting older adults with their medical treatment." "Tool 2. Clear communication" was also frequently selected and usually combined with "Tool 3". Only in one case did a healthcare professional living and working in a rural area favor "Tool 6. Cultural and linguistic differences."

2. *Ways to improve the toolkit.* Participants in the focus group suggested ways to enhance the HL toolkit:
   - to utilize exercises and images to facilitate comprehension of the tools;
   - to include components for older adults with memory deficiencies and dementia in "Tool 3. Teach-back method";
   - to introduce the concept of healthy and active aging;
   - to modify the toolkit for use by people working in the public and private sectors (e.g., banks, supermarkets, post offices);
   - to incorporate suggestions for healthcare professionals working with older adults who are illiterate in "Tool 10. Assisting older adults with their medical treatment";
   - to include a friendly service environment adaptation tool.

3. *HL toolkit usefulness and health organization support.* All the participants in the focus group assessed the HL toolkit as very useful and its resources as comprehensible. They acknowledged that they had to acquire this knowledge through practice with older adults. Participants reported that the toolkit could be a valuable resource for young healthcare professionals starting their careers and for older people to gain new knowledge. They discussed the difficulty in establishing an HL team within their organization because of social distance measures and relevant restrictions imposed by the COVID-19 pandemic (i.e., could not meet regularly with their colleagues). They also had difficulty approaching their experienced colleagues. In addition, frequent changes in supervisors/managers in public healthcare services posed a potential barrier to their efforts to raise HL awareness among the organization's staff. The final adapted toolkit is available in Table 6.

Table 6. Final adapted HLUPT for healthcare professionals working with older adults.

Final Adapted HLUPT Tool After Follow-Up	Content Modification
Tool 1. Raise awareness (path of improvement)	• HLS-EU_Q16 added in annexes • Personal experience from day center for older adults • Planning seminars for older people visiting the day center • Include points of healthy aging as part of the awareness presentation and address society, not only healthcare services
Tool 2. Communicate clearly (spoken communication)	Personal experience from day center for older adults
Tool 3. Teach-back (spoken communication)	Use of teach-back method for people with mild cognitive impairment—facilitate them with clinical appointment
Tool 4. Brown bag medicine reviews (spoken communication)	Personal experience from day center for older adults: facilitate older adults and carers to name their medicines as a memory game
Tool 5. Consider culture, customs, and beliefs, incl. points for language differences (spoken communication)	The role of rural communities and how they might influence older adults' literacy
Tool 6. Assess, select, and create easy-to-understand materials (written communication)	No modification
Tool 7. Use health education material effectively (written communication)	No modification
Tool 8. Welcome patients: helpful attitude, signs, and more	Many healthcare services are not user-friendly; this tool may be useful for them
Tool 9. Encourage questions (self-management and empowerment)	Personal experience from day center and home care for older adults

Table 6. *Cont.*

Final Adapted HLUPT Tool After Follow-Up	Content Modification
Tool 10. Help patients remember how and when to take their medicine (self-management and empowerment)	• Personal experience from day center for older adults • Tips to help older people take their medication when their literacy level is low (e.g., draw images)
Tool 11. Get patient feedback (self-management and empowerment)	Added

4. Discussion

The purpose of the study was the adaptation of a HL toolkit for healthcare professionals working with older adults. This study provided a toolkit written in plain language with examples of everyday clinical practice provided by healthcare professionals. After the 4 h webinars in the framework of the toolkit piloting, healthcare professionals improved their communication self-efficacy and HL knowledge, and this finding remained after the 2-month follow-up for the healthcare professionals who implemented the toolkit in their clinical practice.

There are HL training courses and tools targeting healthcare professionals and physicians [14,23–26], but there is a lack of courses and tools targeting healthcare professionals working with older adults [17]. Older adults are considered an at-risk population with low HL, facing difficulty in adhering to the therapeutic plan and effectively communicating with healthcare professionals [4,5,27]. They face multiple health issues and are usually excluded by healthcare professionals from the decision-making process [28,29].

The findings of this study were valid and reliable. The three stages of the cultural adaptation process model [23] were as follows: setting the scene, planning the adaptation, and proceeding with the adaptation and pilot test. Our findings are in line with Mackert et al.'s [20] findings, according to which, on the one hand, participants overestimated their HL knowledge, and on the other hand, their knowledge improved after a training course. Similar studies assessing self-efficacy in communication found that it was improved after communication skills training of physicians and nurses [29]. Two-thirds of the participants in the present study were aware of and identified aspects of the HL concept (e.g., understanding health information, making health decisions, communication with physicians, and medical adherence).

Healthcare professionals perceived the HL toolkit as a valuable, easy-to-use resource in everyday clinical practice, and they contributed their expertise to the focus groups to improve the toolkit. The most preferred tools included "Tool 1. Raise awareness," "Tool 2. Communicate clearly," "Tool 3. Teach-back method," "Tool 5. Brown bag medication review," and "Tool 10. Assisting older adults with their medical treatment." Callahan et al. [19] recognized the teach-back method and brown bag medication review as the most frequently used tools to raise awareness among staff. Older adults' medication adherence is considered an important dimension of the healthcare professionals' clinical work and usually is reported as the most difficult issue to handle in the older adults' caregiving process [30].

Limitations of this study were the small number of medical professionals in the adaptation process and the small number of participants in the follow-up phase. For this reason, the results of the study concerning the specific sample could not be generalized to other healthcare professionals. The strength of the study included the involvement of healthcare professionals in all phases of the adaptation process and providing a toolkit tailored to the healthcare professionals' needs. During the focus group discussions with older healthcare users regarding their interaction with healthcare professionals, they mostly focused on physicians' input [13], and physicians were the least represented healthcare professional group in our sample. In addition, lack of funding prevented the linguistic adaptation of audiovisual materials that were included in the HLUPT. All video links were added to the toolkit, along with a note instructing users to enable subtitles when applicable.

Primary healthcare in Greece is delivered through public and private services, and healthcare users need to find and appraise healthcare services without any support from the healthcare system [31]. They need to decide on the proper healthcare professional specialty and healthcare department [31]. HL is a concept not fully appraised by health organizations in Greece, even if more and more discussions on the topic have been raised after the COVID-19 pandemic.

Future research could focus on the effectiveness of the HL toolkit within the context of healthcare professional practice and the adaptation of the toolkit to other high-risk populations (e.g., migrants). HL training among healthcare professionals builds networks, promotes HL leadership, empowers professionals, and builds HL organizations [32].

5. Conclusions

Public healthcare services could adopt the HL toolkit to support the training needs of primary care healthcare professionals [32]. We consider that the HL toolkit provides a set of 11 tools tailored to the needs of healthcare professionals working in the Greek context. The HL toolkit could assist healthcare professionals in their everyday clinical work, be part of vocational and educational seminars, and be promoted within the healthcare organizational context. The use of the HL toolkit will facilitate the clinical work of healthcare professionals working with older adults, and indirectly, it is expected to enhance the HL of older adults.

Author Contributions: Conceptualization, A.E.; methodology, A.E. and A.K.; validation, A.E., A.K. and M.R.; formal analysis, A.E.; investigation, A.E. and A.K.; writing—original draft preparation, A.E.; writing—review and editing, A.K. and M.R.; supervision, A.K.; project administration, A.E.; funding acquisition, A.E. All authors have read and agreed to the published version of the manuscript.

Funding: This research was funded by Hellenic Mediterranean University, grant number 67NH46MH2I-IΛ7.

Institutional Review Board Statement: The study was conducted in accordance with the Declaration of Helsinki and approved by the ethics committee of Hellenic Mediterranean University (protocol code 63 and 23 June 2021) for studies involving humans.

Informed Consent Statement: Informed consent was obtained from all subjects involved in the study.

Data Availability Statement: Data are unavailable due to privacy.

Acknowledgments: We would like to acknowledge the healthcare professionals who participated in all phases of the research and provided their valuable feedback on this work.

Conflicts of Interest: The authors declare no conflict of interest.

References

1. World Health Organization (WHO). *Health Literacy: The Solid Facts*; World Health Organization: Geneva, Switzerland, 2013; Available online: https://apps.who.int/iris/bitstream/handle/10665/128703/e96854.pdf (accessed on 17 May 2020).
2. Howard, D.H.; Gazmararian, J.; Parker, R.M. The impact of low health literacy on the medical costs of Medicare managed care enrollees. *Am. J. Med.* **2005**, *118*, 371–377. [CrossRef] [PubMed]
3. VandenBosch, J.; Van den Broucke, S.; Vancorenland, S.; Avalosse, H.; Verniest, R.; Callens, M. Health literacy and the use of healthcare services in Belgium. *J. Epidemiol. Commun. Health* **2016**, *70*, 1032–1038. [CrossRef]
4. Chesser, A.K.; Woods, N.K.; Smothers, K.; Rogers, N. Health Literacy and Older Adults. *Gerontol. Geriatr. Med.* **2016**, *2*, 1–13. [CrossRef] [PubMed]
5. Speros, C. More than Words: Promoting Health Literacy in Older Adults. *OJIN Online J. Issues Nurs.* **2009**, *14*. [CrossRef]
6. Healthy People 2030. Healthy People 2030 Objectives: Older People. U.S. Department of Health and Human Services. Available online: https://health.gov/healthypeople/objectives-and-data/browse-objectives/older-adults (accessed on 26 February 2021).
7. Ford, J.A.; Wong, G.; Jones, A.P.; Steel, N. Access to primary care for socioeconomically disadvantaged older people in rural areas: A realist review. *BMJ Open* **2016**, *6*, e010652. [CrossRef] [PubMed]
8. Wang, L.; Guruge, S.; Montana, G. Older Immigrants' Access to Primary Health Care in Canada: A Scoping Review. *Can. J. Aging/La Rev. Can. Vieil.* **2019**, *38*, 193–209. [CrossRef]
9. Bodenheimer, T.; Pham, H.H. Primary Care: Current Problems and Proposed Solutions. *Health Aff.* **2010**, *29*, 799–805. [CrossRef]
10. Ryskina, K.L.; Shultz, K.; Zhou, Y.; Lautenbach, G.; Brown, R.T. Older adults' access to primary care: Gender, racial, and ethnic disparities in telemedicine. *J. Am. Geriatr. Soc.* **2021**, *69*, 2732–2740. [CrossRef]

11. World Health Organisation. *The Ottawa Charter for Health Promotion*; WHO: Geneva, Switzerland, 1986.
12. Brach, C.; Keller, D.; Hernandez, L.M.; Baur, C.; Parker, R.; Dreyer, B.; Schyve, P.; Lemerise, A.J.; Schillinger, D. Ten Attributes of Health Literate Health Care Organizations. Discussion Paper. Available online: https://nam.edu/wp-content/uploads/2015/06/BPH_Ten_HLit_Attributes.pdf (accessed on 1 March 2023).
13. Efthymiou, A.; Rovithis, M.; Kalaitzaki, A. The Perspectives on Barriers and Facilitators in Communication by the Healthcare Professionals and Older Healthcare Users: The Role of Health Literacy. *J. Psychol. Psychother. Res.* **2022**, *9*, 1–11. [CrossRef]
14. Kripalani, S.; Jacobson, K.L. Strategies to Improve Communication between Pharmacy Staff and Patients: A Training Program for Pharmacy Staff Curriculum Guide. Agency for Healthcare Research and Quality. 2007. Available online: https://www.ahrq.gov/health-literacy/improve/pharmacy/guide/train.html (accessed on 22 February 2021).
15. DeWalt, D.A.; Broucksou, K.A.; Hawk, V.; Brach, C.; Hink, A.; Rudd, R.; Callahan, L. Developing and testing the health literacy universal precautions toolkit. *Nurs. Outlook* **2011**, *59*, 85–94. [CrossRef]
16. Brega, A.; Barnard, J.; Mabachi, N.M.; Weiss, B.D.; DeWalt, D.A.; Brach, C.; Cifuentes, M.; Albright, K.; West, D.R. *Health Literacy Universal Precautions Toolkit*, 2nd ed; AHRQ Publication: Rockville, MD, USA, 2015. Available online: http://www.ahrq.gov/qual/literacy/healthliteracytoolkit.pdf (accessed on 1 March 2023).
17. Efthymiou, A.; Kalaitzaki, A.; Kondilis, B. Health literacy continuing education courses and tools for healthcare professionals: A scoping review. *Gerontol. Geriatr. Educ.* **2022**, 1–36. [CrossRef]
18. Rodríguez, M.M.D.; Baumann, A.A.; Schwartz, A.L. Cultural Adaptation of an Evidence Based Intervention: From Theory to Practice in a Latino/a Community Context. *Am. J. Community Psychol.* **2010**, *47*, 170–186. [CrossRef]
19. Callahan, L.F.; Hawk, V.; Rudd, R.; Hackney, B.; Bhandari, S.; Prizer, L.P.; Bauer, T.K.; Jonas, B.; Mendys, P.; DeWalt, D. Adaptation of the health literacy universal precautions toolkit for rheumatology and cardiology—Applications for pharmacy professionals to improve self-management and outcomes in patients with chronic disease. *Res. Soc. Adm. Pharm.* **2013**, *9*, 597–608. [CrossRef]
20. Mackert, M.; Ball, J.; Lopez, N. Health literacy awareness training for healthcare workers: Improving knowledge and intentions to use clear communication techniques. *Patient Educ. Couns.* **2011**, *85*, e225–e228. [CrossRef]
21. Efthymiou, A.; Rovithis, M.; Kalaitzaki, A. The Healthcare Professionals' Self-reported Communication Skills with Older Healthcare Users in Greece: Validation of the Self-efficacy Questionnaire (SE-12-Gr). *Health Commun.* (in review).
22. Axboe, M.K.; Christensen, K.S.; Kofoed, P.-E.; Ammentorp, J. Development and validation of a self-efficacy questionnaire (SE-12) measuring the clinical communication skills of health care professionals. *BMC Med. Educ.* **2016**, *16*, 1–10. [CrossRef]
23. IMPACCT Erasmus+. Working with Patients with Limited Health Literacy. Future Learn. 2017. Available online: https://www.futurelearn.com/courses/working-health-literacy (accessed on 20 February 2021).
24. University at Albany Centre for Public Health Continuing Education (Organisation), PHTC ONLINE: Health Literacy and Public Health Training. 2006. Available online: https://phtc-online.org/learning/?seriesId=4&status=all&sort=group (accessed on 20 February 2021).
25. Center of Disease Control. Effective Communication for Healthcare Teams: Addressing HL, Limited English Proficiency and Cultural Difference. CDC TRAIN. 2019. Available online: https://www.train.org/cdctrain/course/1077848/ (accessed on 24 February 2021).
26. Centre of Disease Control. Health Literacy for Public Health Professionals—WB4031R. CDC TRAIN. 2018. Available online: https://www.train.org/cdctrain/course/1078759/?activeTab=reviews (accessed on 20 February 2021).
27. Sudore, R.L.; Mehta, K.M.; Simonsick, E.M.; Harris, T.B.; Newman, A.B.; Satterfield, S.; Rosano, C.; Rooks, R.N.; Rubin, S.M.; Ayonayon, H.N.; et al. Limited Literacy in Older People and Disparities in Health and Healthcare Access. *J. Am. Geriatr. Soc.* **2006**, *54*, 770–776. [CrossRef]
28. James, B.D.; Boyle, P.A.; Bennett, J.S.; Bennett, D.A. The Impact of Health and Financial Literacy on Decision Making in Community-Based Older Adults. *Gerontology* **2012**, *58*, 531–539. [CrossRef]
29. Mata, N.D.S.; de Azevedo, K.P.M.; Braga, L.P.; de Medeiros, G.C.B.S.; Segundo, V.H.D.O.; Bezerra, I.N.M.; Pimenta, I.D.S.F.; Nicolás, I.M.; Piuvezam, G. Training in communication skills for self-efficacy of health professionals: A systematic review. *Hum. Resour. Health* **2021**, *19*, 1–9. [CrossRef]
30. Smaje, A.; Weston-Clark, M.; Raj, R.; Orlu, M.; Davis, D.; Rawle, M. Factors associated with medication adherence in older patients: A systematic review. *Aging Med.* **2018**, *1*, 254–266. [CrossRef]
31. Lionis, C.; Papadakis, S.; Tatsi, C.; Bertsias, A.; Duijker, G.; Mekouris, P.-B.; Boerma, W.; Schäfer, W. Informing primary care reform in Greece: Patient expectations and experiences (the QUALICOPC study). *BMC Health Serv. Res.* **2017**, *17*, 255. [CrossRef]
32. Naccarella, L.; Murphy, B. Key lessons for designing health literacy professional development courses. *Aust. Health Rev.* **2018**, *42*, 36. [CrossRef] [PubMed]

Disclaimer/Publisher's Note: The statements, opinions and data contained in all publications are solely those of the individual author(s) and contributor(s) and not of MDPI and/or the editor(s). MDPI and/or the editor(s) disclaim responsibility for any injury to people or property resulting from any ideas, methods, instructions or products referred to in the content.

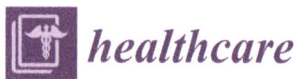

Article

The Effects of the Ukrainian Conflict on Oncological Care: The Latest State of the Art

Emma Altobelli [1,*], Paolo Matteo Angeletti [1,2], Giovanni Farello [1] and Reimondo Petrocelli [3]

1 Department of Life, Public Health and Environmental Sciences, University of L'Aquila, 67100 L'Aquila, Italy
2 Cardiac Surgical Intensive Care Unit, Giuseppe Mazzini Hospital, 64100 Teramo, Italy
3 Public Health Unit, ASREM, 86100 Campobasso, Italy
* Correspondence: emma.altobelli@univaq.it; Tel.: +39-0862-434666; Fax: +39-0862-432903

Abstract: Background: The COVID-19 pandemic has dramatically affected all aspects of the patient's pathway to cancer diagnosis and subsequent treatment. Our main objective was to evaluate the status of cancer trials in Ukraine as of September 2022. Methods: Initially, we examined with a narrative review the state of breast, colorectal, and cervical cancer population-based screening. Subsequently, we assessed each trial status for the years 2021 and 2022. Results: Estimates of participation in breast and cervical cancer screening are different from region to region. Moreover, regarding cervical cancer screening, extremely different participation estimates were reported: 73% in 2003 vs. <10% 2020. Our data show that from 2014 to 2020, despite the pandemic, cancer trials in Ukraine significantly increased from 27 to 44. In 2021 no trials were completed; in fact, we observed that out of 41 trials, 8 were active not recruiting, 33 were recruiting, and 0 were completed or terminated. In 2022 in Ukraine, for oncological pathologies, only 3 trials were registered, while in 2021, 41 trials were registered. The suspension of trials regarded above all concern hematological tissue (66.7%) and the genitourinary tract (60%). Conclusions: Our work has highlighted how the areas most affected by the conflict present criticalities in oncological care.

Keywords: health; randomized clinical trials; RCT; cancers; war; Ukraine

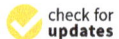

Citation: Altobelli, E.; Angeletti, P.M.; Farello, G.; Petrocelli, R. The Effects of the Ukrainian Conflict on Oncological Care: The Latest State of the Art. *Healthcare* **2023**, *11*, 283. https://doi.org/10.3390/healthcare11030283

Academic Editors: Sofia Koukouli and Areti Stavropoulou

Received: 28 November 2022
Revised: 9 January 2023
Accepted: 14 January 2023
Published: 17 January 2023

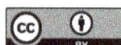

Copyright: © 2023 by the authors. Licensee MDPI, Basel, Switzerland. This article is an open access article distributed under the terms and conditions of the Creative Commons Attribution (CC BY) license (https://creativecommons.org/licenses/by/4.0/).

1. Introduction

Cancers are a major contributor to disease burden worldwide, and projections forecast that global cancer burden will continue to grow for at least the next two decades [1–4]. There is a need for reducing cancer burden by one third and for reducing premature mortality from noncommunicable diseases [NCDs] through prevention and treatment [5]. It is known that population-based screening of breast, colorectal, and cervical cancer are an important secondary prevention means, they have been slowed down globally because of the priorities required by the "pandemic". Therefore, COVID-19 disease has affected in the worldwide all aspects of the patient's pathway to cancer diagnosis and subsequent treatment [6]. It is important to underline that non-communicable diseases in Ukraine represent a total of 80% of mortality and, in the age group between 30 and 69, they represent the leading cause of death. Before the hostilities with Russia, about 13,000 new diagnoses of cancer were diagnosed in Ukraine [7]. The development of the conflict has led to the displacement of a large number of patients to western regions and to foreign countries [8]. The impact of conflicts on the care of people with cancer has highlighted how there is a fragmentation due to the inability of humanitarian aid to cover all needs and the excessive burden that is created in the arrival countries of refugees [8]. The outbreak of the war did not catch regulatory agencies unprepared, even in light of the recent pandemic, which made it possible to make follow-ups more flexible. In particular, patients were reallocated in Europe, where possible, trying to keep the quality of information high [9].

The clinical trial is a fundamental tool for oncologic therapy. Today, free consultation of protocols, funders, and sites where the research is conducted is possible through the clinicaltrial.gov site. The clinicaltrial.gov, managed by the U.S. National Library of Medicine currently records more than 430,000 studies for 222 nations [10]. From 2000 to 2020, the trials steadily increased from 2786 per year to 671,228 per year [11].

A study has shown that about 80% of participants in clinical trials belong to high-income countries [12], while 70% of cancer deaths occur in low and medium-income countries [13]. The choice to conduct a clinical trial in a low-income country involves lower overall costs and it may represent an opportunity to care for the local population. Ukraine is a medium-low-income country and before the Russian invasion, Ukraine was considered an optimal destination for clinical trials. It has, in fact, become an attractive country for companies wishing to carry out clinical trials since 1996 (investigative report by the NGO Public Eye published in 2013) mainly due to its lower costs and some less demanding local legislative practices [14].

The objectives of our research are: (i) to conduct a narrative review of the literature on the art layer of the three tumors subjected to population-based screening; (ii) evaluate the development of cancer trials in Ukraine in the 2014–2022 period; and (iii) assess the impact of the conflict on active trials in Ukraine in the two-year period from 2021 to 2022, and examine the types of cancer for which the trials were most affected by the war.

2. Materials and Methods

Initially, a narrative review of the literature on the art layer of the three tumors subjected to population-based screening (breast, colorectal cancer and cervix) and HPV vaccination was conducted in order to highlight the pre-conflict Russian-Ukraine" situation and identify any changes that occurred during the conflict (Table 1).

Subsequently, we assessed the "state of the art" with regards to clinical trials in Ukraine. A search was conducted using the clinicaltrial.gov portal, using the terms "Cancer" and "Ukraine" as of 18 May 2022. The database was queried starting from 2014 in order to assess the number of trials registered in Ukraine since the beginning of hostilities with Russia in 2022. The resident population in Ukraine was considered, according to world bank data, and the number of active trials with respect to the resident population.

Each trial status was assessed for the years 2021 and 2022 regarding the following: active/suspended/terminated/not yet recruiting/completed/unknow status, the geographic region, the linguistic predominance, according to the last Ukrainian census [15,16] and type of tumor under study.

Table 1. Situation on cancers early detection program in Ukraine before the 2022 war.

Cancer [17]	Incidence [17]	Mortality [17]	Data Quality [17]		Before War
			Incidence	Mortality	
Breast	11.8	8.4%	High	Medium	• An opportunistic screening program is present for woman >50 years old [17]. • A 2018 report showed the capacity of the system to detect an early stage of tumor is widely different among Ukraine regions from 95 % of Vinnytska Region to only 60% Luhanska [18].
Cervical	3.5%	2.5%	High	Medium	• An opportunistic screening program is present. In 2020 Screening participation rates are <10% (WHO) [17], while in 2003 was reported a participation rate 73.7% in all women aged 25–64, screened every 3 y [19]. • No plans for HPV vaccination were implemented [19].
Colorectal	13.1%	14.0%	High	Medium	• No plans for screening were adopted. A large study showed that 50.9% with colon cancer, 60.7% with rectal and anal cancers presented at disease stages 1 and 2 [18]. • The data on Crimea, Donetska, and Luganska Oblast (region) were missing in 2014 and 2015 because of political instability [20].

We also analyzed the 2021 trials status in two different moments (the first in May and the second in September 2022).

Differences between frequencies were assessed using chi-square or Fisher exact tests where appropriated.

Finally, to highlight distribution of trials among the various oblasts we have presented maps according to trials grouped by the following classes: >10; 5–10; 1–5; (Figure 1, Panel A) and number of trials according to status for each Ukrainian oblast' (Figure 1, Panel B).

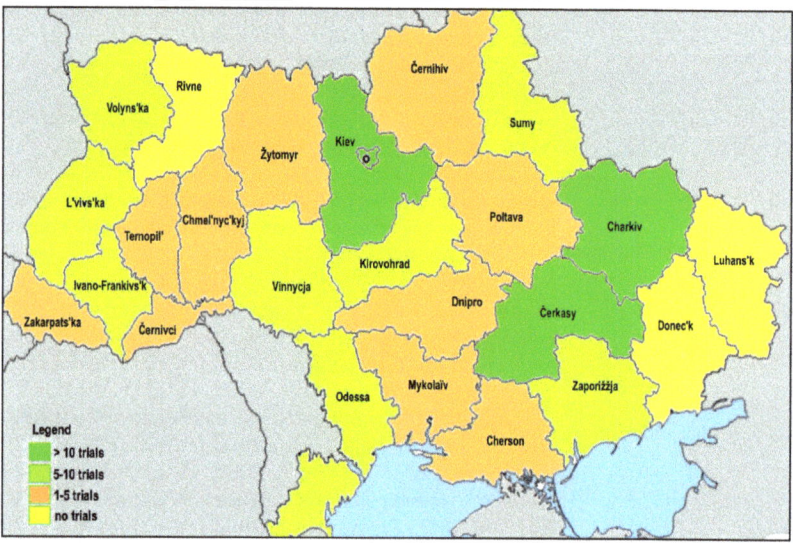

Panel A.

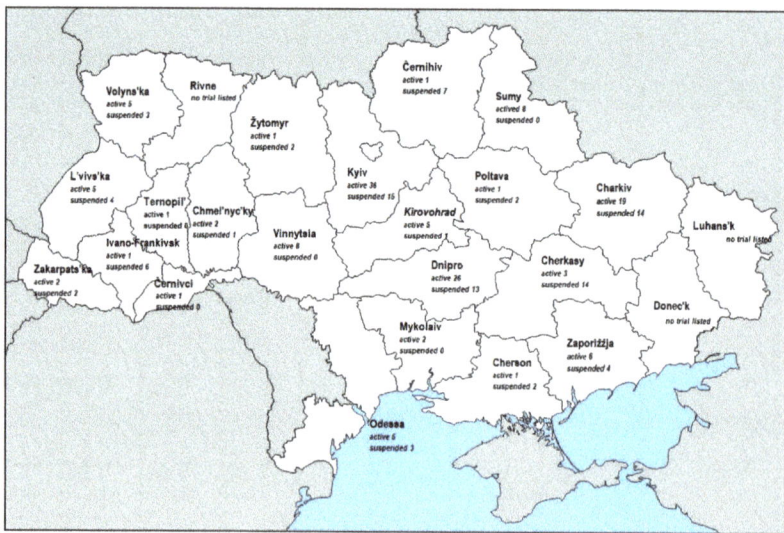

Panel B.

Figure 1. (**A**) Map according to trials grouped by following classes: >10; 5–10; 1–5. (**B**) Number of trials according to status for each Ukrainian oblast' as of 5 May 2022.

3. Results

As reported in Table 1, pre-conflict screening programs in Ukraine were conducted on a spontaneous basis (no population-based screening program). Estimates of participation in breast and cervical cancer screening are different from region to region. Moreover, extremely different participation estimates have been reported for over a decade regarding cervical cancer screening (73% in 2003 vs. <10%) in the WHO data 2020. Yet, with respect to the latter, there are no HPV vaccination campaigns. Primary prevention for colorectal cancer was also absent before the war.

In the period considered, the incidence of cancer in Ukraine remained constant, and on the contrary, mortality decreased (Table S1) [21].

The number of cancer trials registered in Ukraine from 2014 to 2020 has been steadily increasing, going from 27 in 2014 to 44 in 2020. In terms of incidence ratio on the total resident population, it has gone from 0.60 to values of 1.0 compared to the latest proliferation data available in 2020 (Table S1). 275 trials involved adult patients and 16 children (Table S1). It is important to underline that in 2021 no trials were completed; in fact, we observed that out of 41 trials, 8 were active and not recruiting, 33 were recruiting, and 0 were completed or terminated (Table S1). In 2022 in Ukraine, only 3 trials were registered for oncological pathologies, while 41 were registered in 2021.

The comparison between the two periods analyzed showed a reduction of not recruiting trials in May 2022 respect to September 2021 from 4% to 27% (Tables S2 and S3).

Regarding Russian and Ukrainian speaking geographical areas, and furthermore center, east, west and south regions, no statistically significant differences were found (Tables 2 and 3).

Table 2. Numbers of registered trials in 2021 according to different speaking areas and status (active/suspended) as of May and September 2022.

Status as of May and September 2022	Russian Speaking Areas	Ukrainian Speaking Areas	Total	Test
May				
Active	54 (37.2)	91 (62.8)	145	
Suspended	27 (34.2)	54 (65.8)	81	$X^2 = 0.21, p = 0.66$
			224	
September				
Active	69 (38.1)	112 (61.9)	181	
Suspended	23 (28.4)	58 (71.6)	81	$X^2 = 2.32, p = 0.13$
			262	

Table 3. Numbers of registered trials in 2021 according to different geographical areas (center, east, west, south) and status (active/suspended) as of May and September 2022.

Areas	Active	Suspended	Tot	Test
May				
Center	55 (65.5)	29 (34.5)	84	
West	27 (60.0)	18 (40.0)	45	$X^2 = 0.21, p = 0.64$
East	20 (66.5)	12 (37.5)	32	
South	43 (68.3)	20 (31.7)	63	
September				
Center	59 (63.4)	34 (36.5)	93	
West	44 (67.7)	21 (32.3)	65	$X^2 = 3.45, p = 0.33$
East	29 (78.3)	8 (21.7)	37	
South	49 (73.1)	18 (26.9)	67	

Regarding tumor affected sites, the suspension of trials belonged above all to hematological tissue (66.7%) and the genitourinary tract (60%); in fact, there is a statistically significant difference ($p = 0.034$) (Table 4).

Table 4. Numbers of registered trials in 2021 according to status and diagnosis.

Tumors	Active	Suspended	Total
Gender-related	9 (100.0)	0 (0.0)	9
Gastro-intestinal	3 (60.0)	2 (40.0)	5
Hematological	2 (33.3)	4 (66.7)	6
Lung	4 (66.7)	2 (33.3)	8
Urinary tract	2 (40.0)	3 (60.0)	5
$X^2 = 15.74, p = 0.034$			

4. Discussion

With the COVID-19 pandemic, the world population has experienced high levels of stress both from a physical and psychological point of view. The Russian-Ukrainian war is now a new additional stressor. In fact, the impact of the war has repercussions on different areas of life, such as social and economic areas with the increase in the prices of energy, food, and raw materials. The healthcare system has therefore significantly been influenced. Compared to the latter, a significant fact is that only 36.08% of the Ukrainian population received the COVID-19 vaccination and of these, most received only two doses. This means a higher risk of mortality from COVID-19 [22]. Furthermore, children in conflict zones suffer the most since they do not receive necessary vaccinations [23]. In fact, it also is important to underline the Ukrainian polio outbreak from 2014 to 2017 [24] and likewise the measles outbreak in 2016 [25].

Therefore, we can stress that although Ukraine has spent most of its resources defending itself against the Russian invasion, it has now become exposed to multiple infectious diseases [23], some of which are known to be risk factors for the genesis of some cancers.

As highlighted by the review (Table 1) there is no HPV vaccination campaign: in fact, cervical cancer is the fourth most common among women [26].

It is important to underline that the development of the conflict has involved the displacement of a large number of patients to western regions and to foreign countries [8]. With regard to screening, some initiatives in refugee host countries such as the Netherlands should be highlighted [27].

The impact of conflicts on the care of people with cancer has recently been studied in the Syrian and Iraqi conflict: it has been highlighted that there is a fragmentation of care due to the inability of humanitarian aid in countries of refugee arrival [8]. Regarding cancer incidence, it should be remembered that the incidence rates of common cancers in Ukraine increased during 2003–2012, and Ryzhov et al. predicted an overall 18% increase in the number of cancer cases from 2012 to 2022 [24]. In addition, in Ukraine there are no organized screening programs [28–30]. In fact, the absence of screening programs is a feature common to several ex-Soviet countries [31], although in recent decades more progress has been made both at the diagnostic level (by adapting diagnostic techniques with those of other European countries) and organizational level [31].

Our main objective is to provide a report on the status of cancer trials in Ukraine since the beginning of the war in September 2022. Our data show that from 2014 to 2020, despite the pandemic, cancer trials in Ukraine significantly increased from 27 to 44. As van Rosmalen et al. [32] underlined, this growth trend was in line with the worldwide increase in trials. These data are also consistent compared to what is shown by the International Clinical Trials Registry of the WHO Platform (ICTRP), which shows an overall increase in trials in Ukraine from 1999 to 2021: in particular, malignant neoplasms represented 24% of all trials registered [11]. Our work has highlighted how the areas most affected by the conflict present a greater suspension of oncology trials, in particular in Phase 3, in which safety and effectiveness of a new treatment is tested against the current standard treatment. As reported by Ryzohv et al. [31], the incidence of cancer in Ukraine will increase by 14% in males and 21% in females, compared to the previous decade. In light of this, a consideration in our opinion is important. The oncological problem in Ukraine is also linked to the Chernobyl nuclear accident. In fact, Zupunski, et al. [33], showed that in the 5 years following the nuclear accident there was a significant increase in breast cancer in neighboring areas. If the war continues for much longer, the repercussions could be dramatic for people attending Ukrainian studies, for whom a trial is often the last hope against cancer.

5. Conclusions

Despite new therapies and increased awareness of risk factors, it is very likely that there will be a faster increase in new cancer cases in the years to come. Structural factors, such as the aging of the population, and contingent situations such as the pandemic and the war in Ukraine will play a significant role. Nonetheless, this last one did not catch regulatory agencies unprepared (even in light of the recent pandemic which made follow-ups more flexible). In fact, it was possible to reallocate patients to Western Europe, where possible, trying to keep the quality of information high [9]. However, it should be emphasized that it is currently impossible to assess the long-term impacts on drug research because it is difficult to maintain strict clinical trial protocols while hospitals are bombed.

Last but not least, there is the drama of oncological children. With the first bombings, their situation worsened further, since they were transferred from the clinics to basements, which initially, before humanitarian interventions, certainly complicated their treatments.

The future looks very uncertain indeed.

Supplementary Materials: The following supporting information can be downloaded at: https://www.mdpi.com/article/10.3390/healthcare11030283/s1.

Author Contributions: Conceptualization, E.A.; methodology, E.A. and P.M.A.; data curation, R.P. and G.F.; writing—original draft preparation, E.A. and P.M.A.; writing—review and editing, E.A., P.M.A., R.P. and G.F. All authors have read and agreed to the published version of the manuscript.

Funding: This research received no external funding.

Data Availability Statement: Publicly available datasets [2] were analyzed in this study.

Conflicts of Interest: The authors declare no conflict of interest.

References

1. Foreman, K.J.; Marquez, N.; Dolgert, A.; Fukutaki, K.; Fullman, N.; McGaughey, M.; Pletcher, M.A.; Smith, A.E.; Tang, K.; Yuan, C.W.; et al. Forecasting life expectancy, years of life lost, and all-cause and cause-specific mortality for 250 causes of death: Reference and alternative scenarios for 2016-40 for 195 countries and territories. *Lancet* **2018**, *392*, 2052–2090. [CrossRef] [PubMed]
2. Bray, F.; Jemal, A.; Grey, N.; Ferlay, J.; Forman, D. Global cancer transitions according to the Human Development Index (2008–2030): A population-based study. *Lancet Oncol.* **2012**, *13*, 790–801. [CrossRef] [PubMed]
3. International Agency for Research on Cancer. World Cancer Report: Cancer Research for Cancer Prevention. Available online: https://publications.iarc.fr/Non-Series-Publications/World-Cancer-Reports/World-Cancer-Report-Cancer-Research-For-Cancer-Prevention-2020 (accessed on 1 March 2021).
4. Sung, H.; Ferlay, J.; Siegel, R.L.; Laversanne, M.; Soerjomataram, I.; Jemal, A.; Bray, F. Global Cancer Statistics 2020: GLOBOCAN Estimates of Incidence and Mortality Worldwide for 36 Cancers in 185 Countries. *CA Cancer J. Clin.* **2021**, *71*, 209–249. [CrossRef] [PubMed]
5. United Nations. Sustainable Development Goals. Available online: https://sdgs.un.org (accessed on 3 March 2021).
6. Helsper, C.W.; Campbell, C.; Emery, J.; Neal, R.D.; Li, L.; Rubin, G.; van Weert, H.; Vedsted, P.; Walter, F.M.; Weller, D.; et al. Cancer has not gone away: A primary care perspective to support a balanced approach for timely cancer diagnosis during COVID-19. *Eur. J. Cancer Care* **2020**, *29*, e13290. [CrossRef] [PubMed]
7. Sullivan, R. What Impact Does War Have on Ukrainian Cancer Care? King's College London. Available online: https://www.kcl.ac.uk/what-impact-does-war-have-on-ukrainian-cancer-care (accessed on 6 January 2023).

8. Abdul-Khalek, R.A.; Guo, P.; Sharp, F.; Gheorghe, A.; Shamieh, O.; Kutluk, T.; Fouad, F.; Coutts, A.; Aggarwal, A.; Mukherji, D.; et al. The economic burden of cancer care for Syrian refugees: A population-based modelling study. *Lancet Oncol.* **2020**, *21*, 637–644. [CrossRef] [PubMed]
9. Advice to Sponsors on Managing the Impact of the War in Ukraine on Clinical Trials. Available online: https://www.ema.europa.eu/en/news/advice-sponsors-managing-impact-war-ukraine-clinical-trials (accessed on 6 January 2023).
10. NIH, U.S. National Library of Medicine. Available online: https://clinicaltrials.gov/ (accessed on 30 September 2022).
11. World Heatlth Organization Number of Clinical Trial Registrations by Location, Disease, Phase of Development, Age and Sex of Trial Participants (1999–2021). Available online: https://www.who.int/observatories/global-observatory-on-health-research-and-development/monitoring/number-of-trial-registrations-by-year-location-disease-and-phase-of-development (accessed on 30 September 2022).
12. Heneghan, C.; Blacklock, C.; Perera, R.; Davis, R.; Banerjee, A.; Gill, P.; Liew, S.; Chamas, L.; Hernandez, J.; Mahtani, K.; et al. Evidence for non-communicable diseases: Analysis of Cochrane reviews and randomised trials by World Bank classification. *BMJ Open* **2013**, *3*, e003298. [CrossRef] [PubMed]
13. Siegel, R.L.; Miller, K.D.; Fuchs, H.E.; Jemal, A. Cancer statistics, 2022. *CA Cancer J. Clin.* **2022**, *72*, 7–33. [CrossRef] [PubMed]
14. Berne Declaration (Ed.) *Clinical Drug Trials in Ukraine: Myths and Realities*; Public Eye: Lausanne, Switzerland, 2013.
15. State Statistics Service of Ukraine. All-Ukrainian Population Census. Available online: http://www.ukrcensus.gov.ua/eng/ (accessed on 30 September 2022).
16. Limes. Rivista Italiana di Geopolitica. Ucraina: Divisioni Linguistiche ed Etniche. Available online: https://www.limesonline.com/ucraina-divisioni-linguistiche-ed-etniche/60932 (accessed on 30 September 2022).
17. WHO Cancer Ukraine 2020 Country Profile. Available online: https://cdn.who.int/media/docs/default-source/country-profiles/cancer/ukr-2020.pdf?sfvrsn=5d341f5f_2&download=true (accessed on 30 September 2022).
18. Breast Cancer in Ukraine: The Continuum of Care and Implications for Action. Available online: https://openknowledge.worldbank.org/bitstream/handle/10986/30144/127419.pdf?sequence=5&isAllowed=y (accessed on 30 September 2022).
19. Ukraine Human Papillomavirus and Related Cancers, Fact Sheet. 2021. Available online: https://hpvcentre.net/statistics/reports/UKR_FS.pdf (accessed on 30 September 2022).
20. Melnitchouk, N.; Shabat, G.; Lu, P.; Lyu, H.; Scully, R.; Leung, K.; Jarman, M.; Lukashenko, A.; Kolesnik, O.O.; Goldberg, J.; et al. Colorectal Cancer in Ukraine: Regional Disparities and National Trends in Incidence, Management, and Mortality. *J. Glob Oncol.* **2018**, *4*, 1–8. [CrossRef] [PubMed]
21. National Cancer Registry of Ukraine (NCRU), Bulletin of the National Cancer Registry of Ukraine. Available online: http://www.ncru.inf.ua/publications/BULL_23/index_e.htm (accessed on 6 January 2023).
22. Uwishema, O.; Sujanamulk, B.; Abbass, M.; Fawaz, R.; Javed, A.; Aboudib, K.; Mahmoud, A.; Oluyemisi, A.; Onyeaka, H. Russia-Ukraine conflict and COVID-19: A double burden for Ukraine's healthcare system and a concern for global citizens. *Postgrad. Med. J.* **2022**, *98*, 569–571. [CrossRef] [PubMed]
23. European Centre for Disease Prevention and Control. *Operational Public Health Considerations for the Prevention and Control of Infectious Diseases in the Context of Russia's Aggression towards Ukraine*; ECDC: Stockholm, Sweden, 2022.
24. Polio Outbreak Ukraine Report 2015–2016 | the Polio Network. 2017. Available online: https://www.comminit.com/polio/content/polio-outbreak-ukraine-report-2015-2016 (accessed on 30 September 2022).
25. Wadman, M. Measles epidemic in Ukraine drove troubling European year. *Science* **2019**, *363*, 677–688. [CrossRef] [PubMed]
26. Ryzhov, A.; Bray, F.; Ferlay, J.; Fedorenko, Z.; Goulak, L.; Gorokh, Y.; Soumkina, O.; Michailovich, Y.; Znaor, A. Recent cancer incidence trends in Ukraine and short-term predictions to 2022. *Cancer Epidemiol.* **2020**, *65*, 101663. [CrossRef] [PubMed]
27. National Institute for Public Health and the Environment Ministry of Health, Welfare and Sport Cancer Screening Programme for Ukrainian Refugees. Available online: https://www.rivm.nl/en/refugees-ukraine/cancer-screening (accessed on 6 January 2023).
28. Altobelli, E.; Rapacchietta, L.; Profeta, V.F.; Fagnano, R. HPV-vaccination and cancer cervical screening in 53 WHO European Countries: An update on prevention programs according to income level. *Cancer Med.* **2019**, *8*, 2524–2534. [CrossRef] [PubMed]
29. Altobelli, E.; Rapacchietta, L.; Marziliano, C.; Campagna, G.; Profeta, V.F.; Fagnano, R. Differences in colorectal cancer surveillance epidemiology and screening in the WHO European Region. *Oncol Lett.* **2019**, *17*, 2531–2542. [CrossRef] [PubMed]
30. Altobelli, E. Improving cervical cancer screening in Baltic, central, and eastern European countries. *Lancet Oncol.* **2016**, *17*, 1349–1350. [CrossRef] [PubMed]
31. Ryzhov, A.; Corbex, M.; Piñeros, M.; Barchuk, A.; Andreasyan, D.; Djanklich, S.; Ghervas, V.; Gretsova, O.; Kaidarova, D.; Kazanjan, K.; et al. Comparison of breast cancer and cervical cancer stage distributions in ten newly independent states of the former Soviet Union: A population-based study. *Lancet Oncol.* **2021**, *22*, 361–369. [CrossRef] [PubMed]

32. van Rosmalen, B.V.; Alldinger, I.; Cieslak, K.P.; Wennink, R.; Clarke, M.; Ahmed Ali, U.; Besselink, M.G. Worldwide trends in volume and quality of published protocols of randomized controlled trials. *PLoS ONE* **2017**, *12*, e0173042.
33. Zupunski, L.; Yaumenenka, A.; Ryzhov, A.; Veyalkin, I.; Drozdovitch, V.; Masiuk, S.; Ivanova, O.; Kesminiene, A.; Pukkala, E.; Moiseev, P.; et al. Breast cancer incidence in the regions of Belarus and Ukraine most contaminated by the Chernobyl accident: 1978 to 2016. *Int. J. Cancer* **2021**, *148*, 1839–1849. [CrossRef] [PubMed]

Disclaimer/Publisher's Note: The statements, opinions and data contained in all publications are solely those of the individual author(s) and contributor(s) and not of MDPI and/or the editor(s). MDPI and/or the editor(s) disclaim responsibility for any injury to people or property resulting from any ideas, methods, instructions or products referred to in the content.

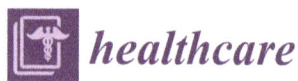

Article

Intensive Care Nurses' Experience of Caring in Greece; A Qualitative Study

Stelios Parissopoulos [1,*], Fiona Timmins [2], Meropi Mpouzika [3], Marianna Mantzorou [1], Theodore Kapadochos [1] and Eleni Papagaroufali [4]

[1] Department of Nursing, School of Health and Care Sciences, University of West Attica, 12243 Athens, Greece
[2] School of Nursing, Midwifery & Health Systems, University College Dublin, Belfield, D04 V1W8 Dublin, Ireland
[3] Department of Nursing, School of Health Sciences, Cyprus University of Technology, Limassol 3036, Cyprus
[4] Department of Social Anthropology, Panteion University of Social and Political Sciences, 17671 Athens, Greece
* Correspondence: spariss@uniwa.gr

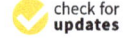

Citation: Parissopoulos, S.; Timmins, F.; Mpouzika, M.; Mantzorou, M.; Kapadochos, T.; Papagaroufali, E. Intensive Care Nurses' Experience of Caring in Greece; A Qualitative Study. *Healthcare* 2023, 11, 164. https://doi.org/10.3390/healthcare11020164

Academic Editor: Luigi Vetrugno

Received: 3 November 2022
Revised: 29 December 2022
Accepted: 3 January 2023
Published: 5 January 2023

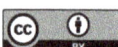

Copyright: © 2023 by the authors. Licensee MDPI, Basel, Switzerland. This article is an open access article distributed under the terms and conditions of the Creative Commons Attribution (CC BY) license (https://creativecommons.org/licenses/by/4.0/).

Abstract: Background: Whilst nurses and critical care services have been at the forefront of the COVID-19 pandemic, it has become more apparent that intensive care nurses are presented with challenging ethical and clinical decisions and are required to care for individuals with critical illnesses under high-pressure conditions. This is not a new phenomenon. The aim of this study, which was conducted before the outbreak of COVID-19, was to explore the experience of caring through the narratives of intensive care nurses in Greece. Methods: A qualitative study was conducted through in-depth, semi-structured interviews with nineteen ICU nurses in Athens. Transcripts were subjected to Braun and Clarke's thematic analysis and organised with Atlas.ti v8 QDA software. Results: The intensive care nurses' experience of caring in Greece encompassed four themes: (A) being *"proximal"*, *"co-present"* and caring with empathy, (B) being *"responsible"* for your patient and *negotiating* with the doctors, (C) technology and *"fighting with all you've got"*, and (D) *"not being kept informed"* and disappointment. Conclusions: The narratives of this study highlight that ICU nurses in Greece provide patient-centred and compassionate care. Nurse leaders should develop appropriate healthcare policies so as to ensure the adequate provision of staff, specialist education, and support to nurses working in critical care. Failure to address these issues may lead to poor quality of care and negative patient outcomes.

Keywords: caring; empathy; technology; negotiation; ICU nurse; thematic analysis; qualitative

1. Introduction

The intensive care unit (ICU) is a technologically advanced microcosm that is physically separated from the rest of the hospital via physical and disciplinary barriers. The ICU presents extra challenges to the ICU nurses, who are expected to not only care for their patients and attend to their physical needs but also care for their psychological and spiritual needs [1–4]. In the recent COVID-19 pandemic, nurses and critical care services were at the center of the media's attention, and it became more apparent to everyone, including peer professionals and lay people, that ICU nurses are continually presented with ethical dilemmas and challenging clinical decisions, and are required to care for individuals with critical illness under extremely high-pressure conditions.

Although caring is a concept that has become synonymous with "nursing care" and "plans of care" [5], it still remains a fuzzy and complex term that has attracted various definitions and conceptualizations [6–8]. According to Leininger [9], who was one of the first theorists to define caring, caring is a term that describes "those actions and activities directed toward assisting, supporting, or enabling another individual or group with evident or anticipated needs to ameliorate or improve a human condition or lifeway" (p.4). More recently, Tang et al. [10] defined caring as participating in reciprocal interactions, embracing the essence of caring, evoking instances of caring, and embodying caring in practice in the contemporary healthcare system. Brilowski and Wendler [11] identified five key aspects under the caring concept, namely "relationship", "action", "attitude", "acceptance", and "variability". Whilst this was tied to the nursing practice, it could also be applicable to other healthcare practitioners. Sebrant and Jong [12] performed a meta-synthesis on the concept of caring and identified four themes: "to be", "to want", "to be able to", and "to do". Caring was understood by nurses as a movement and balance between these four dimensions, while attempting to actualize what they regarded to be a requirement for good care. It goes without saying that the major role of a nurse is to care for patients; therefore, caring for patients revolves around meeting the particular requirements of patients, and the ultimate goal of nursing is to offer high-quality care [13]. However, the experience of caring is experienced differently by nurses.

Caring for critically ill patients in the ICU requires special considerations. The ICU is a high-pressure setting because of the complexities of the work. ICU settings facilitate the delivery of care to patients who are in the midst of a life-threatening physiological crisis [14]. In his or her job, the nurse serves as a key hub for all activities involving the patient [6]. It is important to take into consideration that caring for patients in an ICU can take many forms [6]. It is worth noting that there have been quite a few qualitative studies into critical care, but they have mostly focused on the experience of certain aspects of ICU nursing, such as managing non-invasive ventilation patients [15], nurses' perceptions of patients' thirst in ICU [16], nurses' perceptions of futile care and caring behaviors [13], nurses' experiences of caring for dying patients [17], and others [18–22]. A number of studies during the COVID-19 pandemic specifically explored the extra physical and psychological challenges and strains that nurses had been facing [2,23–27], for example, the experiences of cardiovascular nurses working in a COVID-19 ICU [28] and the spiritual well-being of nurses [29]. However, only a small number of qualitative studies have explored the experience of caring as a whole in the context of the ICU [30–33]. To the best of our knowledge, when this study was conducted, there was no other study that specifically looked at the Greek ICU nurses' experience of caring as a whole.

In the past, the clinical "landscape" of the ICU has offered a unique opportunity to researchers for inductively exploring nurses' views and practices that may shed light on how they "navigate" patients through their trajectory of critical illness [34]. More specifically, those studies looked at how nurses *produce* ICU care and reach clinical decisions in moments of access or exclusion at the hospital [35,36], at how they regulate space and time in order to uphold good care and "produce" patient centered care [37], and at how they exercise power in order to secure "medical orders" and care modalities that are appropriate for their patients [35,38,39].

The aim of this study was to explore the experience of caring through ICU nurses' narratives in Greece. Each interview started with an opening question on what it meant to them to be an ICU nurse and how they experienced what they did. Participants were encouraged to use their own words and share thoughts, feelings, memories, and descriptions. In this study, caring is approached as providing "nursing care" in the context of the ICU. The main researcher (first author), a UK-trained ICU nurse and anthropologist with a Greek background, felt it was important to give the chance to ICU nurses in Greece to share in their own words their experience of caring, as previous studies had suggested that the majority of ICU nurses in Greece were experiencing dissatisfaction, reduced professional autonomy, and reduced participation in their clinical decision-making [1,40–43].

2. Materials and Methods

2.1. Study Design

This is a qualitative study that is part of a larger anthropological PhD study conducted in Greece that looked at nursing practice, clinical decision-making, and power relations in the ICU [44]. A qualitative approach was chosen as it is suitable for examining concepts such as "caring", and it is frequently utilized to highlight the significance of caring from the viewpoints of nurses [45]. Kaba et al. [46] assert that the aim of qualitative research is to explore and achieve a comprehensive knowledge of participants' perspectives, experiences, and attitudes toward a phenomenon of interest. The goal of qualitative researchers is to get a richer, more comprehensive knowledge of the subject that they are studying.

The main researcher looked at ICU nurses' experiences of what they did, thought, and felt during a two-year period at a hospital in Athens. This study was conducted in line with critical medical anthropology [47–50] and phenomenology [51–56]. According to critical medical anthropology, which draws largely from the seminal work of Foucault [57], nurses are individuals who co-exist with other professionals in a space (hospital) and they are subjected to a network of powers unfolding through "technologies" of discipline [47,50,57,58]. Therefore, the study adopted an ethnographic approach through fieldwork in order to uncover the discourses, cultures, and practices that transcended an ICU in Athens [59,60]. In doing this, the main researcher conducted in-depth interviews in addition to ad hoc ethnographic interviews with nineteen participants in order to invoke narratives and approach their experiences and representations surrounding their nursing work. This was the phenomenological element of the study. Phenomenology complements ethnographic research in anthropology, by looking at the individuals' emic perspective and intersubjective experiences of their own world and identity(-ies). This paper reports on particular findings from the analysis of the interviews with nineteen ICU nurses.

2.2. Setting and Participants

Nineteen (n = 19) participants were selected through a purposive and snowball sampling approach. Eleven of them were ICU nurses who worked at an 18-bed general ICU in a public teaching hospital in Athens, and eight of them were added to the sample as they had been identified as experts in ICU nursing. The "expert" nurses (ICU nurses/managers, nurse academics/researchers in critical care) were recognized as such by other peers and nurses in critical care, due to their achievements and reputations in clinical, academic, and research fields. Experts in ICU nursing were included in the sample in order to ensure maximum variation in the data collection. All of the participants, apart from one novice nurse, had >5 years of clinical experience in ICU (Table 1). In qualitative research, certain "informants" are selected because they have firsthand knowledge of the issue being investigated [46]. Purposive sampling is the term used to describe this type of sampling [61], which can produce rich data. The primary goal of sampling in qualitative research is to find what Patton [62] refers to as information-rich instances, which are "presented for in-depth examination" and from which "one may learn a lot about topics of vital relevance for the purpose of research" (p. 230).

2.3. Data Collection

The semi-structured interviews explored the participants' feelings, thoughts, and reflections on being an "ICU nurse", with a particular focus on their experience of caring for critically ill patients. The researcher had prepared exploratory, open-ended questions for the interviews in order to elicit narratives and rich information from the participants (Table 2). Additionally, probing and clarification questions were asked during each interview depending on the participant's responses. Each participant was approached face-to-face to give an interview. The main researcher's previous clinical background in critical care helped establish, from the very beginning of the study, a sense of understanding and a sense of "being one of them" with the participant nurses in the study. All of those who were approached agreed to participate. In some cases, the privacy and "stillness" of time during the interview session offered them a chance to pause, reflect, offload emotions, and share their own intersubjective—but very real to them—embodied experiences of caring. In social anthropology, embodiment is a way of describing enlivened bodily experiences. In other words, the body is more than an object [51,52,55], it "is also a locus from which our experience of the world is arrayed, it is a living entity by which, and through which, we actively experience the world" [63] (p. 89).

Table 1. Participant characteristics.

Pseudonym	Age Group	Gender	Professional Capacity and Education	ICU Experience (Years) at the Time of the Interview	Expert Nurses in Critical Care
Artemis [#1]	25–34	F	ICU nurse, Bachelor's degree	10	
Akrivi (Precious) [#2]	25–34	F	ICU nurse, Bachelor's degree, Master student	7	
Doukissa [#3]	25–34	F	ICU nurse, Bachelor's degree	13	
Galini (Calm) [#4]	25–34	F	ICU nurse, Master's degree	10	
Stefanos [#5]	25–34	M	ICU nurse, Master's degree	6	
Elpida (Hope) [#6]	35–44	F	Former ICU nurse, PhD, Clinical Education	9	Expert #1
Marcella [#7]	35–44	F	Former ICU Sister, Master's degree, Phd(c), Public Health	10	Expert #2
Cleopatra [#8]	45–54	F	ICU Sister, Master's degree, Phd(c)	19	Expert #3
Agne (Pure) [#9]	35–44	F	ICU nurse, Master's degree	10	Expert #4
Erasmia [#10]	35–44	F	Former ICU nurse, Master's degree, PhD(c), Clinical Education	14	Expert #5
Gregoris [#11]	35–44	M	ICU nurse, Bachelor's degree	6	
Monica [#12]	35–44	F	Former ICU Debuty Sister, PhD, Academic	13	Expert #6
Thales [#13]	35–44	M	Former ICU nurse, Master's degree, PhD(c), Academic	10	Expert #7
Olympia [#14]	35–44	F	ICU Debuty Sister, Bachelor's degree	13	
Galenos [#15]	35–44	M	ICU nurse, Bachelor's degree	6	
Sotiris [#16]	45–54	M	ICU Nurse Manager, Bachelor's degree	22	
Elpiniki [#17]	25–43	F	ICU nurse, Bachelor's degree	1,5	
Metaxia [#18]	35–44	F	Former ICU nurse, PhD, Researcher, University	7	Expert #8
Elizabeth [#19]	45–54	F	Matron of Critical Care Division, Bachelor's degree, Master student	20	

The participants selected the place and time of the interviews (home, hospital, work office, or university). Privacy was ensured, and the places were quiet. Each interview lasted approximately one hour, was recorded, and was transcribed verbatim by the main researcher. Finally, interviews were completed once data saturation was reached.

2.4. Ethical Approval

Participants were informed in advance of the purpose and design of the study and signed an informed consent form. Participation was voluntary, and each informant had the right to withdraw at any time. Their willingness to participate in the study was reconfirmed verbally before beginning the interviews. Ethics approval was obtained by the Ethics and Research Committee at the hospital. Particular care was given to protect the participants' identities, by using pseudonyms and sensitive patient information according to the principles of confidentiality.

Table 2. Overview of the questions in the interview guide.

What does it mean to you to be an ICU nurse? Please feel free to use your own words.
If you reflect on your experiences throughout your nursing career, what kind of thoughts could you share with me?
How do you experience what you do? How do you see your role in your unit? Thoughts, feelings, memories, and descriptions.
Could you describe to me a typical shift in the unit? What is it that you do as an ICU nurse?
If I asked you to remember/recollect a particularly difficult/bad shift, what are your thoughts and feelings?
Is there something that bothers you/puts you under stress/presents you with a dilemma in the ICU?
What brings satisfaction to you at work?
Could you please recall a case/patient where you felt you had made a significant contribution?
Clinical decision-making: what kind of decisions do you usually make? Are you having difficulties? Could you mention something that helps/encourages you to reach a decision or participate in a decision? Is there something that makes it harder for you to participate?
Do you think that your professional judgment is considered by the doctors of the unit?
Intensive care unit: what were your first thoughts and impressions of the ICU environment? How did you feel when you started working in critical care? What impressed you, and what scared you?
Would you describe to me your relationship with the doctors of the unit?
Would you describe to me your relationship to the patient?
Let's say that the patient's condition is deteriorating. You are worried about your patient. How would you react/intervene? If medical staff do not act or react the way you had hoped (i.e., they don't take your assessment findings seriously), what do you do?
Have there been times when you thought that the decisions of the treatment team conflicted with your own values/priorities? How do you handle such situations?
How would you describe the ICU environment to someone who is not familiar with it?

2.5. Data Analysis

Interviews were analysed inductively and coded line by line. Coding gradually reached higher levels of abstraction, and the interviews were grouped together to form code groups (categories). The transcripts were subjected to Braun and Clarke's thematic analysis of qualitative data [64]. Braun and Clarke's thematic analysis constitutes an independent qualitative approach for an analysis identifying, analysing, and reporting patterns (themes), but is also characterized by flexibility and compatibility to phenomenological research, which was important in this study [65,66]. The stages of thematic analysis are divided into: (a) familiarity with the data, (b) generation of initial codes, (c) search for codes of higher abstract level and generation of code groups, (d) review of codes, (e) definition and naming of themes, and (f) writing on findings [64,67]. As Braun and Clarke point out in their methodological paper on thematic analysis [64], "A theme captures something important about the data in relation to the research question, and represents some level of patterned response or meaning within the data set... the 'keyness' of a theme is not necessarily dependent on quantifiable measures—but in terms of whether it captures something important in relation to the overall research question." (p. 10). Table 3 presents an example of coding and analysis of an interview transcript. This process of grouping, categorizing, and theorizing the data is very common in qualitative research and helps the researcher "make sense" of the data and reach meaningful interpretations and descriptions. In this study, interviews were analysed simultaneously with the emerging interpretation of the data. The supervisory team of the PhD study discussed, checked, revised, and adjusted "emerging" themes and patterns, on an ongoing basis.

Table 3. An example that illustrates the stages of thematic analysis with operational definitions.

Interview Transcript [a]	Initial Codes [b]	Codes of Higher Abstract Level-Code Groups [c,d]	Themes [e]
Elpida #6: "You give your own fight for your patients, the way I picture it, it is the effort you're making at that time and usually 'fighting' comes to my mind when I think of cardiac arrests, in the cardiology unit we have a lot of arrests, you pick up a lot of tachycardias, a lot of things, a lot of things like that, and when on duty you make use of everything, you use your mind, you use your body, you use the knowledge you had, you use the skills, skills you didn't know you had [she laughs], I mean, it might have taken you the whole shift trying to unscrew a stopcock [fluid flow control valve] and in the event of a cardiac arrest you unscrew it just like that [laughs]… but in the event of emergency you do things that you thought you couldn't do and you use whatever skills you have in this battle, that is, you use your abilities for cooperation, you also use humor, and sometimes to say things you normally wouldn't say. I remember saying to a doctor, "please get going, please get going, do something" [we laugh]. That is because you also need this [humor]. You also have to be authoritarian sometimes, I think what you use is all you've got in terms of skills, every time you use different things, but they all do the same thing. So, you work against time, I mean, you try to catch up, that is, you have things on your mind that you want to get done in your shift-maybe not a lifesaving thing, if it is a quiet shift-but still having a lot of things to do, so you have to manage your time"	*Fighting for your patient* * *The effort* *Fighting* *Emergencies* *Tachycardias and body* *You make use of everything* *Skills* *Mind and body* *Knowledge* *Skills* *Humor* *Emergency-rapid deterioration* *Skills and battle* *Ability to cooperate* *To the doctor: "get going"* *Humor* *Authoritarian* *Skills* *Time management* *Trying to catch up*	11. Responsibility and accountability 12. Communication: nurse-doctor 14. The emergency: body homeostasis 18. Skills, knowledge, and emotions 20. Readiness to act 21. Fighting for your patient	B. Being responsible for your patient and negotiating with the doctors C. Technology and "Fighting with all you've got"

*Red codes → red code groups → theme (C), green codes → green code groups → theme (B). Codes are colored for illustration purposes, as codes may be assigned to more than one code group. The stages of thematic analysis, [64] operational definitions. [a] Familiarizing with your data: transcribing data, reading and re-reading the data, noting down initial ideas. [b] Generating initial codes: coding interesting features of the data systematically across the entire data set, collating data relevant to each code. [c] Searching for codes of higher abstract level and collating all relevant codes into code groups [categories]. [d] Reviewing codes and code groups [categories]. [e] Searching for themes, reviewing them, naming themes: collating code groups into potential themes, gathering all data relevant to each potential theme. Checking if the themes work in relation to the coded extracts.

2.6. Rigor of the Study

Trustworthiness was ensured by satisfying the principles of credibility, confirmability, dependability, and transferability [66,68,69]. Credibility was established through the triangulation of data methods and sources. Firstly, ethnographic fieldnotes were kept during participant observation. The ethnographic part of the study helped the main researcher identify the key informants for interviewing. Secondly, the sample included experts in critical care. Transferability was met by adopting purposive sampling. Confirmability and dependability were satisfied by keeping a research diary, recording methodological decisions for the purposes of audit trail, and member checking. The findings, even at preliminary stage, were discussed with the participants for cross-checking and clarification. The data analysis and revision of the themes carried on well into the write up process of the thesis. The audit trail included reflective writing and ongoing supervisory support from the PhD supervisors. The standards for reporting qualitative research (SRQR criteria) guided the preparation of this paper [70].

3. Findings

The ICU nurses' experience of caring in this study encompassed the following four themes: (a) being *"proximal"*, *"co-present"*, and *"caring with empathy"*, (b) being *"responsible"* for your patient and *negotiating* with the doctors", (c) technology and *"fighting* with all you've got", and (d) *"not being kept informed"* and disappointment (Table 4).

Table 4. Overview of themes and code categories.

	Themes	Code Groups [Categories]
ICU Nurses' Experience of Caring in Greece	A. Being *proximal, co-present,* and caring with empathy	1. The critically ill patient 2. Monitoring and care: ongoing 3. Nurse being fully there 4. Nursing gaze and vigilance 5. Relationship: nurse-patient 6. Proximity 7. Co-presence
	B. Being *responsible* for your patient and *negotiating* with the doctors	8. *My* patient: worrying/stress 9. The "care needs" of the patient 10. Clinical decision-making 11. Responsibility and accountability 12. Communication: nurse-doctor 13. Negotiation 14. The emergency: body homeostasis 15. Observations and the "observation chart"
	C. Technology and *fighting with all you've got*	16. Alarms and equipment 17. Nursing expertise 18. Skills, knowledge, emotions 19. Technology 20. Readiness to act 21. Fighting for your patient 22. "We survive like cockroaches do"
	D. *Not being kept informed* and disappointment	23. Lack of information 24. Absence from doctors' round 25. Clinical decisions: not participating 26. Disappointment and frustration 27. Lack of recognition 28. Lack of supportive environment 29. Heavy workload, too busy

3.1. Theme A: Being "Proximal", "Co-Present", and Caring with Empathy

The participants perceive themselves as individuals who are "proximal" to their patients and continuously "co-present". This type of constant co-presence and closeness describes a nurse-patient relationship that is not just metaphorical but very much physical and embodied. A nurse is always present and available in the patient's area and is vigilant of any physiological changes or alarms going off. This type of nurse-patient relationship can also be described as an empathetic one. "Nursing Gaze and Vigilance" was an important finding (code group 4) and is depicted with its associated codes in Figure 1.

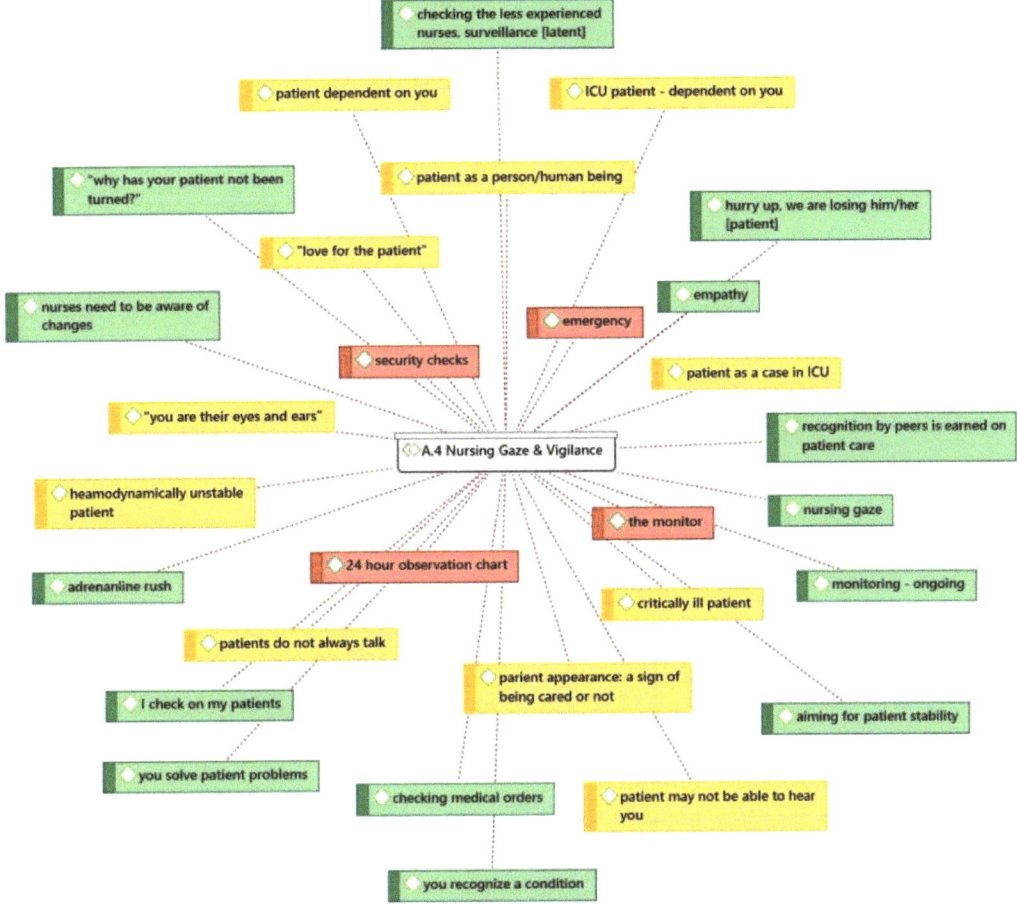

Figure 1. Nursing gaze and vigilance.

ICU nurse Akrivi is "co-present" and "proximal", to her patient, both metaphorically and literally. She constantly has her patient in her mind, "she cares for him", and does what is necessary to keep him alive. Her vigilant eye makes sure that all their bodily functions are monitored and recorded, and that no major functions, such as airway patency, breathing, and blood pressure, are failing the patient. At the same time, she feels the patient's pain and suffering, she speaks to him, supports him, touches him gently with her hands, and reassures him. The participants expressed empathy for their patients' needs and problems, especially when verbal communication with the patient was not possible, due to the threatening critical illness or sedation.

> Akrivi, interview 2: "Sometimes I think of my patients very intensely, I think about their situation, yes, and I think about it very intensely . . . it affects me very badly [. . .] I may be sitting and looking at them and I think 'this man is in bed, motionless, I wonder if he is a little awake, if he is in pain'".

ICU nurse Agne remembers how intensely she had experienced a difficult case, the "Christmas miracle" patient. A multi-trauma 32-year-old woman, mother of a two-year-old girl, had been transferred years ago to the ICU on a Christmas Eve. She had finished work and was waiting to be picked up when two cars collided in front of her. One of the cars hit her and she lost her leg. She was admitted post-op to ICU with one leg amputated from the thigh down, an unstable pelvic fracture and she was in very critical condition. Agne remembers that seven hours had passed since the patient's admission, and that she herself had been stubborn and took it for granted that the patient would do well. She was so involved in her care that she could not accept that her patient would not make it. While the young woman was losing blood non-stop and was being transfused with many units of blood and plasma, Agne and the doctor kept "working on her" with all their physical, cognitive, and emotional resources.

> *Agne [expert nurse] interview 9:* "I remember transfusing her non-stop, I am saying this to you and I am shivering ... I remember both of us (Agne and the doctor) holding the blood units and applying pressure to deliver the blood as fast as possible. I remember a colleague coming on duty and saying 'why give so much blood? since she will not make it.' And I didn't like the sound of it, I remember thinking 'what is she saying? she will survive!'"

Agne was so involved and connected to her patient, that she strongly believed there was a real chance of her survival. The next morning, she was still alive, still critical but still there, and she was discharged from the unit a few weeks later. When she thinks of her, seven years later, she thinks of her as a mom at home, with one leg, but having a life. Her belief that this was a case that had a chance of survival kept her "fighting" on the patient's behalf.

3.2. Theme B: Being "Responsible" for Your Patient and Negotiating with the Doctors

Whilst nurses care for their patients, they engage in creating space for negotiation with the medical team in order to achieve the best possible interventions for their patients. Like most of the participants, one of the reasons nurse Artemis considers herself responsible for the patients assigned to her or under her care is that she is accountable for them at the end of the shift. As in other studies, her sense of responsibility and accountability for her patients is a profound element of her job.

> *Artemis, interview 1:* "As I have to account for the patients assigned to me and I sign off their charts and documentation, I consider myself responsible for these patients. However, if I pick up something wrong with the patients of a colleague, even if he is a senior/experienced one, and I know I just said 'his patients', I will still intervene because the patient comes first! [laughs]"

All participant nurses felt enormously responsible for the patients who were under their care. Interviews revealed the existence of an "intense relationship" with their patient. All participants often referred to their patients as "theirs", as if they "owned" them. However, according to Agne, this sense of responsibility was experienced as an extra burden for them, as their workload was heavy, and they also had to keep an eye on the patients of the less experienced colleagues. Therefore, the participants also "supervised" and exercised some kind of control over their colleagues' work and the patients that had been assigned to them.

For some of the nurses, the sense of responsibility for their patients is so great and heavy that it is embodied as a significant emotional burden. The participants in the current study made themselves available and mobilized their body, their senses, and their "nursing gaze" for the best interest of the patients under their care. All participants utilized basic and advanced clinical skills, and each time they cared for their patient, they produced nursing care that was "culturally" suitable to the lifeworld of ICU.

Although they carefully shielded themselves behind protective personal equipment (PPE) with face masks, gowns, and gloves, every "touch" and act of "care" was carried out with a sense of responsibility, accountability, and intention to heal, such that in a latent fashion it ensured that the patient under their care was not alone in this precarious physical state between life and death. Erasmia tries to make her presence known to her patients, even through a gentle touch.

Erasmia, interview 10: "*yes, I am consciously there . . . this is why you see me touching my patient, you see the 'touch'. I may be passing by my patient and even though I am not verbally communicating to him, because he is sedated, I intentionally touch him. It is my way of telling my patients 'I know and I care for you, I am here for you'*".

Nurses' sense of responsibility for their patients gave rise to the creation of a space for negotiation between nurses and doctors. The analysis of the data in the present study confirms that the daily life in the hospital and in the ICU seems to be organized around a series of negotiations between nurses and doctors. Artemis is in constant negotiations with doctors, especially now that she is experienced and she feels a greater sense of responsibility. Artemis negotiates for almost everything: for the patient's analgesia, whether she will "wake up" the patient or not, or when a new "line" will be inserted in one of her patients. Scheduling invasive procedures and computerized tomography scans by doctors without warning or at least telling nurses was a constant source of tension between nurses and doctors, as the nurses had three patients under their care, and inappropriate scheduling of such interventions meant that they could not keep up with their ongoing "nursing" jobs. While Artemis could not do the same in the first years of her career, she has reached a point where she "controls" the doctors and can have a say in the scheduling of such interventions.

Artemis, interview 1: "*after ten years of experience in critical care, I have the sort of relationship with the doctors where I can tell them what needs to be done, I can control them. It is not like 5 years ago where I would not question their orders. Now I am able to question their decisions and negotiate a timeframe which is possible for me to manage*".

3.3. Theme C: Technology and "Fighting with All You've Got"

Technology in ICU has a prominent place in the provision of care, as it helps nurses and doctors in "invading" and looking at the physiological functions of the body, in the administration of therapeutic interventions, and in reaching clinical decisions based on up-to-date data. The primary concern of the participants was to provide lifesaving and supportive care, to stabilize the patients' clinical condition, to recognize clinical deterioration, and maintain homeostasis in their patients. According to nurse Elpida, nurses can formulate an opinion on the patient's severity just by looking at the number of electronic medication pumps and the type of machines attached to the patient (filter). In the *indigenous* language of ICU nurses, the patient is often described as having "full" or "empty" equipment on his bedside.

Elpida [expert nurse], interview 6: "*I do not think we actually acknowledge the vast number of machines we connect to our patient, because we are so used to this. It is shocking for someone who sees this for the first time, but because we are so used to the image of a patient being attached to IV pumps, monitor, ventilator . . . we do not take much notice*".

Expert ICU nurse Elpida believes that nurses utilize and mobilize "all they've got", such as their knowledge, skills, and humor, in order to achieve patient stability and body homeostasis. The participants also placed particular emphasis on their readiness to act (code group 20) in the event of patient deterioration (Figure 2).

Nurse Elpida describes the experience of caring as a "battle" where the nurses strive with all their "resources" to achieve the best outcome for the patient. At the same time, nurses work closely with the other professionals, they negotiate, they employ their sense of humor, and if needed, they assume a stricter and "authoritarian" approach.

Elpida, interview 6: "*at the time of the cardiac arrest [laughs] . . . at that time you are doing things that you thought you could not do and you are using whatever skills you have in this 'battle', that is cooperation with others . . . humor . . . every time you use different resources*".

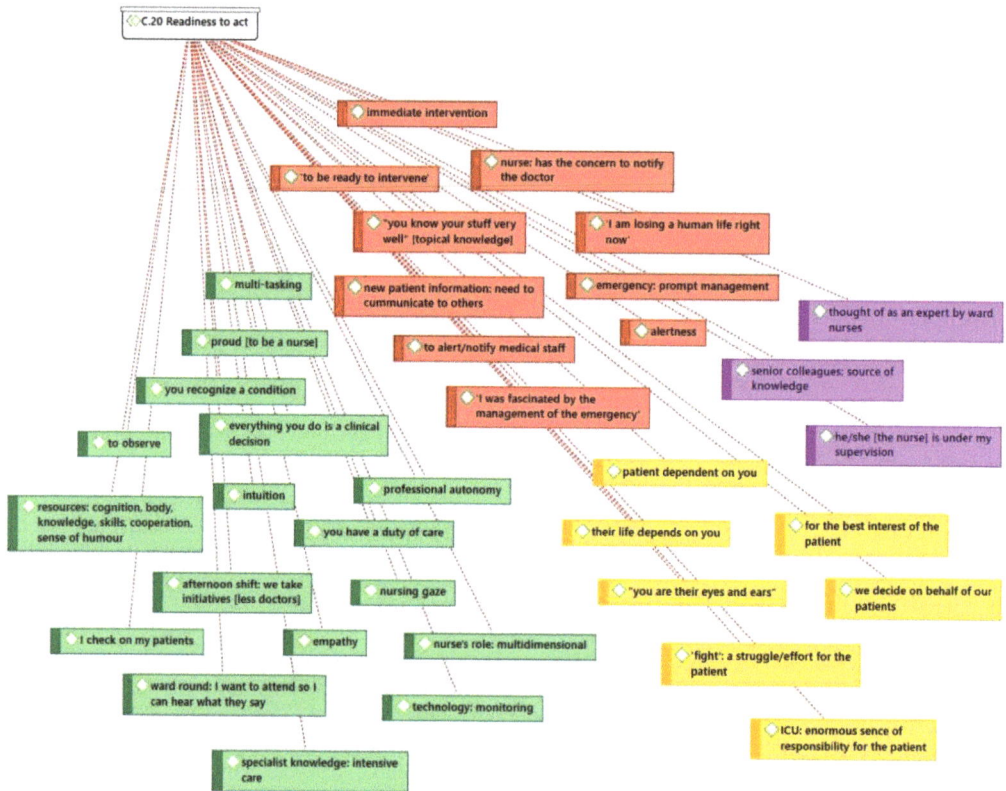

Figure 2. Readiness to act.

Quite often they had to manage faulty and malfunctioning equipment, for example, intravenous cannulas that broke easily, giving sets that "refused" to work, even at a time when their patient was bleeding and "dropped the pressure". At the time of the study, the participants were extremely resourceful in thinking of patients and improvised ways of using this material, as they had to come up with innovative ways in order to provide the best possible treatment. Nurses joked about this, and they described Greek nurses as "cockroaches who survive and manage through tough situations".

3.4. Theme D: "Not Being Kept Informed" and Disappointment

The nurses in this study were sometimes overwhelmed with disappointment and frustration as the medical staff didn't keep them informed of any changes in treatment or patient background. So, even though they were constantly "present" and "close" to their patients and knew the smallest details of their conditions, they often felt that they missed the big picture, and were left out of important clinical decisions. In addition to this, each time the nurses failed to "convince" the doctor that there was something wrong with their patient, they were overwhelmed with frustration, sadness, and anxiety. Therefore, even though some of the participants experienced immense job satisfaction, a strong "sense of helping" the others, a "love for" and, to some degree, an "addiction" for the ICU specialty, some others were very disappointed, frustrated, and felt devalued, and they considered some of the tasks delegated to them of minor importance. Their main complaint was their inability to attend ward rounds due to extreme workload, as each nurse was delegated three patients. Galenos, an experienced nurse, feels like an "intruder" on the few times he has tried to attend the doctors' ward round. He sits somewhere on the edge, listens to them quietly, and when he finds the opportunity, he may ask questions. However, often "there is no time" for Galenos to do so, and he continues with his own work and patient care.

> *Galenos, interview 15: "No there is no time ... we cannot go [to the ward round] ... I cannot afford to sit around for 40–60' for my three patients, right? ... they do not have a set time for the round. As you cannot arrange your work, you cannot be available for ward round without enough warning. If I knew that the round is scheduled for ten o'clock, I would had arranged to finish my jobs by ten o'clock and then join them. But now, you cannot do it".*

In general terms, the nurses in this study disclosed that doctors would not inform them of the details of the patient's previous medical history, investigations, and progress. This made them feel undervalued and unable to participate in both the ward rounds and multidisciplinary clinical decisions. The latter led them to experience a state of nurse invisibility and "absence" from the clinical decisions of the ICU team. Nurse Galene does not hesitate to admit that she, as well as her colleagues, rarely participated in the ward rounds, although she knew it was important for her patients. Galene realized that medical staff would not consult the observation chart to the full extent, and she would like to be part of the ward round and bring areas of concern to the attention of the doctors. Herein lies the frustration of Galene, who, although she sees herself as the "eyes" and "ears" of doctors and as a useful source of information, doctors do not consider her "important" enough to be present at the ward round. Heavy workload (ration 1:3) and fatigue further discourage her from participating in the rounds.

> *Galene, interview 4: "The workload ... because most of the times, when my work is too much and I am thinking of the many pending tasks I don't want to pass on to my colleagues, I don't have the ability to go to the round..."*

According to the participants, the medical team often carried out their ward rounds on their own at ad hoc times and often in their office and the corridor, away from the nurses and the patients. Nurse Akrivi is tired and frustrated that she is distrusted by some of the doctors that she has worked with for so many years. According to her, her fatigue and efforts to provide high-quality care for the three patients under her care went unnoticed. I asked her if there were problems at work.

> *Akrivi, interview 2: "[-] [long pause] there are problems. I .... there are too many ... that disappoint me too much. The disbelief and [....] many times the irony of the doctors towards us... [....] it happens a lot ... [silence] ... I see this, it frustrates me very much and I am very tired in the Unit [....] especially when you know that you do right all the basics and you follow the procedures even though you do not have the resources"*

4. Discussion

The findings of this study capture the experience of caring among ICU nurses in Greece through the analysis of their narratives (Figure 3).

The first theme [A] suggests that the participant nurses in this study ensure that they are *close* (proximal) to their patients, are *co-present,* and demonstrate *empathy* while caring for them. In relation to proximity, in Lundin Gurné's study [71], proximity came up when nurses were described as working more closely with patients than other professions. The participants in that study emphasized that nursing practice was about striving to be in close proximity to the patient. This proximity was not easy to achieve, as nurses were often instructed to perform tasks not traditionally performed by nurses or not clearly perceived as nursing tasks. Nevertheless, they strived to be close to their patients, even though they had less time to care for individual patients due to cuts in healthcare funding [71]. It is worth noting that proximity to the patient enhances the nurses' bargaining role in clinical decision-making [72].

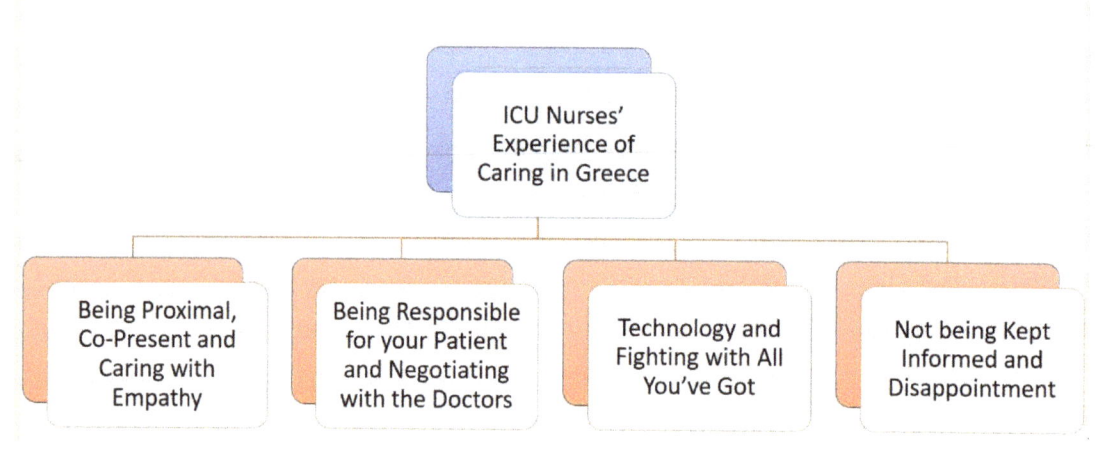

Figure 3. The main themes of the study.

The critically ill patient requires the presence of a trained ICU nurse all the time in order to monitor and detect any rapid changes or deterioration. Being co-present also meant being available for the patient [6,71]. In Lundin Gurné's et al. study [71], the nursing practice was described as being constantly available to patients and their relatives as well as colleagues while also focusing on patients' needs. This was also an important finding in the current study. According to Al-Shamaly [6], the imperative necessity for patient safety demands nurses to be "present with" the patients, "conscious of the non-verbal care demands,", and "sensitive" to the subtle shifting health states of patients. All of these elements are recognized as essential components of patient care in critical care [6]. In the ICU, nurses are concerned with ensuring patient safety for all patients, but especially for the conscious patients who are receiving mechanical breathing [73,74]. When Beeby [30] described the experience of caring among ICU nurses in a UK hospital, the participants experienced caring as "being involved in care" and "sustaining support" but also as "having frustrations". In terms of being involved, they meant that it was important for them to "be close" to the patient, to "be there", and to "do things for the patient". "Sustaining" referred to the nurse's role in providing support to the patient. The nurse provided a foundation of care that allowed the patient to recover by maintaining a stable environment.

According to Rogers, empathy is the ability to momentarily *step into* and *inhabit* another person's life by emotionally and physically *occupying* their personal space with the intention to help [75]. In nursing, caring with empathy also means "I do something for it", "I am available to the patient, I develop a therapeutic relationship and I respond to his needs". Empathy is also required for developing a therapeutic relationship and responding to the needs of others [22,76]. This type of nurse involvement was also found in the phenomenological study on ICU nurses by Vouzavali et al. [20], where the patient-nurse relationship in critical care was described as a "shared world", in other words, as a strong bond/synapse between "neighboring cells" that form a "syncytium". In the study of Stavropoulou et al. [3] on ICU nurses in Greece, care with empathy was described as sustaining communication, providing support, and a necessary condition for maintaining the patient's body homeostasis. ICU patients and their families are well-known for feeling powerless, vulnerable, anxious, and stressed [77]. Empathy in critical care encompasses acting in the best interest of the patient and results in caring with compassion [78].

The second theme of the study [B] demonstrated a profound sense of *responsibility* on the part of the participant nurses, which was linked to *negotiation* with doctors. Nurses negotiate with doctors in order to influence or secure the best possible clinical decision for their patient. Creating space for negotiation was a priority. In the spirit of this, nurses remained vigilant and often took on responsibilities that traditionally belonged to doctors [79] to promote the safety and homeostasis of "their" patients' bodies. The nurses claimed that their responsibility for *their* patients played an important role in this. In Beeby's study [30], caring was also experienced as accepting responsibility for a completely dependent patient and being at the bedside to provide patient care. Caring entailed trying to meet the individual's needs and, despite the gravity of the condition, acting as the patient's advocate within the ICU team. Their obligation to their patients informs their clinical decisions, even when they encounter ethical dilemmas in practice [19,80,81]. In another ethnographic study on the cultural context of an ICU in South Africa, Scholtz et al. [33] argued that nurses "adopt" their patients during their stay in the ICU. That is, they feel that they take full responsibility for them. As a result of this, they took any kind of difficulty or bad outcome very personally. Short pointed out a long time ago [82] that nurses see their bodies as tools of work and the sick bodies of their patients as the work area. Caring is experienced with a sense of responsibility for the monitoring and safety of their patients. For example, sharing both observation responsibility between colleagues and their perception of the patient's clinical condition with other professionals is part of teamwork skills [18]. Responsibility also meant that nurses had to negotiate with doctors on care interventions or drug modification and titration. During negotiation, nurses use communication strategies that encounter issues of concern and problems that cannot be regulated by written rules and institute policies [36]. In Schluter's et al. study [36], competent nurses were considered those who not only were close to their patients but those who effectively negotiated their ideas and opinions with the medical staff.

This study suggests that the participant nurses negotiate with doctors in order to influence or secure the best possible clinical decision for their patient, which also supports the findings of the study by House and Havens [83], where the participants were found to engage in communication and negotiation techniques in order to overcome difficult interdisciplinary collaborations. In other words, it offers support to Coughlin's statement [84], which describes nurses' work as navigating the patient through his/her illness trajectory in the ICU. This is a rather important finding in the Greek context, where the healthcare system has been described as medically centered with no recognized ICU course for nurses in place at the time of the study. Nevertheless, participants described how they engaged in negotiation techniques and tried to overcome difficult interdisciplinary collaborations. A study by Papathanassoglou et al. [42] has revealed moderate autonomy in technical tasks and low decisional autonomy among Hellenic ICU nurses. Overall, the findings offer support to other studies and suggest the existence of what Hasse describes as a person-centered approach [85].

The third theme [C] highlights that technology and resources, such as skills and specialist knowledge, were perceived by the participants as essential tools in achieving the patient's body homeostasis. High-quality care for critically ill patients not only requires humanistic methods of care but also a substantial dependence on the most current technology and knowledge [7,86]. It is a fact that ICU nurses cannot produce nursing care without the use of advanced technology. Price looked at the experience of caring in ICU in relation to technology in the UK [32]. She argued that the technology in the ICU cannot be separated from care, as the ability of nurses to handle technology is considered a profound skill and a prerequisite for care. Technology has changed the way we perceive and look at the human body, resulting in the creation of a new "medicalized" body [87]. It is interesting to note that studies have shown that technology has led to wider responsibilities for nurses in decision-making [88,89]. In other words, ICU nurses were shown to acquire a sense of superiority in their role due to the special knowledge they possessed and their unparalleled familiarity with the technology [32,79]. This enhanced their role in clinical decision-making as they were perceived as technical experts who are called upon to manage patients suffering from severe and threatening disease [88,89]. Since then, nurses have been recognized as an important element in providing a high level of critical care and decision-making [6,90].

Experienced ICU nurses are rather vigilant and look out for minute changes in the patient's condition. Patient monitoring is a key component of modern critical care, and it accounts for a significant percentage of an ICU nurse's work [91]. However, a critical care nurse is not only a technologically competent practitioner but a specialist who has the skills to decipher complicated data, offer therapeutic benefit through presence and comfort measures, create an active program of care for seriously ill patients, and assist other members of staff in providing critical care [92]. However, Pattison points out that the recent implementation of "task-teams" for the delivery of basic care during the COVID-19 pandemic may lead to the "reduction of nursing to tasks and the erosion of what it is to be a critical care nurse" [92] (p. 422). This new phenomenon goes against the notion that critical care nurses should "focus on the tasks that require advanced expert skills, expertise and knowledge of best practice in patient care" [93].

Lastly, the fourth theme [D] suggests that the participants were not valued to the degree they wished by the medical staff of the unit. A heavy workload (nurse-patient ratio 1:3) and their inability to attend the ward rounds made them feel undervalued, as they felt they were unable to participate in the ward rounds. The latter led them to experience a state of nurse "invisibility" and "absence" from the clinical decisions of the ICU team. Reflecting on the responses and accounts of the participants, no differences were noted between male and female nurses. For example, male nurses complained in the same way as their female colleagues about not being able to participate in the doctors' rounds. This might be attributed to both male and female nurses sharing the same values and ethos of care in nursing. Moreover, feelings of disappointment were shared among all the participants, as they recognized they were not participating in the clinical decisions of the ICU team. Clinical decision-making has always been an important aspect of ICU nursing [90]. Whether nurses contribute or not to the clinical decisions of the ICU team is a long-standing issue. Notably, there is evidence of nursing invisibility in clinical decision-making [94–99]. Studies have shown that nurses' assessment findings and judgements are either diminished or ignored [94,100]. When this happens, open confrontation, latent tension, and poor team collaboration can be the result [83,101,102]. This is problematic, as disturbed dynamics in the healthcare team and dysfunctional communications are associated with burnout [103] and low job satisfaction [4,104]. On the other hand, successful patient care and improved outcomes are associated with healthy communication amongst the members of the team [105].

This theme addresses the emotions of the participants. Emotions are important in qualitative research as they may shed light on the culture of a hospital setting. For example, a recent number of qualitative papers brought forward the extra physical and psychological challenges and strains that nurses experienced during the COVID-19 pandemic [2,23–27]. Nurses around the world were facing dread, anxiety, stress, physical tiredness, and a sense of powerlessness in dealing with their patients' situations [106]. Moradi et al. [26] studied the difficulties encountered by 17 ICU nurses while caring for COVID-19 patients. 'Organizational inefficiency in supporting nurses', 'physical exhaustion,', 'living with uncertainty,', and 'psychological load of the disease,' were experienced by the nurses. Nurses are also likely to suffer from psychological issues such as anxiety, depression, sleeplessness, stress [107,108], and burnout [109]. Chronic occupational stressors such as high patient acuity, high levels of responsibility, working with advanced technology, caring for families in crisis, and being involved in morally unpleasant situations are regular features of nursing work [3]. As a result, compassion, fatigue, and burnout may lead to a decline in empathy as a self-protective response. This could make their work more emotionally taxing as they become more engaged or emotionally involved. These issues may result in a "care burden" [19].

5. Limitations and Strengths

This study has some limitations. Data collection took place before the outbreak of COVID-19, and as the clinical landscape in critical care has substantially changed in the last two years, the findings could not be extrapolated to the experiences of nurses working in the era of the COVID-19 pandemic. Nevertheless, as there are very few studies on the whole experience of caring in critical care, the authors feel that the narratives of this pre-COVID-19 study can still contribute meaningfully to the worldwide discussion that focuses on *caring* and the essence of intensive care nursing [92,93]. Caring is a global concept, and this study sheds light on how ICU nurses in Greece care for and "navigate" their patients through their trajectories of critical illness. In retrospect, the inclusion of "expert" nurses in the sample enriched the data with their "expert" perspective and past clinical background and helped contextualize the accounts and narratives of the participants rather than interpret them in isolation. We suggest that further qualitative research should explore the experiences of caring from nurses' and patients' perspective, in order to explore what ICU nursing and care might look like after the COVID-19 pandemic.

6. Conclusions

This study concludes that nurse proximity, co-presence, caring with empathy, and a sense of responsibility are the core qualities that constitute the experience of caring among a group of ICU nurses in Greece. The study highlighted that the participants provided patient-centred care with empathy, engaged in negotiation with medical staff in order to affect clinical decisions in the best interest of the patient, and were resourceful through the use of technology, skills, and knowledge. However, even though they perceived that they engaged in a wide spectrum of interventions that stretched from monitoring to supporting and treating patients, they expressed feelings of disappointment regarding their exclusion from doctors' rounds and non-participation in the clinical decisions of the ICU team. As there has been a long-standing discussion on the power relations between the male-dominated medical and female-dominated nursing professions [58], it is suggested that future research also explore issues of gender regarding the division of therapeutic work between the two professions.

Finally, this paper reveals a strong culture of compassionate care among the participant nurses, even though they provided care under very challenging work conditions with a heavy workload. At times of extreme low nurse staffing levels in critical care across the globe and the recent implementation of "alternative staffing models" by assigning nurses without an ICU qualification [92] (p. 421) to care for ventilated COVID-19 patients, it is imperative to explore and continue the discussion on what actually constitutes ICU nursing and how care is experienced by the nurses in various cultural contexts. The authors suggest further studies that explore ICU nurses' experiences of caring. Such research would not only contribute to the ongoing discussion on the physical and psychosocial dimensions of what constitutes ICU nursing but would also inform and prepare leaders and nurses for future changes in the organization of critical care services and approaches to care.

7. Implications for Practice

This study provides valuable insight into the experience of caring through ICU nurses' narratives in a southern European country. Nurse leaders that aim to support the wellbeing of their nursing workforce should empower and support critical care nurses and allow decision-making freedom so as to encourage autonomous practice. They should encourage empathy, group spirit, mutual respect, trust, and support within the nursing workforce culture. The development of appropriate policies should also consider crucial organizational issues such as workload, resources, and safe staffing levels [110]. The challenges that nurses currently encounter worldwide are begging for the redrafting of social care and health policy. Not only should nurse leaders respond to their concerns, but health policy makers should also ensure the adequate provision of nursing staff, encourage specialist education in critical care, offer adequate resources, and provide in-house support to nurses working in critical care. The failure to address these issues may have an impact on staff retention and the mental health of nursing staff, which may lead to poor quality of care and negative patient outcomes.

Author Contributions: Conceptualization, S.P. and E.P.; methodology, S.P. and E.P.; validation, E.P. and F.T.; formal analysis, S.P. and E.P.; writing—original draft preparation, S.P., M.M. (Meropi Mpouzika) and M.M. (Marianna Mantzorou); writing—review and editing, S.P., F.T., M.M. (Meropi Mpouzika), M.M. (Marianna Mantzorou) and T.K.; visualization, S.P.; supervision, E.P.; funding acquisition, S.P., M.M. (Marianna Mantzorou) and T.K. All authors have read and agreed to the published version of the manuscript.

Funding: This study was funded by the Special Account for Research Grants (ELKE), University of West Attica, Athens, Greece.

Institutional Review Board Statement: The study was conducted in accordance with the Declaration of Helsinki and was approved (a) by the PhD Program at the Department of Social Anthropology, PANTEION University of Social and Political Studies in Athens, and (b) by the Institutional Research and Ethics Committee of a hospital in Athens where the study was conducted (protocol number 7-11/7/12, date 11 July 2012).

Informed Consent Statement: Informed consent was obtained from all subjects involved in the study.

Data Availability Statement: Data generated during the present study cannot be shared due to issues of participants' privacy and confidentiality.

Acknowledgments: The authors are very thankful to the participant nurses of this study for sharing their own stories and experiences with such generosity. The first author is also very thankful to the supervisory team of the doctoral study (Eleni Papagaroufali, Athena Athanasiou and Dimitra Makrinioti) for their ongoing support and expert input.

Conflicts of Interest: The authors declare no conflict of interest.

References

1. Iliopoulou, K.K.; While, A.E. Professional autonomy and job satisfaction: Survey of critical care nurses in mainland Greece. *J. Adv. Nurs.* **2010**, *66*, 2520–2531. [CrossRef]
2. Fernández-Castillo, R.J.; González-Caro, M.D.; Fernández-García, E.; Porcel-Gálvez, A.M.; Garnacho-Montero, J. Intensive care nurses' experiences during the COVID-19 pandemic: A qualitative study. *Nurs. Crit. Care* **2021**, *26*, 397–406. [CrossRef]
3. Stavropoulou, A.; Rovithis, M.; Sigala, E.; Pantou, S.; Koukouli, S. Greek nurses' perceptions on empathy and empathic care in the Intensive Care Unit. *Intensiv. Crit. Care Nurs.* **2020**, *58*, 102814. [CrossRef] [PubMed]
4. Acea-López, L.; Pastor-Bravo, M.D.M.; Rubinat-Arnaldo, E.; Bellon, F.; Blanco-Blanco, J.; Gea-Sanchez, M.; Briones-Vozmediano, E. Burnout and job satisfaction among nurses in three Spanish regions. *J. Nurs. Manag.* **2021**, *29*, 2208–2215. [CrossRef]
5. Karlsson, M.; Pennbrant, S. Ideas of caring in nursing practice. *Nurs. Philos.* **2020**, *21*, e12325. [CrossRef]
6. Al-Shamaly, H.S. A focused ethnography of the culture of inclusive caring practice in the intensive care unit. *Nurs. Open* **2021**, *8*, 2973–2985. [CrossRef] [PubMed]
7. Al-Shamaly, H.S. Patterns of communicating care and caring in the intensive care unit. *Nurs. Open* **2022**, *9*, 277–298. [CrossRef]
8. Cook, L.B.; Peden, A. Finding a Focus for Nursing: The Caring Concept. *Adv. Nurs. Sci.* **2017**, *40*, 12–23. [CrossRef] [PubMed]
9. Leininger, M. Transcultural Care Principles, Human Rights, and Ethical Considerations. *J. Transcult. Nurs.* **1991**, *3*, 21–23. [CrossRef]
10. Tang, F.W.K.; Ling, G.C.C.; Lai, A.S.F.; Chair, S.Y.; So, W.K.W. Four Es of caring in contemporary nursing: Exploring novice to experienced nurses. *Nurs. Heal. Sci.* **2018**, *21*, 85–92. [CrossRef]
11. Brilowski, G.A.; Wendler, M.C. An evolutionary concept analysis of caring. *J. Adv. Nurs.* **2005**, *50*, 641–650. [CrossRef]
12. Sebrant, L.; Jong, M. What's the meaning of the concept of caring?: A meta-synthesis. *Scand. J. Caring Sci.* **2020**, *35*, 353–365. [CrossRef] [PubMed]
13. Rostami, S.; Esmaeali, R.; Jafari, H.; Yazdani-Charati, J. Perception of futile care and caring behaviors of nurses in intensive care units. *Nurs. Ethic* **2017**, *26*, 248–255. [CrossRef] [PubMed]
14. Adam, S.; Osborne, S.; Welch, J. *Critical Care Nursing: Science and Practice*, 3rd ed.; Adam, S., Osborne, S., Welch, J., Eds.; Oxford University Press: Oxford, UK, 2017; ISBN 9780199696260.
15. Sørensen, D.; Frederiksen, K.; Grøfte, T.; Lomborg, K. Practical wisdom: A qualitative study of the care and management of non-invasive ventilation patients by experienced intensive care nurses. *Intensiv. Crit. Care Nurs.* **2013**, *29*, 174–181. [CrossRef]

16. Li, S.; Mi, J.; Tang, Y. A qualitative study of nurses' perception on patients' thirst in intensive care units. *Intensiv. Crit. Care Nurs.* **2022**, *69*, 103184. [CrossRef]
17. Andersson, E.; Salickiene, Z.; Rosengren, K. To be involved—A qualitative study of nurses' experiences of caring for dying patients. *Nurse Educ. Today* **2016**, *38*, 144–149. [CrossRef] [PubMed]
18. Alastalo, M.; Salminen, L.; Lakanmaa, R.-L.; Leino-Kilpi, H. Seeing beyond monitors—Critical care nurses' multiple skills in patient observation: Descriptive qualitative study. *Intensiv. Crit. Care Nurs.* **2017**, *42*, 80–87. [CrossRef]
19. Nasrabadi, A.N.; Wibisono, A.H.; Allen, K.-A.; Yaghoobzadeh, A.; Bit-Lian, Y. Exploring the experiences of nurses' moral distress in long-term care of older adults: A phenomenological study. *BMC Nurs.* **2021**, *20*, 156. [CrossRef]
20. Vouzavali, F.J.; De Papathanassoglou, E.; Karanikola, M.N.; Koutroubas, A.; I Patiraki, E.; Papadatou, D. 'The patient is my space': Hermeneutic investigation of the nurse-patient relationship in critical care. *Nurs. Crit. Care* **2011**, *16*, 140–151. [CrossRef]
21. Morris, K.Y.; Jakobsen, R. Central venous catheter access and procedure compliance: A qualitative interview study exploring intensive care nurses' experiences. *Intensiv. Crit. Care Nurs.* **2022**, *69*, 103182. [CrossRef]
22. Moudatsou, M.; Stavropoulou, A.; Philalithis, A.; Koukouli, S. The Role of Empathy in Health and Social Care Professionals. *Healthcare* **2020**, *8*, 26. [CrossRef]
23. Bergman, L.; Falk, A.; Wolf, A.; Larsson, I.; Rn, C.L.B.; Rn, C.A.W. Registered nurses' experiences of working in the intensive care unit during the COVID-19 pandemic. *Nurs. Crit. Care* **2021**, *26*, 467–475. [CrossRef]
24. Cadge, W.; Lewis, M.; Bandini, J.; Shostak, S.; Donahue, V.; Trachtenberg, S.; Grone, K.; Kacmarek, R.; Lux, L.; Matthews, C.; et al. Intensive care unit nurses living through COVID-19: A qualitative study. *J. Nurs. Manag.* **2021**, *29*, 1965–1973. [CrossRef] [PubMed]
25. Liu, Q.; Luo, D.; Haase, J.E.; Guo, Q.; Wang, X.Q.; Liu, S.; Xia, L.; Liu, Z.; Yang, J.; Yang, B.X. The experiences of health-care providers during the COVID-19 crisis in China: A qualitative study. *Lancet Glob. Health* **2020**, *8*, e790–e798. [CrossRef] [PubMed]
26. Moradi, Y.; Baghaei, R.; Hosseingholipour, K.; Mollazadeh, F. Challenges experienced by ICU nurses throughout the provision of care for COVID-19 patients: A qualitative study. *J. Nurs. Manag.* **2021**, *29*, 1159–1168. [CrossRef]
27. Gordon, J.M.; Magbee, T.; Yoder, L.H. The experiences of critical care nurses caring for patients with COVID-19 during the 2020 pandemic: A qualitative study. *Appl. Nurs. Res.* **2021**, *59*, 151418. [CrossRef]
28. Koken, Z.O.; Savas, H.; Gul, S. Cardiovascular nurses' experiences of working in the COVID-19 intensive care unit: A qualitative study. *Intensiv. Crit. Care Nurs.* **2022**, *69*, 103181. [CrossRef] [PubMed]
29. Alquwez, N.; Cruz, J.P.; Balay-Odao, E.M.; Alquwez, R.N. Nurses' spiritual well-being and the COVID-19 pandemic: A thematic approach. *J. Nurs. Manag.* **2022**, *30*, 604–611. [CrossRef]
30. Beeby, J.P. Intensive care nurses' experiences of caring Part 2: Research findings. *Intensiv. Crit. Care Nurs.* **2000**, *16*, 151–163. [CrossRef]
31. Beeby, J.P. Intensive care nurses' experiences of caring. *Intensiv. Crit. Care Nurs.* **2000**, *16*, 76–83. [CrossRef]
32. Price, A.M. Caring and technology in an intensive care unit: An ethnographic study. *Nurs. Crit. Care* **2013**, *18*, 278–288. [CrossRef]
33. Scholtz, S.; Nel, E.W.; Poggenpoel, M.; Myburgh, C.P.H. The Culture of Nurses in a Critical Care Unit. *Glob. Qual. Nurs. Res.* **2016**, *3*, 1–11. [CrossRef]
34. Turnbull, E.; Flabouris, A.; Iedema, R. An outside perspective on the lifeworld of ICU. *Aust. Crit. Care* **2005**, *18*, 71–75. [CrossRef]
35. White, P.; Hillman, A.; Latimer, J. Ordering, Enrolling, and Dismissing. *Space Cult.* **2012**, *15*, 68–87. [CrossRef]
36. Schluter, J.; Seaton, P.; Chaboyer, W. Understanding nursing scope of practice: A qualitative study. *Int. J. Nurs. Stud.* **2011**, *48*, 1211–1222. [CrossRef]
37. Riley, R.; Manias, E. Foucault could have been an operating room nurse. *J. Adv. Nurs.* **2002**, *39*, 316–324. [CrossRef] [PubMed]
38. Nugus, P.; Greenfield, D.; Travaglia, J.; Westbrook, J.; Braithwaite, J. How and where clinicians exercise power: Interprofessional relations in health care. *Soc. Sci. Med.* **2010**, *71*, 898–909. [CrossRef]
39. Trapani, J. Critical care nurses as dual agents: Enhancing inter-professional collaboration or hindering patient advocacy? *Nurs. Crit. Care* **2014**, *19*, 219–221. [CrossRef]
40. Karanikola, M.N.K.; Papathanassoglou, E.D.E.; Nicolaou, C.; Koutroubas, A.; Lemonidou, C. Greek Intensive and Emergency Care Nurses' Perception of Their Public Image. *Dimens. Crit. Care Nurs.* **2011**, *30*, 108–116. [CrossRef]
41. Merkouris, A.; Papathanassoglou, E.; Pistolas, D.; Papagiannaki, V.; Floros, J.; Lemonidou, C. Staffing and Organisation of Nursing Care in Cardiac Intensive Care Units in Greece. *Eur. J. Cardiovasc. Nurs.* **2003**, *2*, 123–129. [CrossRef]
42. Papathanassoglou, E.D.; Tseroni, M.; Karydaki, A.; Vazaiou, G.; Kassikou, J.; Lavdaniti, M. Practice and clinical decision-making autonomy among Hellenic critical care nurses. *J. Nurs. Manag.* **2005**, *13*, 154–164. [CrossRef] [PubMed]
43. Papathanassoglou, E.D.; Karanikola, M.; Kalafati, M.; Giannakopoulou, M.; Lemonidou, C.; Albarran, J. Professional Autonomy, Collaboration with Physicians, and Moral Distress Among European Intensive Care Nurses. *Am. J. Crit. Care* **2012**, *21*, e41–e52. [CrossRef]
44. Parissopoulos, S. Nursing Praxis in Intensive Care Unit. Clinical Decision Making and Power Relations. Ph.D. Thesis, Panteion University of Social and Political Sciences, Athens, Greece, 2021.

45. Karlou, C.; Papadopoulou, C.; Papathanassoglou, E.; Lemonidou, C.; Vouzavali, F.; Zafiropoulou-Koutroubas, A.; Katsaragakis, S.; Patiraki, E. Nurses' Caring Behaviors Toward Patients Undergoing Chemotherapy in Greece. *Cancer Nurs.* **2018**, *41*, 399–408. [CrossRef]
46. Kaba, E.; Stavropoulou, A.; Kelesi, M.; Triantafyllou, A.; Goula, A.; Fasoi, G. Ten Key Steps to Writing a Protocol for a Qualitative Research Study: A Guide for Nurses and Health Professionals. *Glob. J. Health Sci.* **2021**, *13*, 58. [CrossRef]
47. Good, B.J. *Medicine, Rationality and Experience: An Anthropological Perspective (Lewis Henry Morgan Lectures)*; Cambridge University Press: Cambridge, UK, 2008.
48. Lafaut, D. Beyond biopolitics: The importance of the later work of Foucault to understand care practices of healthcare workers caring for undocumented migrants. *BMC Med. Ethic* **2021**, *22*, 157. [CrossRef]
49. Singer, M.; Baer, H.A. *Critical Medical Anthropology*; Imprint Routledge: Boca Raton, FL, USA, 2018; ISBN 9780415783767.
50. Armstrong, D. Bodies of Knowledge/Knowledge Of Bodies. In *Reassessing Foucault: Power, Medicine and the Body*; Jones, C., Porter, R., Eds.; Routledge: London, UK, 2006; pp. 17–27. ISBN 9780203019481.
51. Duranti, A. Husserl, intersubjectivity and anthropology. *Anthr. Theory* **2010**, *10*, 16–35. [CrossRef]
52. Throop, C.J. Articulating Experience. *Anthropol. Theory* **2003**, *3*, 219–241. [CrossRef]
53. Zahavi, D. The practice of phenomenology: The case of Max van Manen. *Nurs. Philos.* **2020**, *21*, e12276. [CrossRef]
54. Errasti-Ibarrondo, B.; Jordán, J.A.; Díez-Del-Corral, M.P.; Arantzamendi, M. van Manen's phenomenology of practice: How can it contribute to nursing? *Nurs. Inq.* **2019**, *26*, e12259. [CrossRef]
55. Csordas, T.J. *Embodiment and Experience: The Existential Ground of Culture and Self*; Csordas, T.J., Ed.; Cambridge University Press.: Cambridge, UK, 2003.
56. Merleau-Ponty, M. *Phenomenology of Perception*; The Humanities Press: London, UK, 1962.
57. Loudon, J.B.; Foucault, M.; Smith, A.M.S. The Birth of the Clinic: An Archaeology of Medical Perception. *Man* **1974**, *9*, 319. [CrossRef]
58. Allen, D.; Hughes, D.; Jordan, S.; Prowse, M.; Snelgrove, S. *Nursing and the Division of Labour in Healthcare*; Macmillan Education: London, UK, 2002.
59. Ryan, G.S. An introduction to the origins, history and principles of ethnography. *Nurse Res.* **2017**, *24*, 15–21. [CrossRef]
60. Robinson, S.G. The Relevancy of Ethnography to Nursing Research. *Nurs. Sci. Q.* **2013**, *26*, 14–19. [CrossRef] [PubMed]
61. Polit, D.F.; Beck, C.T. *Essentials of Nursing Research Methods, Appraisal, and Utilization*, 6th ed.; Lippincott Williams & Wilkins: Philadelphia, PA, USA, 2006.
62. Patton, M.Q. *Qualitative Research and Evaluation Methods: Theory and Practice*, 4th ed.; Sage Publications: Thousand Oaks, CA, USA, 2015; ISBN 9781412972123.
63. Desjarlais, R.; Throop, C.J. Phenomenological Approaches in Anthropology. *Annu. Rev. Anthr.* **2011**, *40*, 87–102. [CrossRef]
64. Braun, V.; Clarke, V. Using thematic analysis in psychology. *Qual. Res. Psychol.* **2006**, *3*, 77–101. [CrossRef]
65. Vaismoradi, M.; Turunen, H.; Bondas, T. Content analysis and thematic analysis: Implications for conducting a qualitative descriptive study. *Nurs. Health Sci.* **2013**, *15*, 398–405. [CrossRef]
66. Nowell, L.S.; Norris, J.M.; White, D.E.; Moules, N.J. Thematic Analysis: Striving to Meet the Trustworthiness Criteria. *Int. J. Qual. Methods* **2017**, *16*, 1–13. [CrossRef]
67. Maguire, M.; Delahunt, B. Doing a Thematic Analysis: A Practical, Step-by-Step Guide for Learning and Teaching Scholars. *All Irel. J. High. Educ.* **2017**, *9*, 3351.
68. Polit, D.F.; Beck, C. *Nursing Research: Generating and Assessing Evidence for Nursing Practice*, 10th ed.; Wolters Kluwer Health: Philadelphia, PA, USA, 2017; ISBN 1496300238.
69. Sandelowski, M. Using Qualitative Research. *Qual. Health Res.* **2004**, *14*, 1366–1386. [CrossRef] [PubMed]
70. Tong, A.; Sainsbury, P.; Craig, J. Consolidated criteria for reporting qualitative research (COREQ): A 32-item checklist for interviews and focus groups. *Int. J. Qual. Health Care* **2007**, *19*, 349–357. [CrossRef]
71. Gurné, F.L.; Lidén, E.; Ung, E.J.; Kirkevold, M.; Öhlén, J.; Jakobsson, S. Striving to be in close proximity to the patient: An interpretive descriptive study of nursing practice from the perspectives of clinically experienced registered nurses. *Nurs. Inq.* **2021**, *28*, e12387. [CrossRef]
72. Christensen, M.; Hewitt-Taylor, J. Defining the expert ICU nurse. *Intensiv. Crit. Care Nurs.* **2006**, *22*, 301–307. [CrossRef] [PubMed]
73. Karlsson, V.; Bergbom, I. ICU Professionals' Experiences of Caring for Conscious Patients Receiving MVT. *West. J. Nurs. Res.* **2015**, *37*, 360–375. [CrossRef]
74. Karlsson, V.; Bergbom, I.; Forsberg, A. The lived experiences of adult intensive care patients who were conscious during mechanical ventilation: A phenomenological-hermeneutic study. *Intensiv. Crit. Care Nurs.* **2012**, *28*, 6–15. [CrossRef] [PubMed]
75. Rogers, C.R. The necessary and sufficient conditions of therapeutic personality change. *Psychotherapy* **2007**, *44*, 240–248. [CrossRef]
76. Quinn, J.F. The Self as Healer: Reflections From a Nurse's Journey. *AACN Clin. Issues Adv. Pract. Acute Crit. Care* **2000**, *11*, 17–26. [CrossRef] [PubMed]
77. Koukouli, S.; Lambraki, M.; Sigala, E.; Alevizaki, A.; Stavropoulou, A. The experience of Greek families of critically ill patients: Exploring their needs and coping strategies. *Intensiv. Crit. Care Nurs.* **2018**, *45*, 44–51. [CrossRef] [PubMed]
78. Sinclair, S.; McClement, S.; Raffin-Bouchal, S.; Hack, T.F.; Hagen, N.A.; McConnell, S.; Chochinov, H.M. Compassion in Health Care: An Empirical Model. *J. Pain Symptom Manag.* **2016**, *51*, 193–203. [CrossRef]

79. Hov, R.; Hedelin, B.; Athlin, E. Being an intensive care nurse related to questions of withholding or withdrawing curative treatment. *J. Clin. Nurs.* **2007**, *16*, 203–211. [CrossRef]
80. Asadi, N.; Royani, Z.; Maazallahi, M.; Salmani, F. Being torn by inevitable moral dilemma: Experiences of ICU nurses. *BMC Med. Ethic* **2021**, *22*, 159. [CrossRef]
81. Wiegand, D.L.; Funk, M. Consequences of clinical situations that cause critical care nurses to experience moral distress. *Nurs. Ethics* **2012**, *19*, 479–487. [CrossRef]
82. Short, P. Picturing the Body in Nursing. In *The Body in Nursing*; Lawler, J., Ed.; Pearson Professional: South Melbourne, Australia, 1997; pp. 7–9. ISBN 0443052506.
83. House, S.; Havens, D. Nurses' and Physicians' Perceptions of Nurse-Physician Collaboration. *JONA J. Nurs. Adm.* **2017**, *47*, 165–171. [CrossRef] [PubMed]
84. Coughlin, C. An ethnographic study of main events during hospitalisation: Perceptions of nurses and patients. *J. Clin. Nurs.* **2013**, *22*, 2327–2337. [CrossRef] [PubMed]
85. Hasse, G.L. Patient-Centered Care in Adult Trauma Intensive Care Unit. *J. Trauma Nurs.* **2013**, *20*, 163–165. [CrossRef] [PubMed]
86. Limbu, S.; Kongsuwan, W.; Yodchai, K. Lived experiences of intensive care nurses in caring for critically ill patients. *Nurs. Crit. Care* **2019**, *24*, 9–14. [CrossRef] [PubMed]
87. Nettleton, S. *The Sociology of Health and Illness*, 4th ed.; Polity Press: Cambridge, UK, 2021; ISBN 978-1-509-51273-7.
88. Bucknall, T. The clinical landscape of critical care: Nurses' decision-making. *J. Adv. Nurs.* **2003**, *43*, 310–319. [CrossRef]
89. Bucknall, T.K. Critical care nurses' decision-making activities in the natural clinical setting. *J. Clin. Nurs.* **2000**, *9*, 25–36. [CrossRef]
90. Henriksen, K.F.; Hansen, B.S.; Wøien, H.; Tønnessen, S. The core qualities and competencies of the intensive and critical care nurse, a meta-ethnography. *J. Adv. Nurs.* **2021**, *77*, 4693–4710. [CrossRef]
91. Kaya, H.; Kaya, N.; Turan, Y.; Tan, Y.M.; Terzi, B.; Barlas, D.B. Nursing activities in intensive care units in Turkey. *Int. J. Nurs. Pract.* **2011**, *17*, 304–314. [CrossRef]
92. Pattison, N. An ever-thorny issue: Defining key elements of critical care nursing and its relation to staffing. *Nurs. Crit. Care* **2021**, *26*, 421–424. [CrossRef]
93. Bloomer, M.J.; Fulbrook, P.; Goldsworthy, S.; Livesay, S.L.; Mitchell, M.L.; Williams, G.; Friganovic, A. World Federation of Critical Care Nurses 2019 Position Statement: Provision of a Critical Care Nursing Workforce. *Connect. World Crit. Care Nurs.* **2019**, *13*, 3–7. [CrossRef]
94. Liu, W.; Manias, E.; Gerdtz, M. Medication communication through documentation in medical wards: Knowledge and power relations. *Nurs. Inq.* **2014**, *21*, 246–258. [CrossRef]
95. Liu, W.; Manias, E.; Gerdtz, M. Medication communication between nurses and patients during nursing handovers on medical wards: A critical ethnographic study. *Int. J. Nurs. Stud.* **2012**, *49*, 941–952. [CrossRef]
96. Coombs, M. Power and conflict in intensive care clinical decision making. *Intensiv. Crit. Care Nurs.* **2003**, *19*, 125–135. [CrossRef] [PubMed]
97. Coombs, M.; Ersser, S.J. Medical hegemony in decision-making—A barrier to interdisciplinary working in intensive care? *J. Adv. Nurs.* **2004**, *46*, 245–252. [CrossRef] [PubMed]
98. Currey, J.; Botti, M. The influence of patient complexity and nurses' experience on haemodynamic decision-making following cardiac surgery. *Intensiv. Crit. Care Nurs.* **2006**, *22*, 194–205. [CrossRef] [PubMed]
99. Manias, E.; Street, A. The interplay of knowledge and decision making between nurses and doctors in critical care. *Int. J. Nurs. Stud.* **2001**, *38*, 129–140. [CrossRef]
100. Herring, R.; Desai, T.; Caldwell, G. Quality and safety at the point of care: How long should a ward round take? *Clin. Med.* **2011**, *11*, 20–22. [CrossRef]
101. Kozlowski, D.; Hutchinson, M.; Hurley, J.; Rowley, J.; Sutherland, J. The role of emotion in clinical decision making: An integrative literature review. *BMC Med. Educ.* **2017**, *17*, 255. [CrossRef]
102. Parissopoulos, S.; Timmins, F.; Daly, L. Re-exploring the ritual of the ward round. *Nurs. Crit. Care* **2013**, *18*, 219–221. [CrossRef]
103. Mohr, D.C.; Swamy, L.; Wong, E.S.; Mealer, P.M.; Moss, M.; Rinne, S.T. Critical Care Nurse Burnout in Veterans Health Administration: Relation to Clinician and Patient Outcomes. *Am. J. Crit. Care* **2021**, *30*, 435–442. [CrossRef]
104. Tang, C.; Chan, S.; Zhou, W.; Liaw, S. Collaboration between hospital physicians and nurses: An integrated literature review. *Int. Nurs. Rev.* **2013**, *60*, 291–302. [CrossRef] [PubMed]
105. Wang, Y.-Y.; Wan, Q.-Q.; Lin, F.; Zhou, W.-J.; Shang, S.-M. Interventions to improve communication between nurses and physicians in the intensive care unit: An integrative literature review. *Int. J. Nurs. Sci.* **2017**, *5*, 81–88. [CrossRef]
106. Sun, N.; Wei, L.; Shi, S.; Jiao, D.; Song, R.; Ma, L.; Wang, H.; Wang, C.; Wang, Z.; You, Y.; et al. A qualitative study on the psychological experience of caregivers of COVID-19 patients. *Am. J. Infect. Control.* **2020**, *48*, 592–598. [CrossRef]
107. Liu, S.; Yang, L.; Zhang, C.; Xiang, Y.-T.; Liu, Z.; Hu, S.; Zhang, B. Online mental health services in China during the COVID-19 outbreak. *Lancet Psychiatry* **2020**, *7*, e17–e18. [CrossRef]
108. Huang, H.; Xia, Y.; Zeng, X.; Lü, A. Prevalence of depression and depressive symptoms among intensive care nurses: A meta-analysis. *Nurs. Crit. Care* **2022**, *27*, 739–746. [CrossRef] [PubMed]

109. Kelly, L.A.; Johnson, K.L.; Bay, R.C.; Todd, M. Key Elements of the Critical Care Work Environment Associated With Burnout and Compassion Satisfaction. *Am. J. Crit. Care* **2021**, *30*, 113–120. [CrossRef] [PubMed]
110. Moloney, W.; Fieldes, J.; Jacobs, S. An Integrative Review of How Healthcare Organizations Can Support Hospital Nurses to Thrive at Work. *Int. J. Environ. Res. Public Health* **2020**, *17*, 8757. [CrossRef]

Disclaimer/Publisher's Note: The statements, opinions and data contained in all publications are solely those of the individual author(s) and contributor(s) and not of MDPI and/or the editor(s). MDPI and/or the editor(s) disclaim responsibility for any injury to people or property resulting from any ideas, methods, instructions or products referred to in the content.

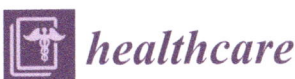

Article

Violence, Harassment, and Turnover Intention in Home and Community Care: The Role of Training

Firat K. Sayin [1,*], Margaret Denton [2], Catherine Brookman [3], Sharon Davies [4] and Isik U. Zeytinoglu [5]

1 Department of Management, Sobey School of Business, Saint Mary's University, Halifax, NS B3H 3C3, Canada
2 Department of Health, Aging & Society, McMaster University, Hamilton, ON L8S 4L8, Canada
3 Catherine Brookman Consulting & Associates, Hamilton, ON L8S 4L8, Canada
4 DeGroote School of Business, McMaster University, Hamilton, ON L8S 4L8, Canada
5 Human Resources and Management Area, DeGroote School of Business, McMaster University, Hamilton, ON L8S 4L8, Canada
* Correspondence: firat.sayin@smu.ca; Tel.: +1-902-420-5781

Abstract: Background: Violence and harassment affect healthcare workers' well-being and career decisions in the home and community care sector. Purpose: The objective of this study is to assess the role of training in alleviating the relationship between violence and harassment at work and turnover intention among personal support workers (PSWs). Methodology/Approach: Cross-sectional survey data from 1401 PSWs in Ontario, Canada are analyzed with structural equation modeling. Utilizing a resource perspective, the associations between job demands (i.e., violence and harassment at work), personal resources (i.e., self-esteem), job resources (i.e., workplace violence training and challenging task training), stress, and intention to stay among personal support workers (PSWs) are examined. Results: Challenging task training is positively associated with self-esteem and negatively associated with stress, whereas workplace violence training does not have a significant association with either variable. Stress has a negative relationship with intention to stay. Self-esteem is the mediator of both associations between violence and harassment at work and stress and between challenging task training and stress. Discussion: The results point to varied degrees of training effectiveness that may be shaping turnover decisions of PSWs who experience violence and harassment in home and community care organizations. Practice implications: There seems to be a need to assess and redesign workplace violence training. Home and community care managers might be able to lower the impact of violence and harassment on PSWs' turnover by providing training that is not directly related to workplace violence and harassment.

Keywords: intention to stay; workplace violence and harassment; conservation of resources theory; job demands–resources theory; workplace training; stress; self-esteem; personal support workers; health support workers; home care organizations; community care organizations

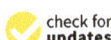

Citation: Sayin, F.K.; Denton, M.; Brookman, C.; Davies, S.; Zeytinoglu, I.U. Violence, Harassment, and Turnover Intention in Home and Community Care: The Role of Training. *Healthcare* **2023**, *11*, 103. https://doi.org/10.3390/healthcare11010103

Academic Editors: Sofia Koukouli and Areti Stavropoulou

Received: 13 November 2022
Revised: 18 December 2022
Accepted: 25 December 2022
Published: 29 December 2022

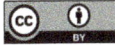

Copyright: © 2022 by the authors. Licensee MDPI, Basel, Switzerland. This article is an open access article distributed under the terms and conditions of the Creative Commons Attribution (CC BY) license (https://creativecommons.org/licenses/by/4.0/).

1. Introduction

Violence and harassment at work is a serious concern in the healthcare sector in Canada and elsewhere. A 2019 report prepared for the House of Commons Canada states that healthcare workers are exposed to workplace violence significantly more than any other profession in Canada [1]. Thus, violence and harassment are increasingly recognized as critical determinants of healthcare workers' well-being and career decisions [2,3]. This paper examines the relationship between personal support workers' (PSWs) job demands that result in violence and harassment at work, personal resource of self-esteem, job resources of workplace violence training and challenging task training, PSWs' well-being of stress, career decisions and organizational outcome of intention to stay in the organization. The analysis utilizes a resource perspective, bringing together job demands and resources theory [4] and conservation of resources theory [5].

Violence and harassment in healthcare workplaces can lead to detrimental worker outcomes related to stress [3] and organizational outcomes of turnover intentions [2]. Training is a job resource used to prevent or alleviate the negative outcomes of violence and harassment in the healthcare sector [6]. Research on workplace violence training in the healthcare sector, however, shows inconclusive results. For example, a study conducted in community care organizations found that there was no difference in workplace violence and harassment exposure among those who received workplace violence training and those who did not [7]. On the other hand, Nachreiner et al. [8] demonstrated that workplace training increased the probability of exposure to workplace violence. Understanding the effectiveness of specialized training related to violence and harassment in the healthcare sector is imperative in reducing stress and retaining PSWs.

While training as a job resource is important in shaping PSWs' experience of violence and harassment at work, the resource perspective argues that violence and harassment at work as work stressors can be ameliorated with the interplay of the personal resource of self-esteem and the job resource of training. Specifically, we examine the buffering roles of self-esteem as a personal resource and workplace violence training and challenging task training as job resources in the relationship between PSWs' exposure to violence and harassment at work, stress, and intention to stay. Furthermore, we investigate the reciprocal relationship among self-esteem, workplace violence training, and challenging task training to apprehend how different resources may be associated with each other. Our data comes from 1401 PSWs in Ontario, Canada.

Our study has important contributions to theory and knowledge. The study contributes to theory by shedding light on the resource perspective. Furthermore, we contribute to practitioner knowledge by examining the effectiveness of two types of training received by PSWs: workplace violence training and challenging task training. It is important to understand the effectiveness of these trainings not only for improving the well-being of PSWs but also for retaining PSWs in their workplaces.

1.1. Background to the Study

There is an increased demand for home and community care services in Canada and most industrialized countries due to demographic shifts and healthcare sector restructuring [9]. PSWs play a key role in addressing the demand for home and community care services. They provide care to individuals such as post-acute patients, older people, and people with disabilities who need support with their everyday tasks to live independently. PSWs are also known in other countries as health support workers, social and healthcare assistants, home healthcare aides, home healthcare workers, and home care workers. PSWs' workplaces include care recipients' dwellings, supportive housing programs, and community care, long-term care, and retirement homes. In accordance with the need for their services, PSWs constitute the largest group of providers in the Canadian home and community care sector.

PSWs, as frontline workers in the home and community care sector, experience violence and harassment at work [10]. Violence and harassment at work can be at least partially avoided by allocating necessary job resources to workers. Thus, human resource policies regarding organizational resources can shape PSWs' exposure to violence and harassment at work. The topic receives extensive attention by all stakeholders, including the health and safety associations providing health and safety training and resources to healthcare employers, unions, and workers, though the extent of training uptake by workers is not known.

The PSWs included in this study work in Ontario, Canada. Ontario has occupational health and safety legislation (e.g., Occupational Health and Safety Act, R.S.O. 1990, c. O.1) that designate responsibilities of healthcare organizations to address workplace violence and harassment. Nevertheless, these responsibilities, including training addressed to alleviate the adverse effect of workplace violence and harassment, are vague and left to employer discretion [6]. Thus, training of PSWs is a high-priority issue for the home care sector in Canada [9], especially because it is an important determinant of retention [11]. The challenges of violence and harassment experienced by the PSWs and the interest of their employing organizations, unions, and professional organizations in assisting the workers, along with the provincial government's interest in documenting this phenomenon, are the impetus for our study.

1.2. Theory

The theoretical foundation of this study is based on the resource perspective, which is the integration of the job demands and resources (JD-R) and conservation of resources (COR) theories [12]. According to the JD-R theory, work environment characteristics can be categorized into two groups, as job demands and job resources [4]. Both job demands and resources can be physical, social, psychological, or organizational [13]. The JD-R theory states that job demands lead to strain but job resources can buffer the impact of job demands on strain. Bakker and Demerouti [4] offer an extended model based on the JD-R theory where personal resources are incorporated into the model. In this model, job resources and personal resources interact and act as a buffer between job demands and strain [4]. According to the COR theory, the prime motivation of human beings is to gain, protect, and accumulate resources such as health, well-being, and personal characteristics that may assist in dealing with stress [5,14]. Furthermore, individuals attempt to acquire resources to recover from losses [15] In the workplace context, workers use their personal resources to cope with job demands [16]. Workers may experience stress when job demands exceed personal resources [5].

The model developed in this paper is guided by the organizational health framework developed by Hart and Cooper [17]. Hart and Cooper's [17] framework argues that organizational and individual characteristics interact to shape employee well-being, which in turn, affects organizational outcomes. We build on this framework using the resource perspective [12] and develop the model of violence and harassment at work, training, self-esteem, stress, and intention to stay relationships for PSWs. The model integrates job demand (violence and harassment at work), job resources (challenging task training and workplace violence training), personal resources (self-esteem), employee well-being (stress), and organizational performance (intention to stay). In applying the JD-R theory to PSWs in our study, we argue that when PSWs experience violence and harassment at work, self-esteem acts as a buffer reducing the effect of violence and harassment at work. The model can be seen in Figure 1.

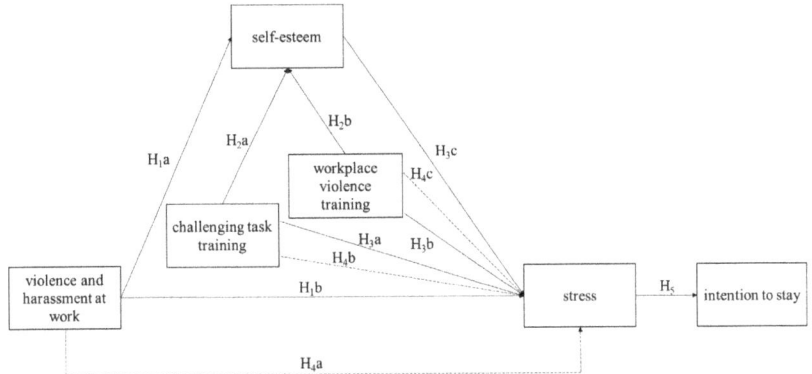

Figure 1. Hypothesized relationships between intention to stay, violence and harassment, challenging task training, workplace violence training, self-esteem, and stress. Notes: Solid lines indicate direct effects; dashes indicate indirect effects.

Self-esteem is one's evaluations of self in life [18] and is a personal resource according to the JD-R theory [13–15,19]. The JD-R theory states that job demands lead to strain [4], which can then manifest itself as stress. The relationship between home care workers' exposure to workplace violence and stress was previously documented in Canada [10]. As presented in our model (see Figure 1), we argue that violence and harassment at PSWs' work increase their level of stress. Thus, we hypothesize that:

Hypothesis 1a (H1a): *Violence and harassment at work is negatively associated with self-esteem.*

Hypothesis 1b (H1b): *Violence and harassment at work is positively associated with stress.*

As PSWs are exposed to violence and harassment at work, they face the risk of losing an important personal resource: self-esteem. We argue that challenging task training and workplace violence training, the types of workplace training examined in this paper, can contribute to self-esteem. Challenging task training is essentially a critical thinking skills training that is broad enough to cover a number of challenging circumstances that PSWs might experience at work and provides skills to identify and resolve those challenges. Challenging tasks training can include assisting with the complex healthcare needs of clients, dealing with irritated clients whose needs are not being met, training to manage too many different tasks at the same time while delivering good quality care, and training to care for clients too sick to be at home. Workplace violence training can help to increase PSWs' awareness of risky situations and prevent problems from happening before they further escalate [20]. Workplace violence training can include recognizing and knowing how to respond to the threat of, attempt to, or exercise of physical strength against the PSW. This may be physical violence (i.e., scratching, pinching, pushing, spitting, slapping/hitting, kicking, biting, punching, restraining) or sexual violence. Workplace violence training can also include recognizing and knowing how to respond to harassing behavior that demeans, humiliates, annoys, alarms, or verbally abuses the PSW or is considered by the PSW as unwelcome. This harassing behavior may be words, gestures, intimidation, bullying, or other inappropriate activities. PSWs who are trained in recognizing workplace violence and harassment and taking measures to prevent the occurrence of violence and harassment have higher self-esteem, with training positively contributing to self-esteem. Thus, training can be an important job resource that enhances PSWs' personal resource of self-esteem. Therefore, we hypothesize that:

Hypothesis 2a (H2a): *Challenging task training is positively associated with self-esteem.*

Hypothesis 2b (H2b): *Workplace violence training is positively associated with self-esteem.*

Stress occurs as a result of interaction between individuals and their environments [5,14]. This implies that job demands, personal resources, and job resources interact to influence stress. According to the JD-R theory, job demands may lead to stress, and job resources and personal resources buffer this relationship [4] The COR theory states that the loss of personal resources such as self-esteem can lead to stress [15]. For example, Yang, Ju, and Lee [21] demonstrated the negative relationship between job stress and self-esteem. Thus, job resources, including challenging task and workplace violence training, are expected to have a negative relationship with stress. Furthermore, the personal resource of self-esteem should have a negative relationship with stress. Therefore, we hypothesize that:

Hypothesis 3a (H3a): *Challenging task training is negatively associated with stress.*

Hypothesis 3b (H3b): *Workplace violence training is negatively associated with stress.*

Hypothesis 3c (H3c): *Self-esteem is negatively associated with stress.*

The JD-R model argues that job resources can act as a buffer between job demands and strains [4]. For example, Xanthopoulou et al. [22] demonstrated the mutual relationship between job and personal resources. However, how job demands, job resources, and personal resources interact to shape strain has not been definitively explained [4]. Demerouti and Bakker [23] suggested that personal resources can be included in the JD-R model as mediator. According to the resource perspective [12], it is possible that personal resources can have a multiple mediator role. Specifically, we argue that the personal resource of self-esteem mediates the relationship between job demands of violence and harassment at work and stress as well as the relationship between the job resources of challenging task training and workplace violence training and stress. As such, we hypothesize that:

Hypothesis 4a (H4a): *Self-esteem mediates the relationship between violence and harassment at work and stress.*

Hypothesis 4b (H4b): *Self-esteem mediates the relationship between challenging task training and stress.*

Hypothesis 4c (H4c): *Self-esteem mediates the relationship between workplace violence training and stress.*

Both job resources and personal characteristics can shape turnover intention in organizations [24]. Intention to stay is a strong indicator of actual turnover behavior [25,26], which is an important outcome considering the potential adverse impact of turnover behavior on organizational outcomes. Previous research showed that stress can lower intention to stay [27]. Furthermore, it was found that stress has a positive relationship with intention to quit [28]. While intention to stay and intention to quit may not be exactly opposite, there is a high level of similarity between them. Thus, we hypothesize that:

Hypothesis 5 (H5): *Stress is negatively associated with intention to stay.*

2. Materials and Methods

2.1. Research Design and Data Collection

The current study is a part of a larger project aimed at examining occupational health and safety of home- and community-based PSWs in Ontario, Canada. Our project is guided by a research advisory committee, which consisted of representatives from home care organization associations, PSW associations, health and safety associations with an expertise in PSWs, unions, and the project research team (see Acknowledgments section). In this study, we use our 2015 cross-sectional survey. The survey was administered online on our project website. Printed mail-out surveys were also sent to respondents upon request. We encouraged participants to complete the entire survey and provided minor incentives such as gift cards to improve the response rate while underlining the voluntary nature of the survey.

2.2. Population and Sample

Our survey respondents are PSWs employed in the home and community care sector in Ontario, Canada. The PSW work is a female-dominated occupation, and similarly, 93.1 percent of our respondents are females. The average age of our respondents is 48.5. Personal support work is not a regulated profession and there is no mandatory registry in Ontario. The number of PSWs working at the home and community care context in Ontario was estimated as 26,000 in 2011 [29]. 1,746 respondents submitted the survey electronically or mailed a completed hard copy of the survey back to us. The sample size of the current study is 1401 after listwise deletion.

2.3. Measures

We used previously published scales in this study. As Table 1 demonstrates, there is a high internal reliability for all scales, ranging from 0.79 to 0.91. Dichotomous variables are coded 1 for agreeing and 0 for disagreeing with the statement. Items are measured on a five-point Likert scale anchored with 5 as 'strongly agree' and 1 as 'strongly disagree'.

Table 1. Means, standard deviations, correlations, and scale reliabilities.

	Variable	Mean	SD	Min	Max	1	2	3	4	5	6	7	8	9	10
1	Intention to stay	11.56	2.76	3	15	0.91									
2	Violence and harassment at work (%)	20.91	-	0	1	−0.13 *									
3	Challenging task training (%)	74.09	-	0	1	0.35 *	−0.21 *								
4	Workplace violence training (%)	72.45	-	0	1	0.16 *	−0.031	0.24 *							
5	Self-esteem	24.60	3.72	6	30	0.18 *	−0.11 *	0.19 *	0.04	0.79					
6	Stress	28.33	7.81	14	57	−0.26 *	0.23 *	−0.24 *	−0.03	−0.65 *	0.86				
7	Tenure (years)	9.80	-	1	38	0.02	0.02	0.00	0.06 *	0.02	−0.02				
8	High school (%)	14.20	-	0	1	0.03	−0.07 *	0.10 *	0.00	0.03	−0.09 *	0.08 *			
9	Trade school (%)	11.64	-	0	1	0.01	0.05 *	−0.11 *	−0.06 *	−0.01	−0.01	−0.01	−0.15 *		
10	College (%)	58.39	-	0	1	−0.02	0.04	−0.01	−0.04	−0.04	0.07 *	0.02	−0.48 *	−0.43 *	
11	University (%)	15.78	-	0	1	−0.02	−0.03	0.02	0.09 *	0.03	−0.00	−0.09 *	−0.17 *	−0.16 *	−0.51 *

Notes: $N = 1401$, * $p < 0.05$, Cronbach's alpha values are in italics on the diagonal. The mean values of the categorical variables are presented as percentage for ease of interpretation.

2.3.1. Dependent Variable

Intention to stay is a three-item scale by Lyons [30]. An example scale item is 'You would like to stay at your organization for a long time'.

2.3.2. Independent Variables

Violence and harassment at work, challenging task training, and workplace violence training are dichotomous variables. Violence and harassment at work is measured with 'In your job as a PSW in the community, in the past 12 months, have you been a victim of physical or sexual violence or harassment at work?' Challenging task training is measured with 'Your organization provides you with the appropriate training to handle challenging tasks'. Workplace violence training is measured with 'What types of health and safety training have you had at your organization? Please choose all that apply: workplace violence training'.

2.3.3. Mediating Variables

Self-esteem and stress are the mediators of this study. We use a global (i.e., general) conceptualization of self-esteem. A global conceptualization of self-esteem has been shown to be related to work conditions such as workplace violence and harassment, job satisfaction, and job rewards [19]. Furthermore, Jex and Elacqua [18] suggest that it can be appropriate to use a global conceptualization of self-esteem if a general stress measure is used. Thus, we use a global conceptualization of self-esteem since we also use a general stress measure. Self-esteem is measured with a six-item scale developed by Pearlin and Schooler [31]. A sample item is "during the past month: on the whole, satisfied with yourself'. The second mediator, stress, is measured with a 14-item symptoms of stress scale by Denton, Zeytinoglu, Davies, and Lian [32]. A sample item is "Below is a list of the ways that some people feel. During the past month: (a) able to sleep through the night (reversed), (b) irritable and tense."

2.3.4. Control Variables

Tenure and education are the control variables. Rodwell and Demir [33] showed that tenure can affect the exposure of workplace violence among healthcare workers. We measured tenure with years working as a PSW in the home and community care sector. Education is included to account for human capital factors besides tenure and categorized into four dichotomous variables: high school (reference), trade school, college, and university.

2.4. Analysis

We used procedural and statistical remedies to alleviate common method bias. We followed procedural remedies such as conducting a pilot study of the survey in both online and print format and balancing positive and negative items as suggested by Podsakoff, MacKenzie, and Podsakoff [34]. As a statistical remedy, we added a first-order factor with all measures and did not find any items with significant factor loadings [35]. We examined multicollinearity by calculating bivariate correlations and variance inflation factors. The strongest bivariate correlation is 0.65, which is lower than the threshold of 0.80 suggested by Meyers et al. [36]. Thus, we believe our analysis does not suffer from multicollinearity.

We used STATA 15 to conduct structural equation modeling (SEM) with maximum-likelihood estimation. We compared the fit indices of full mediation (i.e., no direct effect between violence and stress) and partial mediation (i.e., direct effect between violence and harassment at work) models. The partial mediation model had a better fit than the full mediation model. Thus, we present the partial mediation model as our final model. The goodness-of-fit indices (i.e., root mean square error of approximation, standardized root mean square residual, comparative fit index, Tucker–Lewis index) indicate that our final model has an adequate fit: χ^2 = 2240.48, d.f. 371; RMSEA = 0.06; SRMR = 0.06; CFI = 0.86; TLI = 0.84.

3. Results

3.1. Descriptive Statistics

Table 1 indicates that the PSWs in our sample have a moderately high intention to stay, high self-esteem, and moderately low stress. About one-fifth of the respondents experienced violence and harassment at work in the past 12 months prior to data collection. Most PSWs received challenging task or workplace violence training and hold a college degree or above. Average years of work experience as PSWs approximated to 10 years.

3.2. Correlations

The bivariate correlations can be seen in Table 1. Intention to stay is negatively correlated with violence and harassment at work and stress and positively correlated with challenging task training, workplace violence training, and self-esteem. Violence and harassment at work has a negative correlation with challenging task training and self-esteem, positive correlation with stress, and a statistically non-significant relationship with workplace violence training. Challenging task training is positively associated with workplace violence training and self-esteem and negatively correlated with stress. Workplace violence training does not have a significant correlation with self-esteem and stress. Finally, stress has a strong negative association with self-esteem.

3.3. SEM Analysis

The direct effects can be seen in Figure 2. All coefficients are standardized for ease of interpretation.

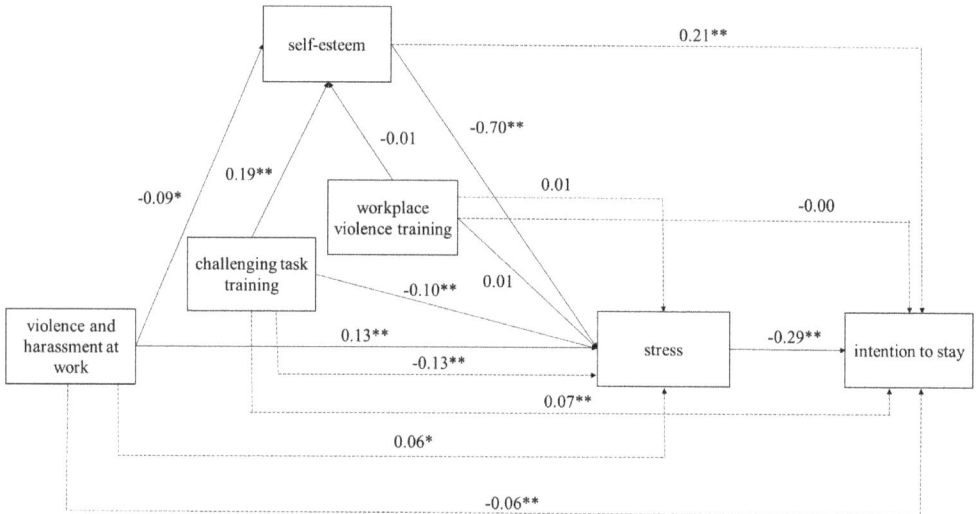

Figure 2. Direct effects between intention to stay, violence and harassment, challenging task training, workplace violence training, self-esteem, and stress. All coefficients are standardized. The control variables are tenure and education (high school or less (reference), trade school, college, university or higher). * $p < 0.01$; ** $p < 0.001$, and $p > 0.05$ for the remaining associations. Notes: N = 1401.

Violence and harassment at work is negatively associated with self-esteem ($\beta = -0.09$, $p < 0.01$) and positively associated with stress ($\beta = 0.13$, $p < 0.001$), supporting Hypotheses 1a and 1b, respectively. Challenging task training is positively associated with self-esteem ($\beta = 0.19$, $p < 0.001$); thus, Hypothesis 2a is supported. Workplace violence training does not have a significant association with self-esteem ($\beta = -0.01$, $p > 0.05$), rejecting Hypothesis 2b. Challenging task training is negatively associated with stress ($\beta = -0.10$, $p < 0.001$), workplace violence training is not significantly associated with stress ($\beta = 0.01, p > 0.05$), and self-esteem is negatively associated with stress ($\beta = -0.70, p < 0.001$). Thus, Hypotheses 3a and 3c are supported and Hypothesis 3b is rejected.

We employ indirect effects to test mediation relationships (i.e., Hypotheses 4a-c) as suggested by Preacher and Hayes [37]. The indirect effects can be seen in Figure 2. The results indicate that stress has an indirect positive association with violence and harassment at work ($\beta = 0.06, p < 0.01$), negative association with challenging task training ($\beta = -0.13, p < 0.001$), and a non-significant association with workplace violence training ($\beta = 0.01, p > 0.05$). Thus, Hypotheses 4a and 4b are supported and Hypothesis 4c is rejected. These results indicate that self-esteem mediates the associations between violence and harassment at work and stress, and challenging task training and stress, but does not mediate the workplace violence training and stress association. Finally, Hypothesis 5 tests the direct association between stress and intention to stay, and it is supported ($\beta = -0.29, p < 0.001$).

The remaining indirect effects indicate that intention to stay is negatively associated with violence and harassment at work, positively associated with challenging task training and self-esteem, and not significantly associated with workplace violence training. These results are in line with our hypotheses, except the non-significant association between workplace violence training and intention to stay.

Most of the control variables do not have statistically significant associations. Among direct effects, stress is positively associated with college ($\beta = 0.08, p < 0.05$) and university ($\beta = 0.08, p < 0.01$). The only statistically significant indirect effect is the negative association between intention to stay and college ($\beta = -0.03, p < 0.05$).

4. Discussion

This study found that violence was related negatively to self-esteem and positively to stress. Self-esteem was positively associated with challenging task training, did not have a significant relationship with workplace violence training, and negatively associated with stress. We showed that stress was not significantly associated with workplace violence training and had a negative association with challenging task training. Furthermore, we demonstrated that self-esteem partially mediated between violence and harassment at work stress and challenging task training/stress relationships. Finally, we found that stress had a negative relationship with intention to stay.

Our theoretical contribution is the extension of the resource perspective by highlighting the relationship between personal resources and job resources. While it was shown before that personal resources and job resources can play a buffer role between job demands and stress and stress-related outcomes (e.g., burnout), the relationship between personal and job resources required further exploration [4,23]. Our findings contribute to this discussion by empirically demonstrating personal and job resource relationship. Specifically, we show that self-esteem as a personal resource partially mediates the relationship between a job demand (i.e., violence and harassment at work) and stress.

Furthermore, we demonstrate that challenging task training as a job resource has a direct and indirect impact on stress with self-esteem as a mediator. Thus, our model indicates that personal resources can mediate both job demand and stress, and job resource and stress relationships. Furthermore, our findings indicate the elevated importance of personal resources in a high job demand–low job resource context. Future studies can further examine the critical role of personal resources in different contexts testing for other personal resources such as self-efficacy, psychological capital, resilience, and autonomy.

Our findings have important contributions to empirical academic knowledge as well. We found that challenging task training can boost PSWs' self-esteem and lower their stress directly and indirectly. Furthermore, challenging task training had a positive indirect relationship with intention to stay. This finding is in line with the results from previous studies that demonstrated the positive relationship between training and intention to stay [38]. On the other hand, we showed that workplace violence training did not have any significant associations with self-esteem, stress, or intention to stay. We conclude that challenging task training can help PSWs to alleviate the adverse impact of workplace violence and harassment, whereas workplace violence training might not be as effective. Thus, our study contributes to establishing conflicting findings [7,8] on workplace violence training effectiveness of healthcare workers.

There can be different factors behind the ineffectiveness of workplace violence training. For example, Kelly [10] indicated that PSW training programs, especially those addressing workplace violence, focused more on long-term care settings and not home care settings. It is also important to underline the structural aspects of training effectiveness as well. Regardless of the amount of training the PSWs received, contextual factors such as staff shortages could render the training programs ineffective [10]. Future research can examine the effectiveness of different types of PSW training for prevention and alleviation of violence and harassment at work.

Although this study has several strengths, it is not without limitations. First, our data is cross-sectional. Thus, our findings should not be interpreted as causal. Future studies can use longitudinal or experimental research design to collect data that allows for determining causality. Second, although our province-wide data has a large sample size, it is not possible to know the exact number of PSWs working in Ontario because PSWs do not have a registry in Ontario. Thus, we cannot provide a response rate and the extent to which our findings are representative of PSWs in Ontario and Canada is not clear. Third, we use an encompassing dichotomous conceptualization of violence and harassment experienced by PSWs at work. While this conceptualization allows us to capture an overview of violence and harassment at work, it comes at the expense of examining the intricacies of violence and harassment at work, such as the source and type of violence and harassment. Future research can examine specific aspects of workplace violence and harassment using continuous variables to provide a more nuanced analysis of the impact of job demands, job resources, and personal resources on intention to stay. Finally, this study uses a self-report approach, which may lead to validity issues. That said, while some of our variables, such as our training and violence and harassment–related variables, could be collected at the organizational level for triangulation purposes, other variables, such as self-esteem, stress, and intention to stay, can only be collected following the self-report approach.

5. Practice Implications

Our results have important implications for home and community care managers and policy makers. Home and community care organizations operate with a limited budget while facing increased demand from an aging population. Considering the majority of PSWs in our sample are receiving both types of training, knowing the effectiveness of training is necessary for home and community care organizations to maximize their efficiency without going over their budget. Furthermore, it has been shown that effective training can improve retention in organizations, which is an important determinant of efficiency in home and community care organizations [39]. Thus, our findings underline the need for ongoing evaluations of PSW training and redesign of training and intervention programs as needed. In doing so, it is important to include all key stakeholders in discussion. For example, Lipscomb and El Ghaziri [40] argued that healthcare workers should be included in the development and implementation of workplace violence training programs. Furthermore, different training delivery methods should be considered to improve the effectiveness of workplace and violence training provided to PSWs. For example, Gillespie, Farra, and Gates [41] found that a hybrid workplace violence training program designed for healthcare workers that includes online and face-to-face classes was effective in knowledge retention.

In conclusion, this study demonstrates that job resources and personal resources can buffer the detrimental impact of violence and harassment on worker and organizational outcomes in an interactive manner. We developed a model using the resource perspective and tested it with data from PSWs in Ontario, Canada. Our findings shed some light on the resource perspective while underlining the mediating role of self-esteem between training and stress, which might be a direct determinant of PSWs' intention to stay in their organizations. These results have important implications for home and community care managers and policy makers.

Author Contributions: Conceptualization, F.K.S. and I.U.Z.; data curation, M.D., C.B., S.D. and I.U.Z.; writing—original draft preparation, F.K.S., M.D., C.B., S.D. and I.U.Z.; writing—review and editing, F.K.S., M.D., C.B., S.D. and I.U.Z.; funding acquisition, M.D., C.B. and I.U.Z. All authors have read and agreed to the published version of the manuscript.

Funding: This research was supported by the Ontario Ministry of Labour, Research Opportunities Program (2014–2016) [grant #13-R-030] and Canadian Institutes of Health Research (CIHR) [funding reference #MOP–142286]. The funder had no role in the design, execution and writing of the study.

Institutional Review Board Statement: The study was conducted in accordance with the Declaration of Helsinki and approved by McMaster University Research Ethics Board (MREB-2014-132).

Informed Consent Statement: Informed consent was obtained from all subjects involved in the study.

Conflicts of Interest: The authors declare no conflict of interest.

References

1. Standing Committee on Health (2019) Violence Facing Health Care Workers in Canada, The House of Commons. Available online: https://www.google.ca/url?sa=t&rct=j&q=&esrc=s&source=web&cd=1&cad=rja&uact=8&ved=2ahUKEwiq7-zsnvfmAhWjmOAKHeXMCWoQFjAAegQIAxAC&url=https%3A%2F%2Fwww.ourcommons.ca%2FContent%2FCommittee%2F421%2FHESA%2FReports%2FRP10589455%2Fhesarp29%2Fhesarp29-e.pdf&usg=A (accessed on 12 December 2020).
2. Houshmand, M.; O'Reilly, J.; Robinson, S.; Wolff, A. Escaping bullying: The simultaneous impact of individual and unit-level bullying on turnover intentions. *Hum. Relat.* **2012**, *65*, 901–918. [CrossRef]
3. Lanctôt, N.; Guay, S. The aftermath of workplace violence among healthcare workers: A systematic literature review of the consequences. *Aggress. Violent Behav.* **2014**, *19*, 492–501. [CrossRef]
4. Bakker, A.B.; Demerouti, E. Job demands–resources theory: Taking stock and looking forward. *J. Occup. Health Psychol.* **2017**, *22*, 273–285. [CrossRef]
5. Hobfoll, S.E. Conservation of resources: A new attempt at conceptualizing stress. *Am. Psychol.* **1989**, *44*, 513–524. [CrossRef] [PubMed]
6. Campbell, A.L. *Invisible Workers, Invisible Hazards: An Examination of Psychological and Physical Safety Amongst Workers in Long-Term Residential Care Facilities in the 'New' Global Economy*; York University: Toronto, ON, Canada, 2016.
7. Anderson, C. Training Efforts to Reduce Reports of Workplace Violence in a Community Health Care Facility. *J. Prof. Nurs.* **2006**, *22*, 289–295. [CrossRef]
8. Nachreiner, N.M.; Gerberich, S.G.; McGovern, P.M.; Church, T.R.; Hansen, H.E.; Geisser, M.S.; Ryan, A.D. Impact of training on work-related assault. *Res. Nurs. Health* **2005**, *28*, 67–78. [CrossRef]
9. Keefe, J.M.; Knight, L.; Martin-Matthews, A.; Légaré, J. Key issues in human resource planning for home support workers in Canada. *Work* **2011**, *40*, 21–28. [CrossRef]
10. Kelly, C. Care and violence through the lens of personal support workers. *Int. J. Care Caring* **2017**, *1*, 97–113. [CrossRef]
11. Saari, M.; Patterson, E.; Killackey, T.; Raffaghello, J.; Rowe, A.; E Tourangeau, A. Home-based care: Barriers and facilitators to expanded personal support worker roles in Ontario, Canada. *Home Health Care Serv. Q.* **2017**, *36*, 127–144. [CrossRef]
12. A Agarwal, U.; Gupta, V. Relationships between job characteristics, work engagement, conscientiousness and managers' turnover intentions. *Pers. Rev.* **2018**, *47*, 353–377. [CrossRef]
13. Xanthopoulou, D.; Bakker, A.B.; Dollard, M.F.; Demerouti, E.; Schaufeli, W.B.; Taris, T.W.; Schreurs, P.J. When do job demands particularly predict burnout? *J. Manag. Psychol.* **2007**, *22*, 766–786. [CrossRef]
14. Hobfoll, S.E. Conservation of resource caravans and engaged settings. *J. Occup. Organ. Psychol.* **2011**, *84*, 116–122. [CrossRef]
15. Westman, M.; Hobfoll, S.E.; Chen, S.; Davidson, O.B.; Laski, S. Organizational stress through the lens of conservation of resources (COR) theory. In *Research in Occupational Stress and Well Being*; Perrewe, P.L., Ganster, D.C., Eds.; Emerald Group Publishing Limited: Bingley, UK, 2004; Volume 4, pp. 167–220. [CrossRef]
16. van Woerkom, M.; Bakker, A.B.; Nishii, L.H. Accumulative job demands and support for strength use: Fine-tuning the job demands-resources model using conservation of resources theory. *J. Appl. Psychol.* **2016**, *101*, 141–150. [CrossRef] [PubMed]
17. Hart, P.M.; Cooper, C.L. Occupational Stress: Toward a More Integrated Framework. In *Handbook of Industrial, Work & Organizational Psychology-Volume 2: Organizational Psychology*; Anderson, N., Ones, D.S., Sinangil, H.K., Viswesvaran, C., Eds.; SAGE: Thousand Oaks, CA, USA, 2001; pp. 93–114. [CrossRef]
18. Jex, S.M.; Elacqua, T.C. Self-esteem as a moderator: A comparison of global and organization-based measures. *J. Occup. Organ. Psychol.* **1999**, *72*, 71–81. [CrossRef]
19. Kuster, F.; Orth, U.; Meier, L.L. High Self-Esteem Prospectively Predicts Better Work Conditions and Outcomes. *Soc. Psychol. Pers. Sci.* **2013**, *4*, 668–675. [CrossRef]

20. Wilkinson, C.W. Violence prevention at work: A business perspective. *Am. J. Prev. Med.* **2001**, *20*, 155–160. [CrossRef]
21. Yang, H.-C.; Ju, Y.-H.; Lee, Y.-C. Effects of job stress on self-esteem, job satisfaction, and turnover intention. *J. Transnatl. Manag.* **2016**, *21*, 29–39. [CrossRef]
22. Xanthopoulou, D.; Bakker, A.B.; Demerouti, E.; Schaufeli, W.B. Reciprocal relationships between job resources, personal resources, and work engagement. *J. Vocat. Behav.* **2009**, *74*, 235–244. [CrossRef]
23. Demerouti, E.; Bakker, A.B. The Job Demands–Resources model: Challenges for future research. *SA J. Ind. Psychol.* **2011**, *37*, 1–9. [CrossRef]
24. Albrecht, S.L.; Marty, A. Personality, self-efficacy and job resources and their associations with employee engagement, affective commitment and turnover intentions. *Int. J. Hum. Resour. Manag.* **2017**, *31*, 657–681. [CrossRef]
25. Mobley, W.H.; Horner, S.O.; Hollingsworth, A.T. An evaluation of precursors of hospital employee turnover. *J. Appl. Psychol.* **1978**, *63*, 408–414. [CrossRef] [PubMed]
26. Steel, R.P.; Lounsbury, J.W. Turnover process models: Review and synthesis of a conceptual literature. *Hum. Resour. Manag. Rev.* **2009**, *19*, 271–282. [CrossRef]
27. Sayin, F.K.; Denton, M.; Brookman, C.; Davies, S.; Chowhan, J.; Zeytinoglu, I.U. The role of work intensification in intention to stay: A study of personal support workers in home and community care in Ontario, Canada. *Econ. Ind. Democr.* **2019**, *42*, 917–936. [CrossRef]
28. Firth, L.; Mellor, D.; Moore, K.; Loquet, C. How can managers reduce employee intention to quit? *J. Manag. Psychol.* **2004**, *19*, 170–187. [CrossRef]
29. Government of Ontario (2011). Ontario Creating Registry for Personal Support Workers. Available online: https://news.ontario.ca/mohltc/en/2011/05/ontario-creating-registry-for-personal-support-workers.html (accessed on 7 February 2020).
30. Lyons, T.F. Propensity to leave scale of 1971. In *Experience of Work: A Compendium and Review of 249 Measures and their Use*; Cook, J.D., Hepworth, S.J., Wall, T.D., Warr, P.B., Eds.; Academic Press: New York, NY, USA, 1981.
31. Pearlin, L.I.; Schooler, C. The structure of coping. *J. Health Soc. Behav.* **1978**, *19*, 2–21. [CrossRef]
32. Denton, M.; Zeytinoglu, I.U.; Davies, S.; Lian, J. Job Stress and Job Dissatisfaction of Home Care Workers in the Context of Health Care Restructuring. *Int. J. Health Serv.* **2002**, *32*, 327–357. [CrossRef] [PubMed]
33. Rodwell, J.; Demir, D. Oppression and exposure as differentiating predictors of types of workplace violence for nurses. *J. Clin. Nurs.* **2012**, *21*, 2296–2305. [CrossRef]
34. Podsakoff, P.M.; MacKenzie, S.B.; Podsakoff, N.P. Sources of method bias in social science research and recommendations on how to control it. *Annu. Rev. Psychol.* **2012**, *63*, 539–569. [CrossRef] [PubMed]
35. Podsakoff, P.M.; MacKenzie, S.B.; Lee, J.-Y.; Podsakoff, N.P. Common method biases in behavioral research: A critical review of the literature and recommended remedies. *J. Appl. Psychol.* **2003**, *88*, 879–903. [CrossRef]
36. Meyers, L.S.; Gamst, G.; Guarino, A.J. *Applied Multivariate Research: Design and Interpretation*; Sage Publications: Thousand Oaks, CA, USA, 2006.
37. Preacher, K.J.; Hayes, A.F. Asymptotic and Resampling Strategies for Assessing and Comparing Indirect Effects in Multiple Mediator Models. *Behav. Res. Methods* **2008**, *40*, 879–891. [CrossRef]
38. Kim, J.; Wehbi, N.; DelliFraine, J.L.; Brannon, D. The joint relationship between organizational design factors and HR practice factors on direct care workers' job satisfaction and turnover intent. *Health Care Manag. Rev.* **2014**, *39*, 174–184. [CrossRef] [PubMed]
39. Dietz, D.; Zwick, T. The retention effect of training: Portability, visibility, and credibility[1]. *Int. J. Hum. Resour. Manag.* **2020**, *33*, 710–741. [CrossRef]
40. Lipscomb, J.A.; El Ghaziri, M. Workplace Violence Prevention: Improving Front-Line Health-Care Worker and Patient Safety. *N. Solut. A J. Environ. Occup. Health Policy* **2013**, *23*, 297–313. [CrossRef]
41. Gillespie, G.L.; Farra, S.L.; Gates, D.M. A workplace violence educational program: A repeated measures study. *Nurse Educ. Pract.* **2014**, *14*, 468–472. [CrossRef] [PubMed]

Disclaimer/Publisher's Note: The statements, opinions and data contained in all publications are solely those of the individual author(s) and contributor(s) and not of MDPI and/or the editor(s). MDPI and/or the editor(s) disclaim responsibility for any injury to people or property resulting from any ideas, methods, instructions or products referred to in the content.

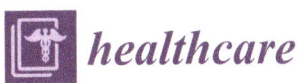

Article

A Longitudinal Study of the Impact of Personal and Professional Resources on Nurses' Work Engagement: A Comparison of Early-Career and Mid-Later-Career Nurses

Satoko Nagai [1,*], Yasuko Ogata [1], Takeshi Yamamoto [2], Mark Fedyk [3] and Janice F. Bell [4]

1. Department of Gerontological Nursing and Healthcare Systems Management, Graduate School of Health Care Sciences, Tokyo Medical and Dental University (TMDU), Tokyo 113-8510, Japan
2. School of Health Sciences, Sapporo Medical University, Sapporo 060-8556, Japan
3. School of Medicine, Betty Irene Moore School of Nursing, University of California, Davis, CA 95817, USA
4. Betty Irene Moore School of Nursing, University of California, Davis, CA 95817, USA
* Correspondence: satoko.nagai212@gmail.com

Abstract: To predict and ensure a healthy and high-performing nursing workforce, it is necessary to identify the antecedents that promote work engagement, especially among early-career nurses. To date no study has focused on this. This longitudinal survey, administered to 1204 nurses working in seven general hospitals with 200 or more beds in four prefectures in Japan at two different times in 2019, aims to examine the causal relationship between the personal and professional resources for nurses to work vigorously (PPR-N) and work engagement among nurses in the early stages of their careers, considering time as a key mediating factor. The analysis of structural equation modeling using the cross-lagged effect model supported that PPR-N had significant and positive effects on work engagement after 3 months among early-career nurses with less than 10 years of nursing experience. The PPR-N is a reliable antecedent of work engagement, which is typical of early-career nurses. These results may be provided guidance for managers in overseeing the work environment to ensure a thriving sustainable nursing workforce.

Keywords: antecedent factors; cross-lagged panel design; early-career nurses; personal resources; professional resources; work engagement

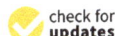

Citation: Nagai, S.; Ogata, Y.; Yamamoto, T.; Fedyk, M.; Bell, J.F. A Longitudinal Study of the Impact of Personal and Professional Resources on Nurses' Work Engagement: A Comparison of Early-Career and Mid-Later-Career Nurses. *Healthcare* 2023, 11, 76. https://doi.org/10.3390/healthcare11010076

Academic Editors: Sofia Koukouli and Areti Stavropoulou

Received: 4 November 2022
Revised: 13 December 2022
Accepted: 17 December 2022
Published: 27 December 2022

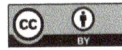

Copyright: © 2022 by the authors. Licensee MDPI, Basel, Switzerland. This article is an open access article distributed under the terms and conditions of the Creative Commons Attribution (CC BY) license (https://creativecommons.org/licenses/by/4.0/).

1. Introduction

The gap between the supply and demand of nurses is widening owing to emerging infectious diseases and epidemics, and the shortage of nurses remains a global challenge [1–3]. A nursing shortage in hospitals reduces the quantity and quality of patient care services. Early-career turnover exacerbates the existing nursing shortages and the cost of recruiting and training new nurses to fill the positions [4].

Nurses—from newcomers to those with 10 years of nursing experience—are generally skilled and critical to patients and organizations as primary providers of nursing care. However, at the start of their careers, nurses must transition through a crucial period [5]. During this period, they are in conflict with their expected roles and the demands of growing as professionals [6]. This critical phase is becoming a problem in the nursing profession. Many nurses' health deteriorates due to the stress caused by this conflict and anxiety about their future careers, leading them to abandon the nursing profession.

Learning more about work engagement may be the key to solving these challenges. Work engagement is a "work-related positive and fulfilling state of mind, characterized by vigor, dedication, and absorption" [7]. It fosters job retention intention, contributing to staff retention. It also positively impacts nurses' health and job satisfaction and can enhance their performance [8]. In other words, work engagement promotes workers' health and organizational performance. Therefore, to ensure a healthy and high-performing nursing workforce, the nurses' antecedents of work engagement need to be identified, particularly as there are limited findings in previous studies on resources promoting work engagement for early-career nurses.

This study aims to identify the antecedents of work engagement using a comparison of early-career and mid-later-career nurses, considering time as a key mediating factor.

2. Background

2.1. The Job Demands-Resources Model

According to the Job Demands-Resources Model, job-related and personal resources are linked to positive job outcomes, with work engagement as a mediating factor; it is also an occupational stress model [7]. The Job Demands-Resources Model includes health impairments and motivational processes. The former is referred to as the "health impairment process" and is a process that can cause physical and mental stress reactions at work (job demands) and negative outcomes with respect to health. It is said to be a stressor when one has to work hard to meet the job demands and keep up with expected performance [9]. In the latter, it is referred to as the "motivational process"; job resources and personal resources explain positive outcomes (behaviors) related to organizational commitment and performance through work engagement [9,10]. Based on this model, it can be shown that creating a healthy workplace with high work engagement involves increasing job and personal resources rather than reducing work demands. Therefore, applying this model in this study allows us to examine the relationship between "job and personal resources" and work engagement and to identify the resources that lead to increased work engagement.

The Job Demands-Resources Model has been validated through the analysis of co-variance (ANCOVA) using cross-sectional and longitudinal data and has good fit to the data [11].

2.2. Work Engagement Outcomes in the Work Environment

Regarding work engagement outcomes in the work environment, we explored the connections between physical and mental health, positive attitudes toward work and one's organization, and work performance. As for physical and mental health, employees with high work engagement experience less psychological distress and have fewer physical complaints [12]. These outcomes are similar for nurses working in healthcare. The higher the work engagement, the more energy nurses have, and the fewer depressive symptoms they experience [13]. In terms of positive attitudes toward work and one's organization, the higher the work engagement, the more nurses demonstrate positive expressive behavior at daily meetings and other events [14], and the more they contribute to the workplace outside of work [15].

Regarding work performance, when work engagement is higher, care-related behavior is more patient-centric [16], the quality of care in the department improves [14], patient satisfaction is greater [17], and turnover intention is lower. Thus, it is vital to identify factors that enhance work engagement regarding nurses' physical/mental health, turnover prevention, and quality of care.

2.3. Work Factors and Individual Antecedents That Promote Work Engagement in Nursing

The determinants of work engagement can be divided into professional and personal resources [9]. Professional resources are found in the workplace; they include managers' leadership [14], support from superiors and colleagues [11], and the organizational climate. Personal resources include self-efficacy [15], self-esteem [18], autonomous motivation [19], and resilience [20]; they serve to maintain and improve individuals' work engagement. Previous studies indicate that the more professional and personal resources a worker has, the more their work engagement is enhanced [21]. However, although reports have investigated the causal relationship between resources and work engagement, factors such as "support from superiors and colleagues" may or may not be significant in each survey [22,23]. One reason is that the results of this study may not be stable because of differences in years of experience and nursing team performance. In Knight's systematic review, to date, about 20 intervention studies have been conducted to improve work engagement. A major challenge is the small effect size of these interventions. A meta-analysis of the effectiveness of interventions to increase work engagement based on 14 controlled studies reported a significant but small overall effect size (Hedges = 0.29, 95%-CI = 0.12–0.46) [24]. One possible reason why these previous studies failed to find large intervention effects on work engagement is that these studies did not employ sufficient strategies to simultaneously improve two important antecedents of work engagement, specifically, job resources and personal resources [9].

Most of the past intervention studies on improving work engagement have focused on programs that focus only on individual resources through cognitive-behavioral approaches [25], and few interventions have focused on job resources. Therefore, research focusing on both job and personal resources is needed. Furthermore, the rankings of the antecedent factors (personal and professional resources) that enhance work engagement differ by occupation [26], reducing the value of extrapolating from other professions to the nursing profession. Hence, it is necessary to identify nurses' unique antecedents (personal and professional resources) of work engagement that match the nursing profession's characteristics and the field of practice.

2.4. Early-Career Nurses

Previous research has underscored that it is difficult for early-career nurses to settle into the workplace quickly and in a healthy manner [27]. An organization's quick and easy workplace transition reduces unnecessary turnover, stabilizes human resources, and leads to high-quality patient care [28]. Prior research [20,29] demonstrate that when nurses have higher work engagement, they have lower turnover intentions. It is assumed that even among early career nurses, higher work engagement results in lower turnover rates [20]. However, no studies have examined early-career nurses' antecedents of work engagement. This seems a critical oversight, as it is imperative to understand how to promote the work engagement of this crucial demographic. Specifically, there is a need to identify the antecedents that enhance nursing professionals' work engagement. This can be done using a prospective research design to estimate potential causal links [4].

The hypothesis and hypothesized model are presented below. (Figure 1.)

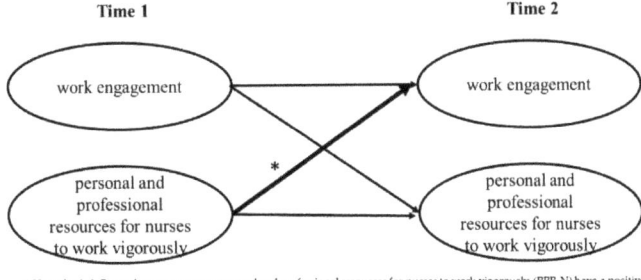

* Hypothesis 1: For early-career nurses, personal and professional resources for nurses to work vigorously (PPR-N) have a positive effect on their subsequent (three months later) work engagement.
Hypothesis 2: For mid- and later-career nurses, PPR-N does not have a direct effect on their subsequent (three months later) work engagement.

Figure 1. Hypothesized model.

Hypothesis 1: *For early-career nurses, personal and professional resources for nurses to work vigorously (PPR-N) have a positive effect on their subsequent work engagement (three months later).*

Hypothesis 2: *For mid-and later-career nurses, PPR-N does not have a direct effect on their subsequent (three months later) work engagement.*

3. Methods

3.1. Design

We used a longitudinal research design the core of which is a cross-lagged effect model. Two surveys were administered to the nurses in 2019, and data from these surveys were used to estimate the model.

3.2. Participants

Using snowball sampling, we selected seven general hospitals with more than 200 beds in four prefectures in Japan. All staff nurses working in the hospitals were surveyed (n = 1204). Of the seven hospitals, three were in urban areas, and four were in rural areas. The inclusion criteria were staff nurses with at least 10 months of work experience. Nurse managers, such as division directors, assistant division directors, head nurses, and assistant head nurses were excluded from the study. A total of 956 staff nurses returned the first survey (response rate: 79.4%), and 507 of those who returned the first survey returned the second one (response rate: 53.0%) (see Figure 2).

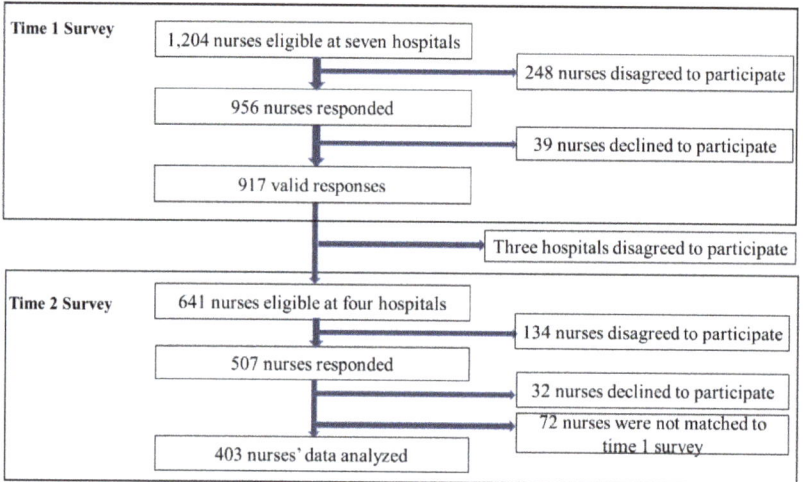

Figure 2. Data collection flow chart.

3.3. Data Collection

We collected data using an anonymous questionnaire. In the first survey (February–March 2019), the questionnaires were distributed to nurses by the collaborators (head nurse or deputy) of each hospital, who then collected the sealed questionnaire after completion. The second survey (May–June 2019) was conducted similarly and sent only to nurses who had responded to the first survey. The sealed questionnaires were also collected via the hospital collaborators. Each participant was assigned a unique identifier used on both surveys so that the surveys could be linked without identifying the participant. The cross-lagged design requires that we assess the correlation between variables measured at two different times. To this end, we used PPR-N as a predictor of work engagement among nurses, measured in two different surveys administered three months apart. In the following, Time1 corresponds to measures derived from data collected from February–March 2019, and Time2 corresponds to measures derived from data collected from May–June 2019. In addition, in prior studies, job crafting [29] and a web-based stress and depression literacy [30] interventions were reported to significantly improve work engagement after three or four months. Therefore, we surveyed twice after a time frame of three months later for this study, based on these studies.

3.4. Pilot Study

Prior to the pilot study, surface validity was ensured by checking the wording of the questionnaire and the ease of answering. There were six participants: four graduate students majoring in nursing and two nurses working at a hospital. We revised the text and structure of the questions in the questionnaire, as indicated by the participants.

The pilot study was conducted from April to May 2018, and 88 staff nurses returned the questionnaire (collection rate: 32.0%). The data from this survey were used to confirm the reliability and validity of items and to verify the analysis method used in the main survey.

In addition to the pilot studies, we applied the total design method [31] to improve the mail survey's response rate by using the cumulative response proportion [32].

3.5. Instruments
3.5.1. The Utrecht Work Engagement Scale

We used the Japanese version of the Utrecht Work Engagement Scale to measure work engagement [33]. The scale's items are rated on a 7-point Likert scale ranging from 0 = *never* to 6 = *every day*. The nine work engagement items consist of three subscales: vigor, dedication, and absorption. The score is calculated as the average of all the that comprising each factor. The higher the score, the higher the level of engagement. Confirmatory factor analysis supports the scale's 3-factor structure. The validity and reliability of the scale have been tested in various occupations and are very useful as they can be employed for inter-occupational and global comparisons [33].

3.5.2. Personal and Professional Resources for Nurses to Work Vigorously (PPR-N)

This study's main construct of interest—PPR-N—was derived from a content analysis of interviews with ten nurses, from which a set of items was derived [34]. In these interviews, they described their work resources (workplace characteristics) and personal resources (e.g., their position in the workplace) as antecedents to work engagement.

Four nurses with nursing education experience examined these items to determine whether the terminology was easy to understand, whether the wording was appropriate in actual use, and also whether the wording of the items was refined (surface validity was confirmed). Subsequently, as a pilot test, a questionnaire survey of 275 nursing staff at a medium-sized general hospital in Japan was conducted on the PPR-N items (Medical Research Ethics Committee of Tokyo Medical and Dental University, approval number: M2017-321). The results of the ceiling effect, floor effect, and item-total correlation analysis indicated that none of the items deviated from the reference values. Exploratory factor analysis (EFA) revealed a three-factor structure (KMO = 0.64). The alpha coefficient was 0.89, confirming internal consistency. Through these processes, PPR-N was confirmed to have certain validity.

Specifically, the PPR-N consists of 14 items, each rated on a 7-point Likert scale ranging from 0 = *never* to 6 = *always*. It has three subscales: "work environment with peace of mind" (6 items), "efforts that lead to good outcomes" (5 items), and "prospects for moving forward" (3 items). Its scores are calculated by summing and averaging the item scores for each factor and then calculating the scores for "job resources" and "personal resources" (Appendix A).

3.5.3. Early/Mid-and Later-Career Nurses

In the career development process, Schein [5] considers a career to be one's work experience throughout life and divided the career cycle into nine stages according to how general or specific the problems an individual typically faces and has the skills or resources to overcome. Early-career individuals share a set of problems common to all the individuals, while later-career individuals face much more specific problems. The process from entry-level to approximately ten years of work experience is the early stage of a career [35], with career development challenges such as "successfully performing one's job", "acquiring specialized skills and knowledge to lay the foundation for cross-disciplinary career growth", and "seeking to develop the skills and knowledge needed to succeed in the workplace" and other career development issues [5].

Furthermore, the duration of approximately ten years of work experience, beginning with a new employee, is a critical period in the career development of nurses, as this duration shapes the career orientation of nurses as well as their identities [36,37].

Based on Schein's (1991) career classification, this study defined nurses in the early stages of their career as "having less than 10 years of experience" [5,35], while nurses in the middle or later stages were defined as "having more than 10 years of experience".

3.6. Data Analysis

To test whether a model exhibits a cross-lagged effect—and thus whether a causal relationship exists between two or more time-separated variables—we must first construct a structural equation model of the data [38]. We accomplished this with a model employing maximum likelihood estimation. Specifically, we modeled work engagement as a latent variable and used the subfactors (vigor, dedication, and absorption) as reflective indicators. We modeled PPR-N as a latent variable and used the subfactors ("work environment with peace of mind", "efforts that lead to good outcomes", and "prospects for moving forward") as reflective indicators. We set the critical values of the comparative fit index [39] and the Tucker–Lewis index to 0.90. Root mean square error of approximation evaluates the degree to which a model does not fit; if it is smaller than 0.06, the model has good fit [40]. Descriptive statistics were performed using SPSS version 27 (IBM). This structural equation model then allows us to assess whether a cross-lagged effect exists in our data. To do this, we used AMOS 25.0 to analyze our data.

3.7. Validity, Reliability, and Rigor of Measurement Scales

The Cronbach's alpha was 0.935 on work engagement. An exploratory factor analysis of the PPR-N items revealed a 14-item, 3-factor structure with a Cronbach's alpha of 0.930. Work engagement and PPR-N showed high internal consistency.

3.8. Ethical Considerations

This study was approved by the Medical Research Ethics Committee of Tokyo Medical and Dental University (approval number: M2017-321; M2018-215). Requests were made to the person in charge of the nursing department of the relevant hospitals inviting their nurses to participate. They were invited to participate by distributing flyers to all eligible nurses through collaborators at each hospital. We explained to the participants the purpose and method of the study, privacy policy, the voluntary nature of participation, and that they would not be disadvantaged by not participating or withdrawing their consent after completing the survey. Consent was obtained from all study participants.

4. Results

Table 1 outlines the demographic characteristics of the sample according to work experience. Four hundred three staff nurses were included in the study (see Figure 1). On average, respondents were 40.1 years old (SD = 11.9) and had 15.7 years of experience (SD = 10.5). The majority were female (90.6%), with 80.6% graduating from a vocational school or junior college and over 90% working full-time. They worked in various patient care facilities (e.g., acute, specialty, sub-acute, long-term care, etc.) On average, early-career nurses had 5.7 years of work experience (SD = 2.7) and were in their 20 s (61.0%) and 30 s (34.0%). Most early-career nurses had gone to vocational school or junior college (92.2%). The mid-career nurse participants had an average of 22.3 years of work experience (SD = 8.2). Nurses aged in their 40 s (41.8%) were most common in this group.

Table 2 outlines the descriptive statistics for work engagement and personal and professional resources for nurses to work vigorously by years of work experience.

Table 1. Demographic traits of the participants according to years of work experience (Time 1).

Variables	Categories	Total (n = 403) Mean ± SD	n	%	0–10 Years (n = 159) Mean ± SD	n	%	10 Years and More (n = 244) Mean ± SD [†]	n	%
Age		40.1 ± 11.9	403		29.5 ± 6.1	159	100.0	46.8 ± 8.7	244	100.0
	20–29		98	24.3		97	61.0		1	0.0
	30–39		110	27.3		54	34.0		56	23.0
	40–49		106	26.3		4	2.5		102	41.8
	50–59		63	15.6		3	1.9		60	24.6
	60-		26	6.5		1	0.6		25	10.2
Sex	Male		38	9.4		24	15.1		14	5.7
	Female		365	90.6		135	84.9		230	94.3
Years of experience in nursing		15.7 ± 10.5	403		5.7 ± 2.7	159		22.3 ± 8.2	244	
Years of experience at the hospital		12.1 ± 13.4	403		5.9 ± 13.2	159		14.7 ± 12.3	244	
Education	Vocational school or junior college		325	80.6		100	63.7		225	92.2
	Undergraduate or graduate school		73	18.1		57	36.3		16	6.6

[†] SD: Standard deviation. 0–10 years: $n = 159$, 10 years and more: $n = 244$.

Table 2. Descriptive statistics for work engagement and personal and professional resources for nurses to work vigorously by years of work experience.

Years of Work Experience	All (n = 403)		0–10 Years (n = 159)		10 Years and More (n = 244)	
Variables	Time 1 Mean ± SD [†]	Time 2 Mean ± SD	Time 1 Mean ± SD	Time 2 Mean ± SD	Time 1 Mean ± SD	Time 2 Mean ± SD
UWES [‡] [range: 0–6]	2.51 ± 1.02	2.44 ± 0.88	2.28 ± 0.99	2.24 ± 0.88	2.65 ± 1.01	2.57 ± 0.86
Vigor [range: 0–6]	2.25 ± 1.10	2.21 ± 1.05	2.04 ± 1.03	1.96 ± 1.01	2.39 ± 1.12	2.37 ± 1.04
Dedication [range: 0–6]	2.97 ± 1.04	2.86 ± 1.01	2.72 ± 1.01	2.64 ± 1.05	3.13 ± 1.03	3.00 ± 0.95
Absorption [range: 0–6]	2.30 ± 1.17	2.26 ± 0.83	2.09 ± 1.13	2.13 ± 0.83	2.44 ± 1.17	2.34 ± 0.83
[§] PPR-N [range: 0–6]	4.08 ± 0.76	3.97 ± 0.75	4.09 ± 0.81	3.94 ± 0.80	4.07 ± 0.73	3.98 ± 0.71
Work environment with peace of mind [range: 0–6]	4.32 ± 1.01	4.18 ± 0.94	4.38 ± 1.05	4.23 ± 0.99	4.27 ± 0.98	4.15 ± 0.91
Efforts that lead to good outcomes [range: 0–6]	3.73 ± 0.84	3.64 ± 0.86	3.70 ± 0.92	3.59 ± 0.92	3.75 ± 0.78	3.67 ± 0.82
Prospects for moving forward [range: 0–6]	4.19 ± 0.76	4.08 ± 0.74	4.15 ± 0.75	3.95 ± 0.73	4.22 ± 0.76	4.16 ± 0.74

[†] SD: Standard deviation, [‡] UWES: Utrecht Work Engagement Scale, [§] PPR-N: personal and professional resources for nurses to work vigorously.

4.1. Work Engagement Scores Based on Years of Work Experience at Time 1 and Time 2

The mean work engagement score of the 403 staff nurses at Time1 was 2.51 (SD = 1.02). The highest scoring work engagement factor was "dedication", and the lowest was "vigor". Nurses with a minimum of 10 years of experience had significantly higher total work engagement scores than nurses with less than 10 years of experience (mean: 2.65 and 2.28, respectively, $p < 0.001$). The mean scores for the three work engagement factors were higher for nurses with more experience. The mean scores for the three-work engagement subfactors were higher at Time1 than at Time2 for both the early- and mid-career nurse cohorts. However, the "absorption" factor for early-career staff nurses was lower at Time1 (mean: 2.09 [SD: 1.13]) than at Time2 (mean: 2.13 [SD: 0.83]).

4.2. Item Group Scores for Factors Preceding Work Engagement Based on Years of Work Experience at Time 1 and Time 2

The 403 staff nurses had a mean PPR-N score of 4.08 (SD = 0.76) at Time1. The total PPR-N score at Time1 was significantly higher ($p < 0.001$) for early-career staff nurses (mean: 4.09 [SD: 0.81]) than for mid- and later-career staff nurses (mean: 4.07 [SD: 0.73]). The mean score for each PPR-N factor was significantly higher at Time1 than at Time2 for both groups of nurses in the early- and mid-career stages ($p < 0.001$). The mean scores for the PPR-N factors, "efforts leading to good outcomes", and "prospects in the profession" were higher in the group with more years of work experience, while the mean score for "work environment with peace of mind" was lower in the same group.

4.3. Hypothesis Testing: Cross-Lagged Effects Model

We tested two models (model a, b) that included a stability effect and a cross-lagged relationship between PPR-N and work engagement in a cohort of early-career nurses and mid-later-career nurses. For early-career nurses, 159 were included, and the results of the analysis are shown in Figure 3 (model a); for mid- to late-career nurses, 244 were included, and the results are shown in Figure 4 (model b). As can be seen in Figures 3 and 4, all estimated structural models fit well (Figure 3: CFI = 0.986, NFI = 0.961, RMSEA = 0.058, Figure 4: CFI = 0.986, NFI = 0.967, RMSEA = 0.055).

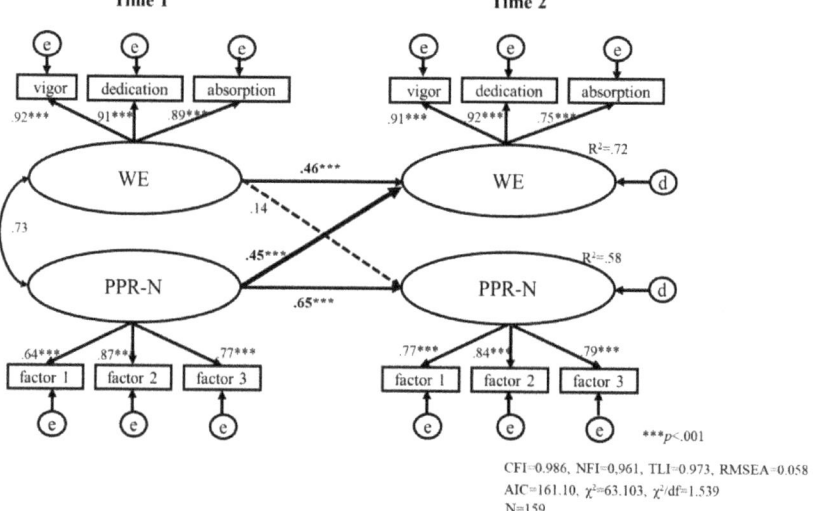

Note. The dotted line denotes a non-significant relationship. WE: work engagement; PPR-N: personal and professional resources for nurses to work vigorously.

Figure 3. Model (a). The causal relationship between work engagement and personal and professional resources for nurses to work vigorously using a cross-lagged effects model in nurses with less than 10 years of work experience (early-career nurses).

The PPR-N at Time1 was positively correlated with work engagement at Time 2 ($\beta = 0.45, p < 0.001$) for the early-career nurses. Work engagement at Time1 was independent of PPR-N at Time2 ($\beta = 0.14$, ns) for the early-career nurses (see Figure 3). From these we test Hypotheses 1; PPR-N has a positive (cross-lagged) effect on their subsequent (three months later) work engagement, and there is no direct effect of work engagement on PPR-N held for the early-career nurses' population. In brief, it is clear that PPR-N is an antecedent resource of work engagement, and work engagement is not an antecedent of PPR-N among early-career nurses.

The PPR-N at Time1 was unrelated to work engagement at Time 2 ($\beta = 0.00$, ns), and work engagement at Time1 was positively correlated with PPR-N at Time2 for mid- and later-career nurses ($\beta = 0.35, p < 0.001$) (see Figure 4). From these, we test Hypothesis 2; there is no direct effect of PPR-N on their subsequent (three months later) work engagement for mid- and later-career nurses. In addition, there is direct effect from work engagement to PPR-N for nurses in mid-career and beyond.

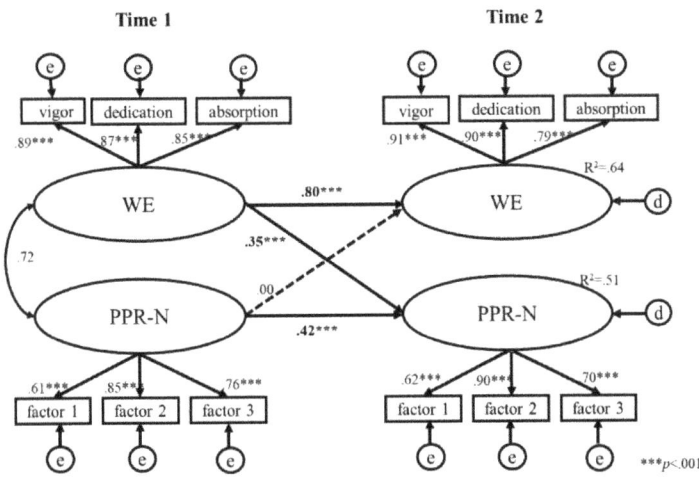

Figure 4. Model (b). The causal relationship between work engagement and personal and professional resources for nurses to work vigorously using a cross-lagged effects model in nurses with more than 10 years of work experience (mid- and later-career nurses).

In brief, for early-career nurses, by comparing with mid- and later-career nurses, PPR-N influenced work engagement and was a predictor of work engagement. In contrast, PPR-N did not directly affect work engagement among mid- and later-career nurses.

5. Discussion

The present study is the first to investigate the concept of predicting work engagement among early-career nurses, by comparing nurses in the early-career stage to those in later stages. Our data support the conclusion that for nurses at the beginning of their career, their commitment and dedication (i.e., the strength of their work engagement) will be enhanced by work environments that supply adequate professional resources.

5.1. The Characteristics of Nurses' Work Engagement

The mean work engagement score of all participants in this study was 2.51 points, lower than the mean score of 3.96 points in the US [41], 4.1 points in Saudi Arabia [42], 3.13 points in China [43], and scores reported in previous studies. The low work engagement in Japan may be related to nurses' workload rather than a shortage of nurses. In addition, this study took place in Japan, where it is culturally desirable to suppress positive emotions and attitudes [12]. This may have led to a similar tendency in this study, and the work engagement scores may have been lower than for nurses outside Japan.

The highest score among the three subscales was "dedication", consistent with a national survey of 1194 registered nurses in Japan [44]. Similarly, in a work engagement survey of registered nurses ($n = 747$) providing direct patient care at five rural acute care hospitals in the US, the highest subscale for any generation of nurses was "dedication". For early-career nurses in the present study, the next highest score on the three subscales after dedication was "absorption", and the lowest was "vigor". Previous literature has found that employees with low dedication and vigor have strong turnover intention, especially when the workload is high. Therefore, nurse managers need to be aware of subordinates' potential intent to leave when the total score of it is relatively low. Vigor is the lowest of the subfactors, as found in the participants of this study.

Participants with more than 10 years of experience had significantly higher work engagement scores than those with less than 10 years of experience, consistent with an earlier study of 1194 registered nurses in Japan [44]. Past studies indicate that work engagement scores rise as years of experience increase. Nurses with more than 10 years of experience may be less likely to feel burdened by their workload due to their proficiency in their roles, which may have increased work engagement.

The mean of the total work engagement scores was higher at Time1 than at Time2. This outcome is similar to the findings of a longitudinal study involving Chinese female nurses with a six-month gap between surveys [45] and a longitudinal study of Canadian nurses with a one year gap between surveys [19]. Possible reasons for this have not been mentioned in prior studies and require further investigation.

5.2. Comparison of Resources to Promote Work Engagement for Early-Career and Mid-Later Career Nurses

In this study, the PPR-N was indicated to be effective for work engagement after three months among nurses with less than ten years of experience, and the PPR-N was not found to be effective in work engagement among nurses with more than ten years of experience. This may have been due to the fact that the PPR-N was a group of items obtained through qualitative analysis of interviews with nurses with almost exclusively less than ten years of experience. Furthermore, compared to nurses with less than ten years, nurses with more than ten years are in what Schein describes as the "mid-career crisis" stage [5,36], which involves career challenges such as "reaffirming the position of their career in their overall life" and "accepting reality and deciding to continue working. This may have affected the difference in results between the two groups because the challenges are different in the "early career" stage, which is to "perform tasks successfully" and "remain in the organization or seek harmony between organizational constraints/opportunities and one's own desires", compared to the mid-career stage, where the challenges are different.

Nurses with more than ten years of experience had higher work engagement scores after three months than nurses with less than ten years of experience, and their work engagement remained relatively stable after three months ($\beta = 0.80$, $p < 0.001$). In addition, work engagement affects PPR-N among this mid-and later-career nurses. These suggest the possibility that nurses with more than ten years of experience may have a job and personal resources other than PPR-N that promote work engagement. For example, a prior study [44,46] has stated that veteran nurses with ten or more years of experience have a higher degree of confidence in their work due to their greater experience and that these personal resources increase work engagement.

5.3. The Usefulness of Personal and Professional Resources for Nurses to Work Vigorously in the Nursing Field

Although the period between Time1 and Time2 in this study was brief (three months, as noted), it was a time of fluctuation due to nursing staff turnover because it spanned the entire fiscal year. Some staff members and new nurses were not yet accustomed to their work, and the PPR-N may have been implemented during a busy period. Regardless, it was still a leading factor in work engagement. In other words, PPR-N may be a stable antecedent of work engagement not substantially impacted by the degree of activity in the ward.

5.4. Relevance for Clinical Practice

Our results suggest that strengthening the support provided for nurses in areas linked to our PPR-N construct could enhance the work engagement of early-career nurses with less than ten years of experience. Enhancing nurses' work engagement is a complex issue for organizations. However, our data suggest that this complexity can be simplified using a career cycle (time of career) focused approach to enable the deployment of targets and resources [41]. Nurse managers are best positioned to improve the work-life of their subordinates as they are more familiar with the problems and conditions faced in the unit. Therefore, in the future, managers can employ resources that enhance the work engagement of early-career nurses, implement these resources at the appropriate time, and prepare a supportive work environment in which nurses can work vigorously. Ultimately, early-career nurses can continue to work without interruptions in their careers. They can improve their performance, enhance the quality of care provided by the nursing profession, and nurture a better medical and healthcare environment.

5.5. Limitations of the Study and Future Research

This study has several limitations. First, the PPR-N was limited only to the nursing work environment in Japan. As such, the roles of nurses in Japan may be different from those of other countries. For future studies, it is necessary to examine to confirm the cultural applicability of the model. Second, this study only considered the point of view on the work engagement effectiveness of PPR-N. To examine the effects of work engagement more comprehensively, future research should consider other antecedent factors as well, such as staff nurses' performance. Third, the design was longitudinal, and causality was estimated in two intervals. In the future, it will be necessary to change the time period and further design the study at a different time point (Time3) and at a medium- to long-term interval to test the usability of the model.

6. Conclusions

We aimed to determine the antecedents of work engagement using a comparison of early-career and mid-later-career nurses considering, using time as a mediating effect. Our results supported the hypotheses and indicated that in early-career nurses, PPR-N has a significant and positive effect on work engagement. However, PPR-N in mid- and later-career nurses with more than ten years of experience did not promote work engagement. It may also be an antecedent to work engagement among early-career nurses with less than ten years of work experience. Increasing PPR-N resources increases the possibility of promoting promote work engagement. Our results can guide managers in predicting and implementing beneficent work environment measures to enable nurses to work more effectively.

Author Contributions: Conceptualization, S.N. and Y.O.; methodology, S.N., Y.O., T.Y., M.F. and J.F.B.; software, S.N., Y.O. and T.Y.; validation, S.N., Y.O., T.Y. and M.F.; formal analysis, S.N., Y.O. and T.Y.; investigation, S.N. and Y.O.; resources, S.N. and Y.O.; data curation, S.N., Y.O. and T.Y.; writing—original draft preparation, S.N.; writing—review and editing, Y.O., T.Y., M.F. and J.F.B.; visualization, S.N. and Y.O.; supervision, S.N. and Y.O.; project administration and funding acquisition, S.N. All authors have read and agreed to the published version of the manuscript.

Funding: This research was funded by the Michi Takahashi Scholarship for Postgraduate Education (Nursing Management) in 2018 (grant number T181005).

Institutional Review Board Statement: The study was conducted in accordance with the Declaration of Helsinki and approved by the Medical Research Ethics Committee of Tokyo Medical and Dental University (approval nos. M2017-321; date of approval, 22 March 2018 and M2018-215; date of approval, 22 January 2019).

Informed Consent Statement: Informed consent was obtained from all subjects involved in the study.

Data Availability Statement: Data sharing is not applicable to this article because we have not obtained approval of the participants or the Ethics Committee to release the data.

Acknowledgments: We deeply thank all staff nurses who participated in this survey.

Conflicts of Interest: The authors declare no conflict of interest.

Appendix A

Personal and professional resources for nurses to work vigorously

The following 14 statements describe how you may feel about your job: read each statement carefully, and rate how you feel about each statement. Choose the option that best describes your experience at your work. If you cannot relate to the statement, please circle the number 0, if you relate to the statement, please circle the number from 0 to 6 depending on how often.

Items of personal and professional resources for nurses to work vigorously

---

Factor 1: Work environment with peace of mind (6 items)
I am surrounded by coworkers who will support me in times of difficulty.
There are positive relationships within the workplace.
The workplace environment is accepting and tolerant toward anybody to speak up.
I feel comfortable talking to other staff members.
I feel a sense of belonging at my workplace.
There is a positive atmosphere at the workplace.
Factor 2: Efforts that lead to good outcomes (5 items)
There are jobs that stimulate my interest.
I receive feedback on the accomplishments that I have worked for.
My efforts lead to good outcomes.
I can use my strengths and abilities to assist others.
I feel that my efforts and works are going well.
Factor 3: Prospects for moving forward (3 items)
I am able to predict what I need to do next based on what I have learned in the past.
I am making progress towards becoming the nurse that I strive to be in the future.
I have a sense of ownership in the workplace.

Note. Choices 0: never, 1: rarely, 2: occasionally, 3: sometimes, 4: often, 5: usually, 6: always.

References

1. Jackson, D.; Bradbury-Jones, C.; Baptiste, D.; Gelling, L.; Morin, K.; Neville, S.; Smith, G.D. Life in the pandemic: Some reflections on nursing in the context of COVID-19. *J. Clin. Nurs.* **2020**, *29*, 2041–2043. [CrossRef] [PubMed]
2. Marć, M.; Bartosiewicz, A.; Burzyńska, J.; Chmiel, Z.; Januszewicz, P. A nursing shortage: A prospect of global and local policies. *Int. Nur. Rev.* **2019**, *66*, 9–16. [CrossRef] [PubMed]
3. World Health Organization. *State of the World's Nursing 2020: Investing in Education, Jobs and Leadership*; World Health Organization: Geneva, Switzerland, 2020. Available online: https://apps.who.int/iris/rest/bitstreams/1284585/retrieve (accessed on 12 August 2022).
4. Keyko, K.; Cummings, G.G.; Yonge, O.; Wong, C.A. Work engagement in professional nursing practice: A systematic review. *Int. J. Nurs. Stud.* **2016**, *61*, 142–164. [CrossRef] [PubMed]
5. Schein, E.H. *Career Dynamics: Matching Individual and Organizational Needs*; Addison-Wesley: Boston, MA, USA, 1978; pp. 36–48.
6. Oyamada, K. A literature review of the characteristics of nurses in mid-career and professional development methods in Japan. *J. Jpn. Acad. Nurs. Admin. Policy* **2009**, *13*, 73–80. [CrossRef]
7. Schaufeli, W.B.; Bakker, A.B. Job demands, job resources, and their relationship with burnout and engagement: A multi-sample study. *J. Organ. Behav.* **2004**, *25*, 293–315. [CrossRef]
8. Jenaro, C.; Flores, N.; Orgaz, M.B.; Cruz, M. Vigour and dedication in nursing professionals: Towards a better understanding of work engagement. *J. Adv. Nurs.* **2011**, *67*, 865–875. [CrossRef]
9. Bakker, A.B.; Demerouti, E. The Job Demands-Resources model: State of the art. *J. Manag. Psychol.* **2007**, *22*, 309–328. [CrossRef]
10. Hakanen, J.J.; Schaufeli, W.B.; Ahola, K. The Job Demands-Resources model: A three-year cross-lagged study of burnout, depression, commitment, and work engagement. *Work Stress* **2008**, *22*, 224–241. [CrossRef]
11. Hakanen, J.J.; Bakker, A.B.; Schaufeli, W.B. Burnout and work engagement among teachers. *J. School Psychol.* **2006**, *43*, 495–513. [CrossRef]
12. Shimazu, A.; Schaufeli, W.B.; Miyanaka, D.; Iwata, N. Why Japanese workers show low work engagement: An item response theory analysis of the Utrecht Work Engagement scale. *Biopsychosoc. Med.* **2010**, *4*, 17. [CrossRef]
13. Laschinger, H.K.S.; Finegan, J. Empowering nurses for work engagement and health in hospital settings. *J. Nurs. Admin.* **2005**, *35*, 439–449. [CrossRef] [PubMed]
14. Wong, C.A.; Spence Laschinger, H.K.; Cummings, G.G. Authentic leadership and nurses' voice behavior and perceptions of care quality. *J. Nurs. Manag.* **2010**, *18*, 889–900. [CrossRef] [PubMed]

15. Salanova, M.; Lorente, L.; Chambel, M.J.; Martínez, I.M. Linking transformational leadership to nurses' extra-role performance: The mediating role of self-efficacy and work engagement. *J. Adv. Nurs.* **2011**, *67*, 2256–2266. [CrossRef] [PubMed]
16. Abdelhadi, N.; Drach-Zahavy, A. Promoting patient care: Work engagement as a mediator between ward service climate and patient-centered care. *J. Adv. Nurs.* **2012**, *68*, 1276–1287. [CrossRef] [PubMed]
17. Bacon, C.T.; Mark, B. Organizational effects on patient satisfaction in hospital medical-surgical units. *JONA* **2009**, *39*, 220–227. [CrossRef]
18. Xanthopoulou, D.; Bakker, A.B.; Demerouti, E.; Schaufeli, W.B. The role of personal resources in the job demands-resources model. *Int. J. Stress Manag.* **2007**, *14*, 121–141. [CrossRef]
19. Austin, S.; Fernet, C.; Trépanier, S.; Lavoie-Tremblay, M. Fatigue in new registered nurses: A 12-month cross-lagged analysis of its association with work motivation, engagement, sickness absence and turnover intention. *J. Nurs. Manag.* **2020**, *28*, 606–614. [CrossRef]
20. Cao, X.; Chen, L. Relationships among social support, empathy, resilience and work engagement in haemodialysis nurses. *Int Nurs. Rev.* **2019**, *66*, 366–373. [CrossRef]
21. Van Bogaert, P.; Kowalski, C.; Weeks, S.M.; Clarke, S.P. The relationship between nurse practice environment, nurse work characteristics, burnout and job outcome and quality of nursing care: A cross-sectional survey. *Int. J. Nurs. Stud.* **2013**, *50*, 1667. [CrossRef]
22. Van Bogaert, P.; Wouters, K.; Willems, R.; Mondelaers, M.; Clarke, S. Work engagement supports nurse workforce stability and quality of care: Nursing team-level analysis in psychiatric hospitals. *J. Psychiatr. Ment. Health Nurs.* **2013**, *20*, 679–686. [CrossRef]
23. Walker, A.; Campbell, K. Work readiness of graduate nurses and the impact on job satisfaction, work engagement and intention to remain. *Nurse Educ. Today* **2013**, *33*, 1490–1495. [CrossRef] [PubMed]
24. Knight, C.; Patterson, M.; Dawson, J. Building work engagement: A systematic review and meta-analysis investigating the effectiveness of work engagement interventions. *J. Organ. Behav.* **2017**, *38*, 792–812. [CrossRef] [PubMed]
25. Coffeng, J.K.; Hendriksen, I.J.; Duijts, S.F.; Twisk, J.W.; van Mechelen, W.; Boot, C.R. Effectiveness of a combined social and physical environmental intervention on presenteeism, absenteeism, work performance, and work engagement in office employees. *J. Occup. Environ. Med.* **2014**, *56*, 258–265. [CrossRef] [PubMed]
26. Bakker, A.B.; Demerouti, E.; Sanz-Vergel, A.I. Burnout and work engagement: The JD–R approach. *Annu. Rev. Organ. Psychol. Organ. Behav.* **2014**, *1*, 389–411. [CrossRef]
27. Suzuki, E.; Itomine, I.; Kanoya, Y.; Katsuki, T.; Horii, S.; Sato, C. Factors affecting rapid turnover of novice nurses in university hospitals. *J. Occup. Health* **2006**, *48*, 49–61. [CrossRef]
28. De Simone, S.; Planta, A.; Cicotto, G. The role of job satisfaction, work engagement, self-efficacy and agentic capacities on nurses' turnover intention and patient satisfaction. *Appl. Nurs. Res.* **2018**, *39*, 130–140. [CrossRef]
29. Sakuraya, A.; Shimazu, A.; Imamura, K.; Kawakami, N. Effects of a job crafting intervention program on work engagement among Japanese employees: A randomized controlled trial. *Front. Psychol.* **2020**, *11*, 235. [CrossRef]
30. Imamura, K.; Kawakami, N.; Tsuno, K.; Tsuchiya, M.; Shimada, K.; Namba, K.; Shimazu, A. Effects of web-based stress and depression literacy intervention on improving work engagement among workers with low work engagement: An analysis of secondary outcome of a randomized controlled trial. *J. Occup. Health* **2017**, *59*, 46–54. [CrossRef]
31. Dillman, D.A.; Smyth, J.D.; Christian, L.M. *Internet, Phone, Mail, and Mixed-mode Surveys: The Tailored Design Method*; John Wiley & Sons: Hoboken, NJ, USA, 2014.
32. Wakabayashi, C.; Hayashi, K.; Nagai, K.; Sakamoto, N.; Iwasaki, Y. Effect of stamped reply envelopes and timing of newsletter delivery on response rates of mail survey: A randomized controlled trial in a prospective cohort study. *BMJ Open* **2012**, *2*, e001181. [CrossRef]
33. Shimazu, A.; Schaufeli, W.B.; Kosugi, S.; Suzuki, A.; Nashiwa, H.; Kato, A.; Sakamoto, M.; Irimajiri, H.; Amano, S.; Hirohata, K.; et al. Work engagement in Japan: Validation of the Japanese version of the Utrecht Work Engagement Scale. *Appl. Psychol.* **2008**, *57*, 510–523. [CrossRef]
34. Nagai, S.; Okawara, C.; Yumoto, Y.; Ogata, Y. Personal and professional-related factors influencing staff nurses' experiences of work vigorously: A semi-structured interview-based content analysis. *J. Jpn. Soc. Healthcare Admin.* **2022**, *59*, 168–176.
35. Nakamoto, A.; Yada, M.; Mitani, R.; Katayama, M.; Hosona, M. Career development process of clinical nurses over 10 years of occupational experiences. *J. Jpn. Acad. Nurs. Admin. Policy* **2018**, *22*, 1–11. [CrossRef]
36. Seki, M. A consideration on stagnation in career development of mid-career nurses. *J. Jpn. Acad. Nurs. Sci.* **2015**, *35*, 101–110. [CrossRef]
37. Shirataki, M.; Jono, H.; Ikeuchi, M. Factors influencing the full-fledged employee degree in early career nurses. *J. Jpn. Soc. Nurs. Adm. Manag.* **2021**, *3*, 1–9. [CrossRef]
38. Little, T.D.; Preacher, K.J.; Selig, J.P.; Card, N.A. New developments in latent variable panel analyses of longitudinal data. *Int. J. Behav. Dev.* **2007**, *31*, 357–365. [CrossRef]
39. Bentler, P.M.; Bonett, D.G. Significance tests and goodness of fit in the analysis of covariance structures. *Psychol. Bull.* **1980**, *88*, 588–606. [CrossRef]
40. Hu, L.; Bentler, P.M. Cutoff criteria for fit indexes in covariance structure analysis: Conventional criteria versus new alternatives. *Struct. Equ. Model.* **1999**, *6*, 1–55. [CrossRef]

41. Sullivan Havens, D.; Warshawsky, N.E.; Vasey, J. RN work engagement in generational cohorts: The view from rural US hospitals. *J. Nurs. Manag.* **2013**, *21*, 927–940. [CrossRef]
42. Aboshaiqah, A.E.; Hamadi, H.Y.; Salem, O.A.; Zakari, N.M.A. The work engagement of nurses in multiple hospital sectors in Saudi Arabia: A comparative study. *J. Nurs. Manag.* **2016**, *24*, 540–548. [CrossRef]
43. Wang, X.; Liu, L.; Zou, F.; Hao, J.; Wu, H. Associations of occupational stressors, perceived organizational support, and psychological capital with work engagement among Chinese female nurses. *Biomed Res. Int.* **2017**, *2017*, 5284628. [CrossRef]
44. Sato, Y.; Miki, A. Influences of job stress, coping profile and social support on work engagement among hospital nurses: A comparative analysis according to their years of clinical experience. *Labor. Sci.* **2014**, *90*, 14–25. [CrossRef]
45. Lu, C.-Q.; Siu, O.-L.; Chen, W.-Q.; Wang, H.-J. Family mastery enhances work engagement in Chinese nurses: A cross-lagged analysis. *J. Vocat. Behav.* **2011**, *78*, 100–109. [CrossRef] [PubMed]
46. Huber, P.; Schubert, H. Attitudes about work engagement of different generations—A cross-sectional study with nurses and supervisors. *J. Nurs. Manag.* **2019**, *27*, 1341–1350. [CrossRef] [PubMed]

Disclaimer/Publisher's Note: The statements, opinions and data contained in all publications are solely those of the individual author(s) and contributor(s) and not of MDPI and/or the editor(s). MDPI and/or the editor(s) disclaim responsibility for any injury to people or property resulting from any ideas, methods, instructions or products referred to in the content.

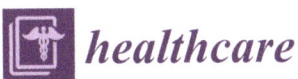

Article

Hospital Management and Public Health Role of National Hospitals after Transformation into Independent Administrative Agencies

Yoshiaki Nakagawa [1], Kaoru Irisa [2], Yoshinobu Nakagawa [3] and Yasuhiro Kanatani [1,*]

1. Department of Clinical Pharmacology, School of Medicine, Tokai University, 143 Shimokasuya, Isehara 259-1193, Japan
2. Department of Respiratorology, Tokyo Medical Center, 2-5-1 Higashigaoka, Meguro-ku, Tokyo 152-8902, Japan
3. Emeritus President, Shikoku Medical Center for Children and Adults, 2-1-1 Senyu, Zentsuji 765-8507, Japan
* Correspondence: kanatani.yasuhiro.f@tokai.ac.jp

Abstract: The development of medical care, technological advances, and the ageing of society have led to rising medical costs. As a result, there is a demand to improve the efficiency of healthcare delivery systems, including public healthcare institutions, in order to ensure the sustainability of healthcare functions. In 2004, as part of national civil service reform in Japan, national hospitals were merged in order to form the National Hospital Organization (NHO). The NHO used new public management methods and was required to be self-financing and to maintain critical functions under a five-year management plan. The objective of this study was to examine whether the NHO was able to maintain its key function in the national infrastructure in terms of management. An analysis of the business conditions of the NHO was performed based on the financial statements from FY 2004 to FY 2018 using evaluation indexes. In the first and second periods, the NHO achieved its targeted management improvements. However, since FY 2014, even with the utmost restrictions on capital investment, the profits have not increased, and the free cash flow has been negative. Our results suggest that further organizational reforms are needed in order to sustain the NHO infrastructure in the long term and to withstand health crisis management during periods such as the COVID-19 pandemic.

Keywords: hospital management; financial management; independent administrative agency; infrastructure; health crisis

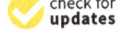

Citation: Nakagawa, Y.; Irisa, K.; Nakagawa, Y.; Kanatani, Y. Hospital Management and Public Health Role of National Hospitals after Transformation into Independent Administrative Agencies. *Healthcare* 2022, 10, 2084. https://doi.org/10.3390/healthcare10102084

Academic Editors: Sofia Koukouli and Areti Stavropoulou

Received: 15 September 2022
Accepted: 15 October 2022
Published: 19 October 2022

Publisher's Note: MDPI stays neutral with regard to jurisdictional claims in published maps and institutional affiliations.

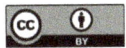

Copyright: © 2022 by the authors. Licensee MDPI, Basel, Switzerland. This article is an open access article distributed under the terms and conditions of the Creative Commons Attribution (CC BY) license (https://creativecommons.org/licenses/by/4.0/).

1. Introduction

Rapid changes in the social environment, i.e., the rapid ageing of society, the changes in the structure of disease, and the advances in medical science and technology, have led to rapidly rising healthcare costs, and the sustainability of healthcare delivery systems has become an issue in Japan and in other countries [1–3]. Various hospital reforms have been implemented in Asia, particularly in public hospitals. One of these is the reform of public hospitals using the new public management approach, which has been introduced in Japan and in several other countries [3–5]. The largest group of public hospitals that have been reformed using this method in Japan is the National Hospital Organization (NHO), which includes about 140 hospitals.

In 2004, as a part of national civil service reform, the National Hospital Organization (NHO) was formed from national hospitals and sanatoriums in Japan as an independent administrative agency, with the aim of improving the management and the efficiency of medical care through the use of an independent accounting system that is used in most private hospitals [4,5]. The main differences with private hospitals are the management restrictions that are based on salary schedules and staffing, which are based on the standards of the national civil service era; the control of projects that compete with private hospitals, which are considered to put pressure on the private sector; a five-year plan as a medium-term target management corporation; and the operation and management under state supervision based on the plan. In addition, while the government has the authority to assign the President and the Vice-President, the hospital director can appoint the hospital staff with the approval of the President and the Vice-President. The personnel structure is the same as that of the private hospitals in Japan, except that the government appoints the ultimate management head.

In particular, in terms of management, under the Act on General Rules for Independent Administrative Agencies, the NHO is required to formulate a medium-term plan covering five years, to formulate an annual plan that is in line with this medium-term plan, and to manage their operations following the plan that was approved by the competent minister [4,6]. In addition, the NHO is obliged to report their business to the competent minister every fiscal year. Article 15 of the Act on the National Hospital Organization, Independent Administrative Agency stipulates the following four purposes for establishing the NHO and the scope of their operations [6]:

(i) To provide medical care;
(ii) To conduct surveys and research on medical care;
(iii) To provide training for medical technicians;
(iv) To perform services that are incidental to the services that were listed in the preceding three items.

The NHO must fulfil the objectives of the scope of its operations in this law and prepare the mid-term plan and the reports for the mid-term plan. In other words, the management plan that is drawn up is regulated and approved by the government. This includes all of the investment plans and the plans for establishing beds and hospitals; management is carried out in order to fulfil these items. This is a management style that differs significantly from that of private hospitals. The mid-term and annual plans include the following four items, which can be further divided into three to five sub-items [6]:

I. Matters concerning the improvement of the quality of services and other operations that are provided to the public;
II. Matters that are related to the efficiency of business management;
III. Matters that are related to the improvement of the financial status;
IV. Other matters.

The three items that are considered to be within the scope of the NHO operations are listed in (I). These qualities of services are separately monitored as "Clinical Services", "Clinical Research Business", and "Education and Training Business" by the government [7–9]. This means that, although it is formally independent from the government in terms of its management, its policies as a healthcare organization are always regulated by the government.

Under the national insurance system, the hospital management in Japan is subject to maintenance standards for insurance reimbursement. The only way to reduce management costs is to reduce the portion of the hospital that is not in operation. In particular, the standard number of nurses in hospital wards is strictly regulated according to the amount of reimbursement. At least one nurse must be assigned for 24 h daily for every seven patients in order to receive the highest reimbursement. In other words, if a hospital reduces its staffing too much, it will be audited by the Ministry of Health, Labor and Welfare (MHLW), even if it is a private hospital, and its fees will be refunded, or its license will be revoked. Thus, in Japan, everything is controlled by staffing, and no outcome data have been obtained in order to allow for a comparison of the benefits of treatment. Even in the private sector, the personnel costs are highly constrained, and the personnel cost ratio is the most significant cost item, at around 50%, which is unavoidable under the insurance system. In addition, medical safety issues, such as nosocomial infections, are subject to supervision by the local health department. The establishment permit will be revoked if the hospital does not take action. As has been described above, the medical institutions are treated equally and legally, regardless of their organizational form. The most significant difference is that the management objectives require permission from the minister with the jurisdiction (Table 1).

Table 1. Governance structures of health organizations; for more detailed information see Supplementary Material Table S1.

Classification by Type of Establishment	National	NHO	Public Hospital	Private
Act on Basis for Establishment	Law for Establishing Jurisdiction	Act on the National Hospital Organization, Independent Administrative Agency.	Local Public Enterprise Act/Articles of Incorporation	Medical Care Act.
Establishers	The competent minister	Chairman of the board of directors	Head of the local government/Business Manager	Hospital Administrator
Appointing authority of the establisher	The competent minister	Minister of Health, Labor and Welfare, National	Head of the local government	Hospital Administrators
Status of the establisher	Specialized National Public Servants	Non-government officer	Local government officer	Non-government officer
Director Appointee	-	The competent minister	-	Establishers
Method of Election of Executive Board Members	-	The competent minister	-	Board of directors/Establishers
Management organization	The ministry in charge	Board of directors	Hospital Organization	Board of directors/Establishers
Operation Plans	The ministry in charge	Board of directors	Hospital Organization/Local government that has established	Board of directors/Establishers
Approval of operating plan	The competent minister	The competent minister	Local government that has established	Board of directors/Establishers
Approval of Management Report	The competent minister/Council in charge	The competent minister/Council in charge	Local government that has established	Board of directors/Establishers
Sponsor of a capital	National government	National government	Local government that has established	Own private financial resources
Budget Approval	Congress	Board of directors	parliament	Board of directors/Establishers
Financial Repor	Congress	The competent minister	Ministry of Internal Affairs and Communications/Established local governments	Board of directors/Establishers
Advisory board	Council of Ministries and Agencies	Committee on the system of evaluating incorporated administrative agencies	Local Self-Governance Committee	Consultant firms, etc.
Investment funds	Special Accounts	FILP system/Own Assets	Municipal accounting	Own Assets/Bank
Hospital Administrator (Hospital Director)	A person who has been registered under Article 16-6, paragraph (1) of the Medical Practitioners' Act as stipulated in Article 7, paragraph (1) of the Medical Care Act.			

Table 1. Cont.

Classification by Type of Establishment	National	NHO	Public Hospital	Private
Hospital administrator's appointee	The competent minister	Chairman of the board of directors	Head of the local government	Chairman of the board of directors/Hospital Administrator
Licensor for the establishment of hospitals	Prefectural Governor			
Limitations of opening	Prefectural Governor			
Authority to limit the number of hospital beds	Prefectural Governor			
Status of Employees	Government officer	Private	Local government officer	Private
Status under the Criminal Code	Government officer	Public officer	Local government officer	Private
Government's right to command and control	Has command and control authority.	The Minister of Health, Labor and Welfare may request the implementation of operations in the event of a disaster or public health crisis.	-	-
Operational Supervisory Authority	The competent minister	Prefectural Governor		
Public audits on insurance treatment	Regional Bureau of Health and Welfare (Ministry of Health, Labour and Welfare)			
Surplus Profit	Surpluses must in principle be paid into the national treasury	Surpluses after the end of the medium-term target period are managed by the agency for the next medium-term target period if they are approved by the competent minister, and if permission is not granted, the part of the surplus that has not been planned for use in the next plan must be returned to the national treasury.	Local government	Transfer of assets

The independent administrative agency system in Japan was adopted with reference to the agency system in the United Kingdom, with the aim of separating the functions that are related to policy planning from those that are related to the implementation in order to ensure that the implementation functions are carried out efficiently and effectively [10]. However, from its inception, there were major concerns that the Japanese-style independent administrative agency system was a new form of government corporation that would lead to strengthened political control [11,12].

The most important reason for the reorganization into an independent administrative agency was to reduce or to eliminate the transfer of funds from the national budget to the national hospitals [5,10]. For example, as shown in Figure 1, about USD 1 billion

(USD 1 = JPY 110) was transferred from the national general account in 2003 and about USD 2.35 billion at the peak in 1994 [13–16]. Therefore, improving the management and the efficiency of medical care (i.e., increasing healthcare "sales" and operating on a low budget) became the most important mission of the NHO. The NHO achieved a surplus for five consecutive years by restricting the new investment and securing the human resources, with the aim of increasing the medical treatment profit in the first five-year period (April 2004 to March 2009) [17]. In the second period, the investment was gradually resumed, with a further reduction in hospital beds and attempts to reduce the costs of materials, etc.; the current account balance exceeded 100% each year [4,18]. In the third period, increasing the number of medical staff in order to obtain higher reimbursement without changing the business structure led to an imbalance between the labor costs and the medical business income gradually becoming apparent. These results were evaluated by the Independent Administrative Institution System Evaluation Committee and were published as evaluation results by the competent minister, the Minister of Health, Labor and Welfare [7–9]. As a result, the "III. Matters Related to Improvement of Financial Condition" was rated "S" (much above target) or "A" (target achieved) in the first and second periods, but "B" (treated as achieved but some targets did not achieve) in the third period. To the best of our knowledge, no further detailed investigation of these issues has been conducted. In this study, we focused our analysis and review on the financial relations that were rated the final score of "B" in the third period. (Table 2).

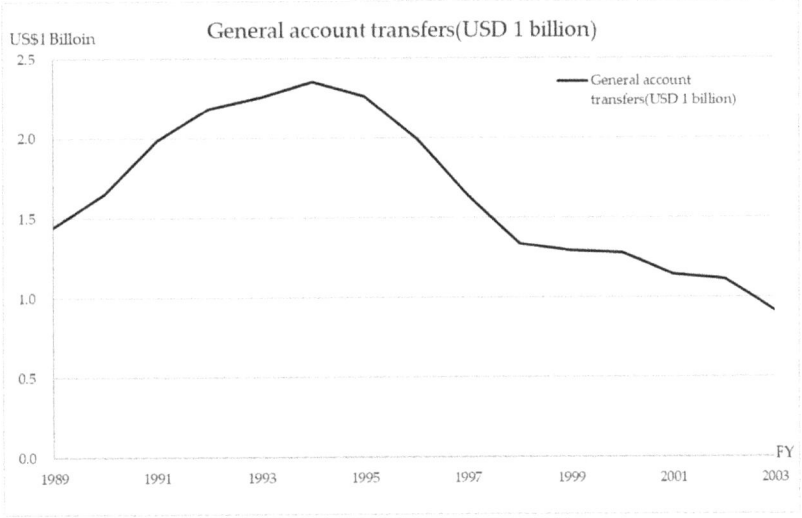

Figure 1. General account transfers (USD 1 billion).

The NHO hospitals provide medical care from the chronic to the acute phases and can be considered to be a microcosm of the Japanese healthcare system. The management analysis in this study was conducted by classifying the NHO by healthcare function in order to identify the managerial problems in the healthcare system in Japan. In addition, the NHO has an important function in the national infrastructure for health risk management, such as that required in the event of a pandemic, such as COVID-19, or in a large-scale disaster, such as the 2011 great East Japan earthquake [18]. This function is a permanent role that has to be fulfilled in the long term as infrastructure. On the other hand, if the NHO is to become operationally independent, the most important issue is its potential viability in terms of the balance of payments. Therefore, in this study, the management status of each NHO hospital group has been analyzed using an original index in order to examine the problems that were brought about by the efficiency improvement of medical management after the establishment of the NHO as an independent administrative agency.

Table 2. Final review of the medium-term management plan; for more detailed information see Supplementary Material Table S2.

Target item			Final review of medium-term		
Medium-term plan			1	2	3
I. Matters concerning the improvement of the quality of services and other operations provided to the public					
	Clinical Services				
		Providing Medical Care	A	A	B
		Providing Safe and Reliable Medical Care	A	A	
		High-Quality Medical Care	S	S	Reclassified.
		Contribution to National Health Care Policy	—	—	A
		Contribution to Local Medical Services	—	S	A
	Clinical Research Business		S	S	A
	Education and Training Business		A	S	B
II. Matters related to the efficiency of business management					
	Efficient Business Operation Structure		A	A	B
	Improvement of Efficiency of Business Operation, etc.		A	A	
	Effective Utilization of Medical Resources		S	S	
	Reduction of Expenses Related to Businesses Other Than Clinical Services, etc.		A	—	
	Promotion of Information Technology		A	—	
	Securing Revenue		—	A	
III. Matters Related to Improvement of Financial Status					
	Budget, Income and Expenditure Plan and Financial Plan		—	—	B
	Improvement of Management		S	A	
	Improvement of Fixed Liabilities Ratio		S	S	
IV. Other matters					
	Other Matters Concerning Business Operation as Provided for in the Ordinance of the Competent Ministry		A	A	B

The result of the rated score. "S": much above target, "A": target achieved, "B": treated as achieved but some targets did not achieve. And there are even worse scores that the NHO has not received. "C": failed to achieve targets overall, "D": Improvements, including the discontinuation of operations, are required.

2. Materials and Methods

The study covered three periods (15 years) from April 2004 to March 2019. The business conditions were analyzed for each period by using financial statements that were published by the NHO, especially the profit and loss (PLS) and the cash flow statement (CFS) [19]. The items used in the PLS were limited to the medical service revenue and medical service cost portions. The CFS was not categorized by business, therefore, the entire cash flow was used. The financial statements were for 142 hospitals (141 in FY 2018, after one hospital was discontinued). For the analysis, these hospitals were categorized into six groups, using the NHO classification, as follows: hospitals offering acute-phase medical care with <349 beds (group 1), 350–499 beds (group 2), and >500 beds (group 3); hospitals offering medical care for disabilities (group 4); hospitals offering psychiatric medical care (group 5); and hospitals offering mixed medical care (group 6).

The following indicators were used in the analysis. From the PLS, the rate of increase in the medical revenue was based on the revenue that was shown in the medical service section. The growth rate was obtained by calculating the medical revenue per hospital bed for each hospital and then calculating the average for each group by determining the difference from the previous year's figures and dividing by the amount of the previous year. The same method was used for the growth rate in the previous year. The rate of increase in each group was calculated as the rate of increase = (average value per hospital bed − average value per hospital bed in the previous fiscal year)/average value per hospital bed in the previous fiscal year × 100%. The rates of increase in personnel-related expenses, material costs, and capital investment expenses were obtained using the salaries and outsourcing costs, material costs, and equipment-related costs, respectively, in the medical service costs. The five-year averages were calculated for each group for the growth rates of the medical revenues, personnel-related expenses, material expenses, and equipment-related expenses.

The management index that we developed in 2010 was used for the analysis of the PLS. In this approach, the ratio of marginal profit after personnel cost to personnel cost (RMP), the ratio of investment per personnel cost (RIP), and the operating profit per personnel cost (OPP) were converted into USD 1 of labor cost [17,20,21]. These indicators can be expressed as follows from the relationship between the cost of medical expenses and medical income A in the PLS of the hospital shown in Figure 2:

A: (Medical) Revenue					
	B: Fixed cost			C: Variable cost	
α	a	b	c	d	e
	D: Indirect cost			E: Direct cost	

Figure 2. PL structure A: (Medical) Revenue, B: Fixed cost, C: Variable cost, D: Indirect cost, E: Direct cost, α: Medical profit, a: Depreciation for a hospital, b: Maintenance cost for a hospital, c: Labor costs, d: Cost of medical materials, e: Food expenses. A = α + B + C = α + D + E, B = a + b + c, C = d + e, D = a + b, E = c + d + e.

Indicator 1: Ratio of the marginal profit after personnel cost per personnel cost (RMP), as follows: $\mathbf{RMP} = \frac{A-E}{c} = \frac{\alpha+a+b}{c}$

Indicator 2: Ratio of investment (= indirect cost) per personnel cost (RIP), as follows: $\mathbf{RIP} = \frac{D}{c}$

Indicator 3: Operation profit per USD 1 of personnel cost (OPP) (difference between the RMP and the RIP), follows: $\mathbf{OPP} = \frac{\alpha}{c} = \mathbf{RMP} - \mathbf{RIP}$

The indicator OPP represents the efficiency of medical management.

These indicators are generally expressed in relation to labor costs, which are the largest cost item in Japanese healthcare, accounting for around 50% of costs, and can be used for management benchmarking between healthcare organizations [20,21].

First, the break-even point (BEP) is α = 0, i.e., zero medical profit. In other words, when the OPP = α = 0, from the OPP formula, RIP = RMP is the BEP. This means that the BEP can also be determined using the following formula [20,21]:

$$\mathbf{BEP} = \frac{\text{Fixed cost}}{1 - \left(\frac{\text{Variable cost}}{\text{Revenue}}\right)} = \frac{B}{1 - \frac{C}{A}} = \frac{a+b+c}{\frac{A-C}{A}} = \frac{A(a+b+c)}{\alpha+a+b+c} = \frac{A\left[c\left(\frac{a+b}{c}\right)+c\right]}{c\left[\left(\frac{\alpha+a+b}{c}\right)+1\right]} = \frac{A(c \times \text{RIP} + c)}{c(\text{RMP}+1)}$$
$$= \frac{Ac(\text{RIP}+1)}{c(\text{RMP}+1)} = \frac{A(\text{RIP}+1)}{\text{RMP}+1}$$

Then, using the indicators RMP, RIP, and BEP, the break-even ratio (BER) can be expressed as follows:

$$\mathbf{BER} = \mathbf{BEP} \times \frac{1}{A} = \frac{A(\text{RIP}+1)}{\text{RMP}+1} \times \frac{1}{A} = \frac{\text{RIP}+1}{\text{RMP}+1}$$

$$\mathbf{BER}(\%) = \mathbf{BER} \times 100(\%) = \frac{\text{RIP}+1}{\text{RMP}+1} \times 100(\%)$$

The relationship between the RMP and the RIP can also be expressed using the BEP, as follows: $\text{RIP} = \text{BEP}(\text{RMP}+1) - 1$

The relationship between the RMP, the RIP, the OPP, and the break-even line is shown in Figure 3.

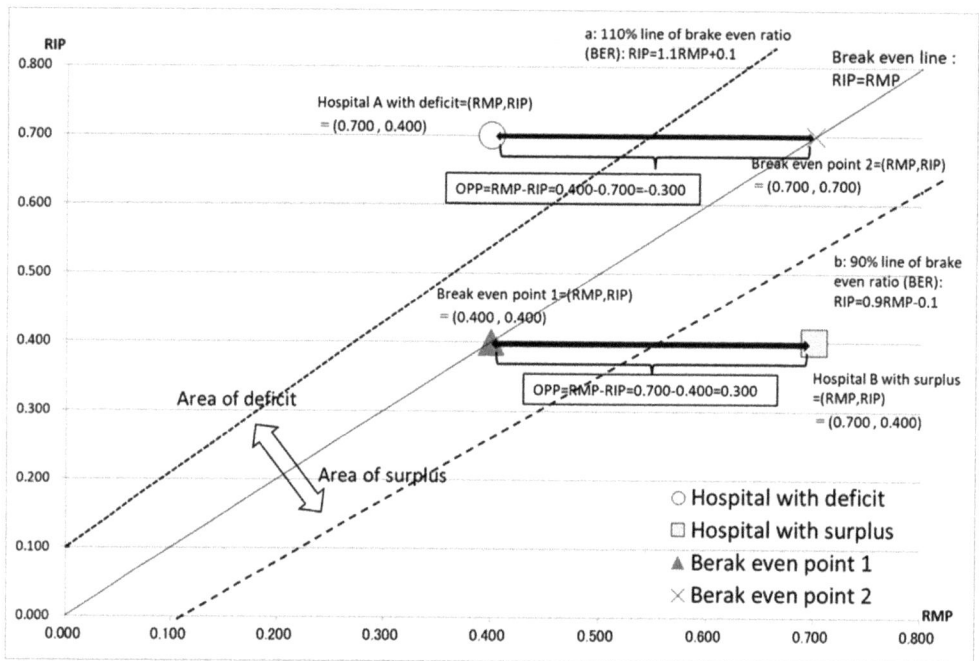

Figure 3. The relationship between RMP, RIP, OPP, and the break-even line. Hospital A, with a deficit, is shown as (RMP, RIP) = (0.400, 0.700). Hospital B, with a surplus, is shown as (RMP, RIP) = (0.700, 0.400). The line RIP = RMP is the break-even line. Line "a" represents 110% of the break-even ratio (BER): RIP = 1.1RMP + 0.1, calculated by the formula: RIP = BER (RMP + 1) − 1. Line "b" represents 90% of the BER: RIP = 0.9RMP − 0.1. The width between hospital A and BEP of $0.400 - 0.700 = -0.300$ shows the operating profit per USD 1 of personnel cost (OPP) of hospital A. The width between hospital B and BEP of $0.700 - 0.400 = 0.300$ shows the operating profit per USD 1 of personnel cost (OPP) of hospital B. The area over the BER line is the deficit area and that below the BER line is the surplus area.

Using the CFS, the free cash flow (FCF) was obtained from the sum of the cash flow (CF) from the operating activities and investment activities, and the average value over five years was calculated for each group.

3. Results

3.1. Medical Revenue

The medical revenues increased from 1.1% to 2.9% in the third five-year period but were 1–2% lower than in the first and second periods (Table 3). The increases were lowest in 2016, at <1%, except in groups 1 and 6. These groups increased by 3.3% and 3.2% in 2016, respectively; however, these values were not reflected in the RMP. This suggests an increase in the labor costs beyond the increase in the medical revenues. In the third period, the increase for all of the NHO hospitals was 1.9%, and the medical revenues in the acute care groups 1, 2, and 3 increased by >2%.

Table 3. Management indicators in the 15 years of the study.

	Group	2004	2005	2006	2007	2008	2009	2010	2011	2012	2013	2014	2015	2016	2017	2018	Average of 1st Period	Average of 2nd Period	Average of 3rd Period
Rate of increase in medical revenue	Group 1	-	−0.1%	0.3%	6.3%	2.6%	6.2%	9.1%	5.1%	2.7%	2.4%	0.8%	1.3%	3.3%	0.3%	4.3%	2.3%	5.1%	2.0%
	Group 2	-	3.3%	0.4%	6.7%	1.2%	5.9%	9.6%	4.3%	4.5%	2.5%	1.9%	5.1%	0.5%	3.6%	5.0%	2.9%	5.4%	3.2%
	Group 3	-	6.4%	2.3%	8.5%	2.7%	3.8%	7.8%	2.3%	3.7%	4.2%	1.8%	3.2%	0.9%	3.4%	3.8%	5.0%	4.3%	2.6%
	Group 4	-	5.9%	−2.4%	2.9%	3.3%	2.1%	2.9%	1.1%	0.4%	3.7%	2.2%	2.2%	−0.7%	0.6%	4.9%	2.4%	2.1%	1.8%
	Group 5	-	5.6%	2.7%	11.7%	7.0%	1.5%	2.4%	3.6%	−0.6%	2.3%	2.6%	−0.8%	−1.0%	3.5%	1.7%	6.7%	1.8%	1.2%
	Group 6	-	−0.8%	0.3%	3.6%	9.1%	2.6%	5.6%	2.5%	3.3%	8.3%	0.0%	3.1%	3.2%	4.1%	−3.1%	3.1%	4.5%	1.5%
	Total	-	3.4%	0.0%	5.6%	4.0%	3.7%	6.4%	2.9%	2.7%	4.0%	1.3%	2.2%	1.1%	2.1%	2.9%	3.3%	4.0%	1.9%
Rate of increase in personnel-related expenses	Group 1	-	1.7%	2.8%	6.9%	7.1%	4.2%	4.1%	5.6%	0.8%	2.9%	2.1%	5.9%	3.1%	0.7%	3.0%	4.6%	3.5%	2.9%
	Group 2	-	6.0%	1.5%	5.7%	3.1%	8.2%	4.4%	5.0%	4.0%	3.2%	4.0%	9.2%	2.2%	3.7%	4.9%	4.1%	4.9%	4.8%
	Group 3	-	8.9%	4.1%	8.2%	4.1%	5.3%	3.8%	4.4%	2.5%	5.9%	4.6%	7.2%	2.8%	2.0%	2.4%	6.3%	4.4%	3.8%
	Group 4	-	5.4%	−3.1%	1.7%	1.1%	1.6%	2.0%	1.8%	0.6%	2.6%	4.4%	7.1%	0.8%	0.9%	4.6%	1.3%	1.7%	3.6%
	Group 5	-	12.5%	2.6%	6.8%	−0.2%	1.4%	1.3%	1.1%	0.9%	2.7%	3.3%	5.4%	1.6%	1.6%	1.3%	5.4%	1.5%	2.6%
	Group 6	-	−1.0%	1.8%	3.1%	7.3%	3.9%	1.4%	3.4%	1.7%	7.5%	1.6%	8.4%	3.5%	2.8%	−3.2%	2.8%	3.6%	2.6%
	Total	-	4.6%	0.8%	4.5%	3.8%	4.1%	2.8%	3.5%	1.9%	4.1%	3.3%	7.0%	2.2%	1.7%	2.4%	3.4%	3.3%	3.3%
Rate of increase in material costs	Group 1	-	−3.1%	2.1%	4.2%	1.1%	7.5%	7.0%	4.2%	−1.7%	4.7%	−0.1%	1.0%	4.4%	−0.3%	4.0%	1.1%	4.3%	1.8%
	Group 2	-	3.9%	−0.1%	6.1%	0.0%	7.5%	4.4%	5.5%	2.0%	5.3%	3.1%	9.1%	2.1%	4.9%	5.5%	2.5%	4.9%	4.9%
	Group 3	-	6.9%	3.1%	7.1%	3.2%	6.2%	5.5%	4.0%	3.5%	7.0%	5.8%	7.5%	1.9%	2.9%	2.9%	5.1%	5.2%	4.2%
	Group 4	-	4.2%	−4.7%	4.0%	4.2%	5.1%	1.7%	1.0%	2.5%	6.1%	4.3%	5.4%	−1.5%	−0.5%	4.4%	1.9%	3.3%	2.4%
	Group 5	-	5.6%	−2.1%	4.9%	3.0%	0.8%	−0.5%	5.4%	4.5%	2.4%	−0.4%	5.7%	−3.5%	−3.0%	3.8%	2.9%	2.5%	0.5%
	Group 6	-	1.4%	0.8%	3.5%	11.2%	3.5%	4.0%	2.4%	2.7%	10.5%	1.9%	9.0%	7.8%	2.7%	−3.4%	4.2%	4.6%	3.6%
	Total	-	3.2%	0.3%	5.2%	3.6%	6.0%	4.4%	3.8%	2.0%	6.3%	2.8%	5.6%	2.8%	1.7%	2.8%	3.1%	4.5%	3.1%
Rate of increase in capital investment expenses	Group 1	-	−7.5%	−6.5%	1.0%	4.3%	26.7%	8.8%	4.4%	3.8%	13.2%	3.7%	−7.2%	0.8%	0.2%	−0.8%	−2.2%	11.4%	−0.6%
	Group 2	-	11.4%	0.3%	−1.0%	4.5%	44.3%	8.2%	1.6%	6.1%	3.9%	3.8%	−8.0%	−1.3%	1.7%	7.2%	3.8%	12.8%	0.7%
	Group 3	-	2.6%	−11.6%	−0.7%	1.2%	32.8%	8.7%	0.8%	5.9%	11.9%	−0.1%	−11.7%	−3.4%	−3.7%	−1.1%	−2.1%	12.0%	−4.0%
	Group 4	-	13.2%	−14.0%	−2.5%	3.1%	24.4%	6.3%	1.6%	4.2%	12.2%	4.0%	−7.8%	−2.1%	4.3%	4.9%	0.0%	9.7%	0.7%
	Group 5	-	18.0%	−7.5%	−4.4%	1.6%	27.7%	7.4%	−10.9%	11.0%	8.0%	0.7%	−6.5%	−5.9%	0.7%	3.5%	1.9%	8.6%	−1.5%
	Group 6	-	1.3%	−10.4%	−1.4%	7.6%	27.9%	2.6%	2.3%	4.3%	19.6%	−3.6%	−8.3%	6.2%	6.2%	−3.7%	−0.7%	11.3%	−0.7%
	Total	-	6.0%	−8.9%	−1.4%	4.1%	31.1%	6.6%	1.3%	5.2%	11.5%	1.3%	−8.8%	−0.3%	2.0%	2.0%	0.0%	11.1%	−0.8%

Table 3. *Cont.*

	Group	2004	2005	2006	2007	2008	2009	2010	2011	2012	2013	2014	2015	2016	2017	2018	Average of 1st Period	Average of 2nd Period	Average of 3rd Period
FCF (US$1 million)	Group 1	−34.4	11.2	1.4	6.3	−6.8	−12.5	−26.4	−24.5	−7.7	−8.0	−51.6	−39.9	3.3	−4.9	36.0	−4.5	−15.8	−11.4
	Group 2	36.7	−22.8	25.6	72.4	−103.5	−142.2	52.5	130.2	131.8	112.3	38.6	−31.1	18.7	2.2	−151.1	1.7	56.9	−24.5
	Group 3	45.7	113.4	139.3	141.5	123.9	78.7	145.4	96.0	97.3	119.0	81.2	89.7	−19.9	71.7	22.0	112.8	107.3	48.9
	Group 4	−23.6	24.2	75.2	71.8	74.0	75.6	73.3	58.9	31.0	−27.8	−63.5	−18.7	33.0	−34.4	−61.4	44.3	42.2	−29.0
	Group 5	−14.4	−1.5	−7.8	9.6	21.4	23.8	17.2	27.4	4.1	3.6	−21.0	−51.5	−2.1	−4.0	−3.1	1.5	15.2	−16.3
	Group 6	4.4	42.9	52.7	53.1	51.3	37.8	39.6	56.8	71.7	−47.4	−49.0	−51.6	−77.9	−118.2	−6.7	40.9	31.7	−60.7
	Total	14.4	167.4	286.5	354.6	160.2	61.3	301.7	344.7	328.3	151.8	−65.3	−103.0	−44.9	−87.6	−164.3	196.6	237.6	−93.0
Number of Beds	Group 1	4854	4708	4558	4352	4014	3922	3899	3884	3929	3693	3793	4187	4187	4274	4222	4408	3865	4133
	Group 2	9454	9751	9858	9767	9784	9631	9728	9775	9735	9744	9725	9295	9271	8851	8711	9790	9723	9171
	Group 3	8420	8412	8384	8357	8357	8369	8350	8324	8299	8164	8103	8051	8019	7984	7832	8378	8301	7998
	Group 4	13,934	13,881	13,986	13,819	13,601	13,529	13,388	13,331	13,235	13,218	13,570	14,747	14,851	14,761	14,846	13,822	13,340	14,555
	Group 5	4963	4816	4838	4574	4555	4554	4458	4459	4386	4322	4306	4312	4362	4291	4284	4696	4436	4311
	Group 6	13,263	13,727	13,450	13,164	12,724	12,493	12,639	12,501	12,366	12,471	11,968	10,641	10,648	10,975	10,795	13,266	12,494	11,005
	Total	54,888	55,295	55,074	54,033	53,035	52,498	52,462	52,274	51,950	51,612	51,465	51,233	51,338	51,136	50,690	54,359	52,159	51,172

3.2. Personnel-Related Expenses

There were very few years in which the expenses that were related to labor costs decreased (Table 3). The only decreases were in group 4 by 3.1% in 2006, in group 5 by 0.2% in 2008, and in group 6 by 1% in 2005 and by 3.2% in 2018. The acute care groups 1 to 3 had increased personnel expenses in all of the years. The overall average increase over the 15 years was 3.3% and was almost the same for the three five-year periods. The highest increase of 7.0% occurred in 2015 and the highest group increase of 9.2% occurred in group 2.

3.3. Material Costs

The average cost of the medical materials for all of the NHO hospitals increased in all periods (Table 3). However, the rate of growth was lower in the third period compared to the first and second periods. In the third period, the rate of increase was <3%, except in 2015, but groups 2, 3, and 6, which provide acute care, showed large increases of 4.9%, 4.2%, and 3.6%, respectively. Group 3, in particular, did not have a single year of decline in 15 years. However, since 2016, the growth rate of material costs has been <3%.

3.4. Capital Investment Expenses

As shown for the RIP (Figure 4), little capital investment was made in the first period, but this increased by 11.1% in the second period (Table 3). This impact continued until 2014. The RMP also increased from FY 2010, but this was presumably due to the effects of capital and personnel investment. In the third period, investment was curtailed again from 2015, which was triggered by increased labor costs in 2015, and both the RIP and the RMP decreased. These effects continued until the end of the third period. There was a significant decline in all of the groups in 2015, with an average of -8.8% for the year, and the impact is shown in the subsequent changes in the RIP.

3.5. RMP, RIP, OPP, and BER

Figures 5 and 6 demonstrate the relationship between the RIP, the RMP, and the rate of increase in the personnel-related expenses in each group.

Group 1 includes the acute-phase medical care hospitals with less than 350 beds. In the first period, the investment was restrained and both the RIP and the RMP decreased in line with the growth in labor costs (Figure 5a). In the second phase, significant capital investment was made in 2009, and this trend continued throughout the second period (Table 3). Both the RIP and the RMP increased accordingly, showing the effects of the investment. In the third period, the capital investment was restrained, but the impact of increased capital investment in the second period continued after 2014 and the RIP remained high in 2018. On the other hand, the labor costs increased in all periods, especially in FY 2015 in the third period, which increased the gap between the RIP and the RMP (increasing the deficit).

Group 2 includes the acute-phase medical care hospitals with 350–499 beds. The increase in the capital investment started in the first period, with a particularly large increase in capital investment in 2009 in the second period, and continued until 2014 in the third period (Table 3). The labor costs increased during the whole period and, finally, in the third period both the RIP and the RMP decreased at the same time, in line with the growth in labor costs. The capital investment was strongly reduced in FY 2015, but the capital investment from the second period and the continuous increase in the labor costs could not be absorbed, resulting in a deficit (negative OPP) from FY 2016 (Figure 5b).

A clear difference between the first, second, and third periods is apparent in the acute groups since group 1 has had a negative OPP (deficit) since FY 2013 and group 2 since FY 2016 (Figure 5a,b).

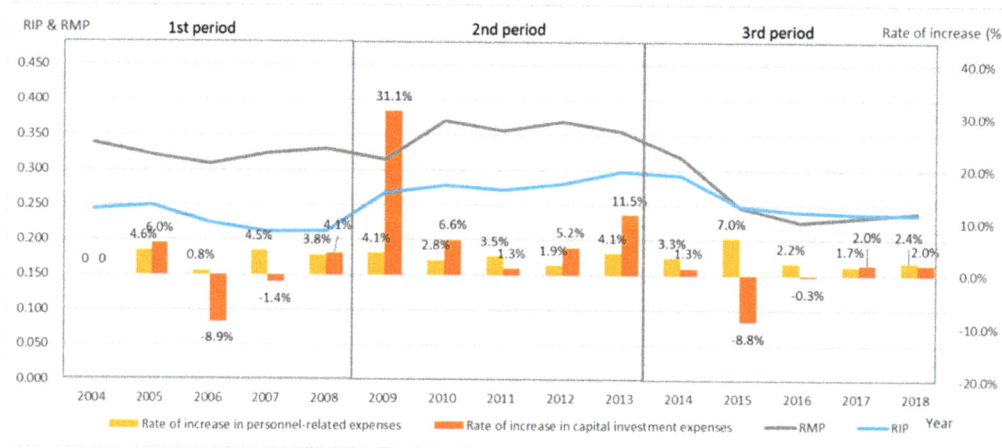

Figure 4. Relationship between RIP and the rate of capital investment expenses of all NHO hospitals. The RIP remained high, above 0.25, for the second period from FY 2009 to FY 2014. This indicates that the NHO had sustained investment during this period. The rate of change, which shows the rate of growth from the previous year, showed an increase of over 30% in FY 2009 and sustained that investment until FY 2014; the investment was restrained in the third period from FY 2015 onwards.

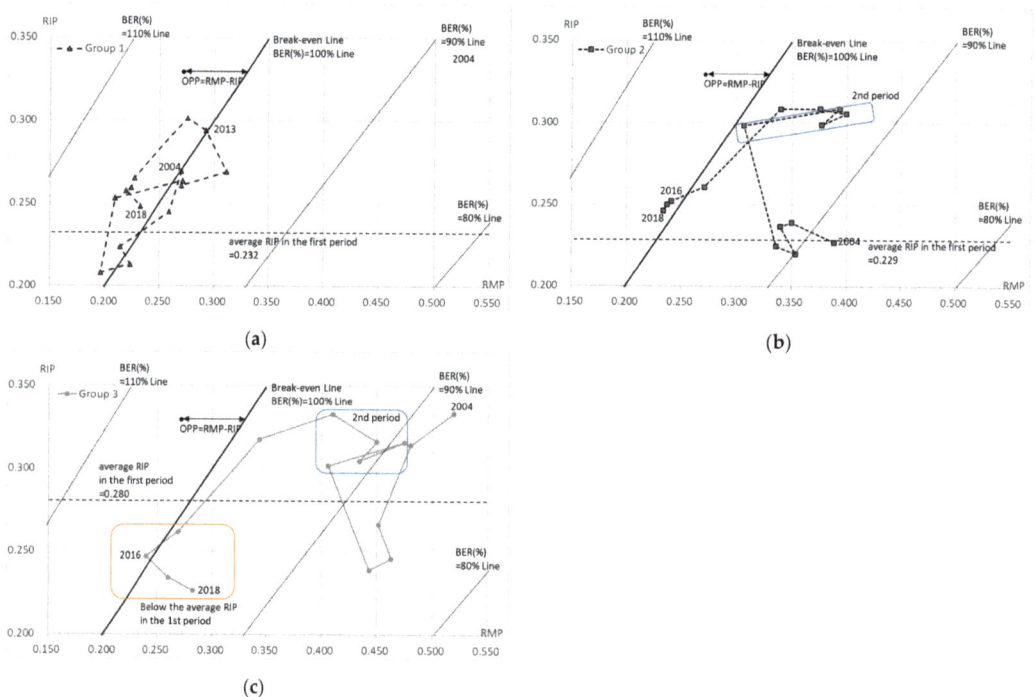

Figure 5. RMP, RIP, OPP, and BER in hospitals offering acute-phase medical care. (**a**) Group 1 (<350 beds); (**b**) group 2 (350–499 beds); (**c**) group 3 (>500 beds). The OPP shows the difference

between RMP and RIP; OPP = RMP − RIP. Break-even Line; RIP = RMP. 90% of break-even ratio (BER (%)): RIP = 0.9RMP − 0.1, calculated by RIP = BER (RMP + 1) − 1. 80% of BER (%): RIP = 0.8RMP − 0.20. 110% of BER (%): RIP = 1.1RMP + 0.10.

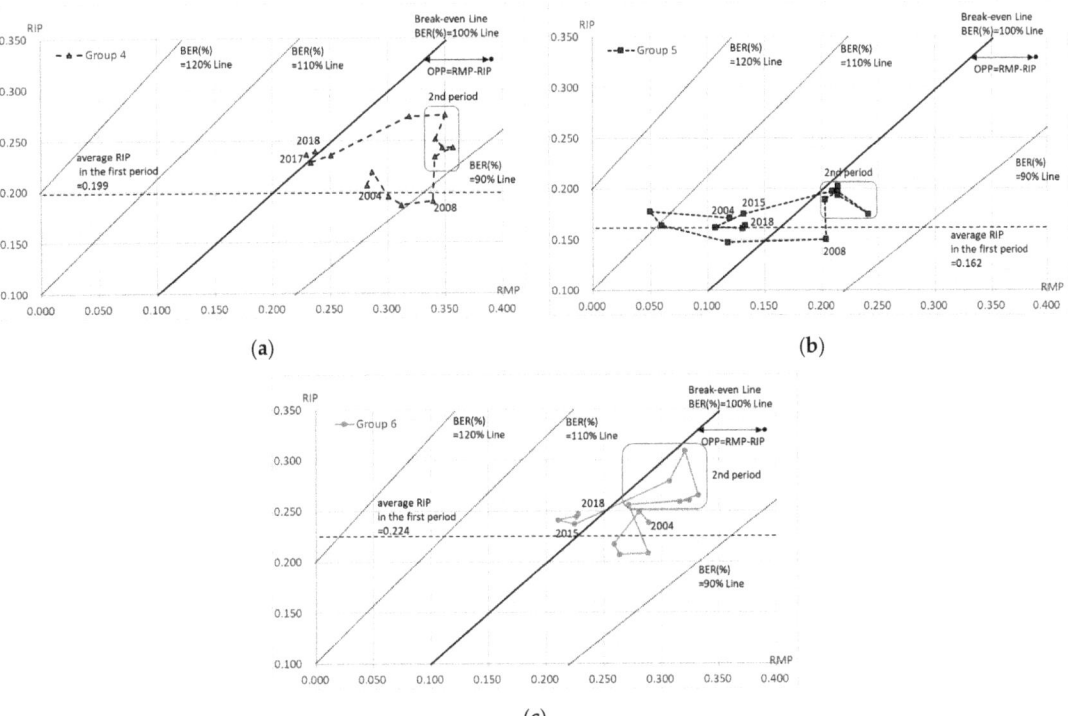

Figure 6. RMP, RIP, OPP, and BER in hospitals offering chronic-phase medical care. (**a**) Group 4 (hospitals offering medical care for disabilities); (**b**) group 5 (hospitals offering psychiatric medical care); (**c**) group 6 (hospitals offering mixed medical care). The OPP shows the difference between RMP and RIP; OPP = RMP − RIP. Break-even Line; RIP = RMP. 90% line of break-even ratio (BER (%)): RIP = 0.9RMP − 0.1, calculated by the formula: RIP = BER (RMP + 1) − 1. 110% line of BER (%): RIP = 1.1RMP + 0.10. 120% line of BER (%): RIP = 1.2RMP + 0.20.

Group 3 includes the acute-phase medical care hospitals with more than 500 beds. In the first period, the capital investment was restrained and both the RIP and the RMP decreased in line with the growth in labor costs (Table 3, Figure 5c). In the second period, a significant capital investment was made in 2009, which continued throughout the second period, and the RIP also increased. After the significant capital investment in FY 2009, the RMP increased significantly from FY 2010 and remained high until FY 2013. In the third period, the capital investment became more restrained from FY 2015, while the labor costs continued to increase, resulting in a decline in both the RIP and the RMP, but the labor costs grew significantly in FY 2015 and the OPP became negative (deficit) for the first time in FY 2016. However, the RMP subsequently increased and was above 0.25, resulting in a positive (surplus) OPP. Thus, group 3 increased its RIP in the second period due to capital investment, but this was balanced by high RMP being maintained. However, its RMP declined sharply in the third period, and it was in deficit (negative OPP) for the first time in FY 2016 (Figure 5c).

Group 4 includes the hospitals offering medical care for disabilities. In the first period, the capital investment was restrained, except in 2005 (Table 3). The labor costs were also restrained, with little increase, except in 2005 (Table 3). As a result, the OPP was positive (surplus). In the second period, a significant capital investment was made in 2009, and this trend continued until 2014 in the third period (Figure 6a). Along with this, the RIP also increased and had an impact until FY 2018. The RMP continuously showed high values, but both the RIP and the RMP had started to decrease in line with the increased labor costs and the decreased capital investment in FY 2015. In the third period, both the RIP and the RMP were relatively stable; however, from FY 2017 they were in deficit (negative OPP).

Group 5 includes the hospitals offering psychiatric medical care. In the first phase, significant personnel and capital investment were made in 2005, but the capital investment was subsequently reduced (Table 3). On the other hand, the investment in labor costs continued during the whole period (Table 3). The business turned into a surplus in 2008, and a significant capital investment was made again in 2009 (Figure 6b). The capital investment was temporarily curbed in 2011, but the RIP also rose again as a result of the increased capital investment in 2012 and 2013. In the third period, while there was a significant increase in human rights expenditure in 2015, the capital investment remained reduced or restrained from 2015, and the RIP decreased. However, the RMP decreased further, causing a significant deficit (negative OPP) to continue from 2015.

Group 6 includes the hospitals offering mixed medical care. In the first phase, both the capital investment and the labor costs were controlled until 2008, and the RIP continued to decline, while the RMP was maintained or showed an upward trend (Table 3, Figure 6c). Both the capital investment and the labor costs increased from 2008, with a significant capital investment in 2009, which was a trend that continued throughout the second period. The RIP increased accordingly, and its impact continued until FY 2018. The RMP has been high since 2010, but the RMP decreased sharply in line with the increase in labor costs in 2015. The impact of increased labor costs was observed over the entire third period, with a deficit (negative OPP) from FY 2015.

The BER (%) can also be read in Figures 5 and 6. It is shown as the range of each BEP, which is indicated by RIP=BEP (RMP+1) -1. Furthermore, Figure 7 shows the BER (%) for each group for each year, where a BER (%) above 100% means a deficit and a BER (%) below 100% means a surplus. Period one was the best situation in total, although the second period was seen to be in a better business position. In total, the BER (%) was worse in periods one, two, and three. In addition, all but group 3 were in the red in FY 2017 and FY 2018.

The BER was calculated for each RMP for the acute care hospitals and the chronic care hospitals (Figures 8 and 9). The BER decreased as the RMP increased. The number of hospitals that were in surplus was higher than the number that were in deficit when the RMP was ≥ 0.25 for the acute hospitals and ≥ 0.21 for the chronic hospitals (Figures 8 and 9).

3.6. Free Cash Flow (FCF)

In terms of FCF, only group 3 had positive averages for all of the three periods, amounting to approximately USD 112.8 million, USD 107.3 million, and USD 48.9 million, respectively. In particular, only group 3 was positive in the third period and was negative only in FY 2016 (Table 3). However, the total for all of the NHO hospitals was negative for the fifth consecutive year, since 2014. The situation was particularly bad for group 1, which was negative in all but FY 2005, FY 2006, FY 2007, FY 2016, and FY 2018. Groups 5 and 6 had negative results for all five years of the most recent period, with five-year averages of approximately USD -16.3 million and USD -60.7 million, respectively.

3.7. Number of Hospital Beds

After the formation of the NHO, the number of hospital beds has been steadily reduced in order to decrease the fixed costs and secure profits. The average numbers of beds were 54,359, 52,159, and 51,172 in the first, second, and third five-year periods, respectively, showing a decrease of about 3200 from the first to the third periods (Table 3).

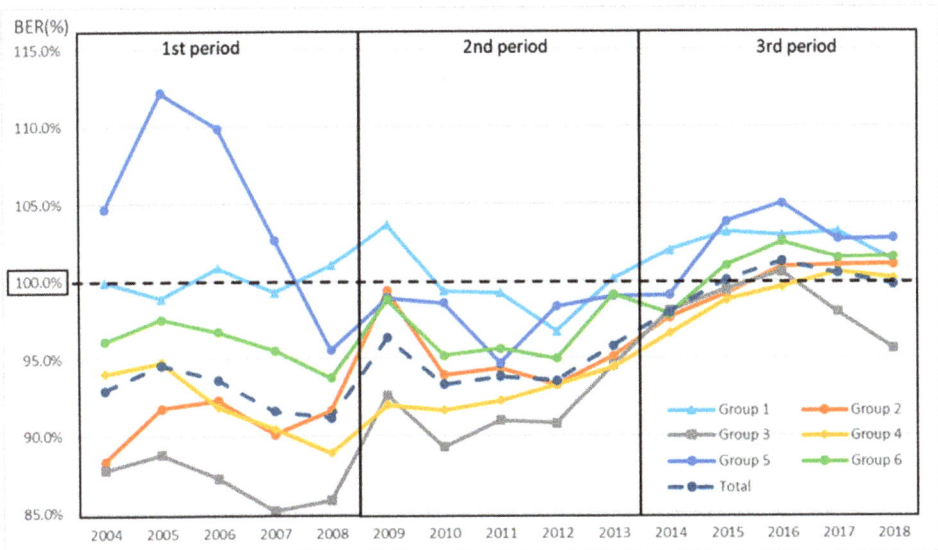

Figure 7. Calculation of BER (%) for each group. BER (%) above 100% means a deficit and a BER (%) below 100% means a surplus; in 2017 and 2018, all but group 3 were in deficit.

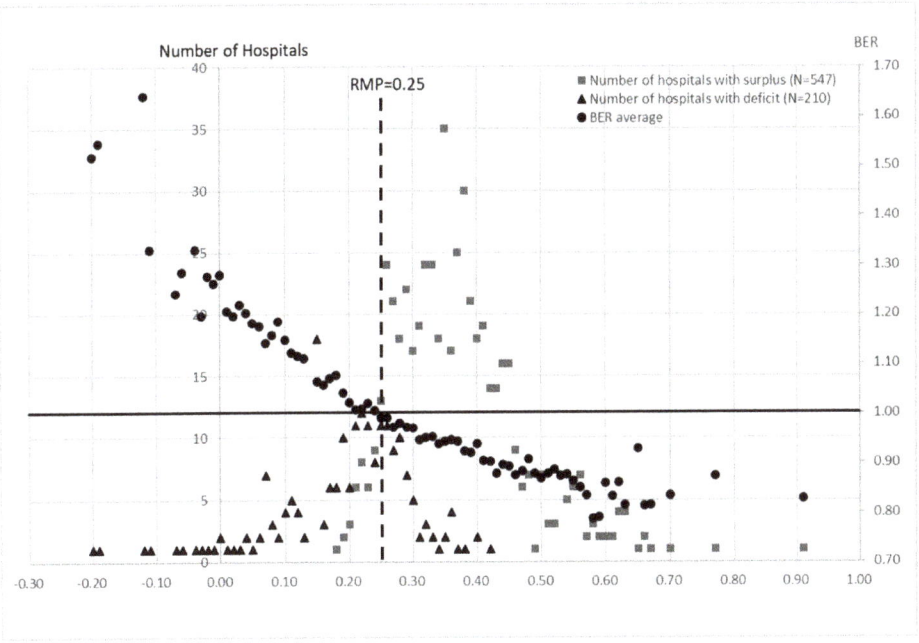

Figure 8. Calculation of BER for each RMP in groups 1, 2, and 3 for all 15 years. The BER shows the average of all hospitals with each RMP value. The number of deficit and surplus hospitals for all years was disaggregated by the RMP value. Most surplus hospitals were located above RMP = 0.25, while most deficit hospitals were located below 0.25. On the other hand, the average BER crosses the line of RMP = 0.25 between surplus and deficit hospitals. This indicates that RMP = 0.25 is a critical point in terms of management.

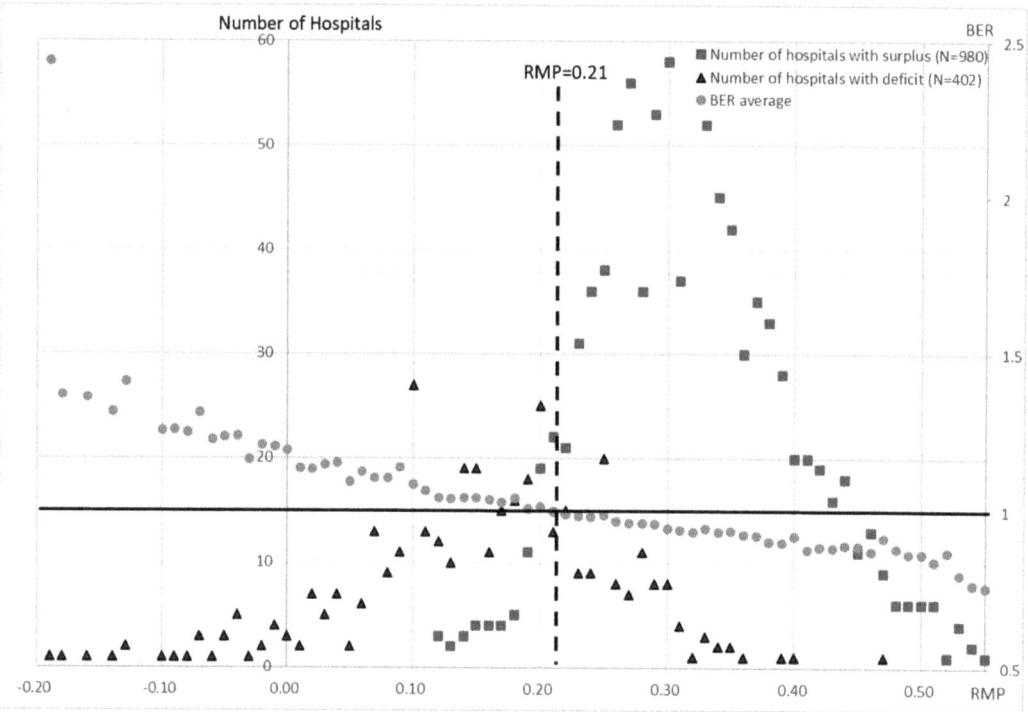

Figure 9. Calculation of BER for each RMP in groups 4, 5, and 6 for all 15 years. The number of deficit and surplus hospitals for all years was disaggregated by RMP value. The BER shows the average of all hospitals with each RMP value. Most surplus hospitals were located above RMP = 0.25, while most deficit hospitals were located below 0.21. On the other hand, the average BER crosses the line of RMP = 0.21 between surplus and deficit hospitals. This indicates that RMP = 0.21 is a critical point in terms of management.

4. Discussion

The healthcare system in Japan is characterized by universal health coverage, in which the price of the medical treatment is uniformly determined by the official prices, and, in principle, medical care is provided to the patients in kind [1,2]. At the same time, the source of a hospital's income from reimbursement is not entirely from insurance premiums, but from the national treasury, insurance premiums, and approximately 30% of the patient's co-payment [2]. In addition, there is no distinction between public and private hospitals, including the NHO hospitals, in terms of hospital medical income and the competitive drive to recruit more patients, and the reimbursement is balanced against the amount of capital investment [22]. Therefore, in order to maintain good hospital management, there is a tendency to increase the hospital functions and to prioritize the availability of the medical services that can provide a high number of patients and a high unit cost per treatment in order to ensure a profit margin.

As part of the monitoring of such services, the NHO has created and started using clinical evaluation indicators since FY 2006 for the purpose of evaluating the quality of medical care. Ver. one (FY2006–FY2009) introduced 26 indicators, which were revised every few years, and Ver. two (FY2010–FY2014) used 87 indicators (including 63 process indicators and 7 outcome indicators), while Ver. three (FY2015–FY2010) used 115 indicators (including 102 process indicators and 13 outcome indicators). The Ministry of Health, Labor and Welfare (MHLW) launched a research project known as the "Project to Promote

Evaluation and Publication of the Quality of Medical Care" in FY 2010, with the aim of improving the quality of medical care, and it is accepting applications from all over Japan. The project aims to visualize the medical care that is provided by each hospital and to equalize and improve the quality of medical care. However, most of the indicators are process indicators and are not outcome indicators corresponding to the process; they have not yet reached the point where they can be used to evaluate performance.

The other clinical evaluation indicator is an evaluation indicator of business performance that is in line with the mid-term goals. In regard to the evaluation of the mid-term plan, the first to the third period is reported to the minister of MHLW and is rated on five levels of "S", "A", "B", "C", and "D", with "S" being the highest rating. The evaluation results show that, except for an increase in the number of items that were rated as "B", i.e., "treated as achieved but some targets did not achieve" in the third period, the results were rated as "S" or "A" as "significantly above" or "above target", respectively [7–9]. As a result, the agency is rated as "treated as achieved but some targets did not achieve " in the third period, but the reality is that the number of items that can be monitored numerically for medical functions did not fall much lower than that in the second period, but the increase disappeared (Table 2).

Medical reimbursement is defined in detail in all of the areas by each activity function and, as mentioned above, the conditions of provision are described for each item. However, the healthcare organizations themselves do not conduct the audits or the monitoring of the treatment outcomes that are related to benefits. On the other hand, the number of patients, the state of the medical equipment, and the specialist index, which was removed the advertising restrictions that are set by the MHLW, are published on a commercial basis. The healthcare system in Japan allows patients to visit any hospital if they wish. We have the highest number of beds and hospitals in the world, the management of hospitals is constantly in a competitive environment, and it is highly necessary to keep the service environment up-to-date in order to continue earning high profits. Therefore, the more proactive healthcare organizations will be more attentive to these commercial factors, while focusing their investments on areas where they can earn higher profits more efficiently.

Furthermore, the medical reimbursements, which define the price for the services and the delivery system, are revised every two years, with various conditions being removed or added repeatedly in order to suit the situation [1,23]. With the system that is related to the 'medical fee schedule' as the key in Japan's healthcare policy, the healthcare delivery environment, which is mostly private, is constantly being induced to be cheaper and maintained at a higher level. As a result of these policy inducements, while the healthcare expenditure as a percentage of GDP is in the top group of OECD countries at around 11%, per capita the healthcare expenditure is not high, and Japan has maintained health outcomes that make it the country with the longest life expectancy in the world [24,25]. This also indicates that the policy has induced the continuous provision of healthcare of a certain level of quality. Furthermore, this approach means that healthcare that has little or no track record of this provision will not be reimbursed itself, inducing voluntary downsizing of functions and concentrating resources in the more general and high-demanded areas. In other words, it can be considered a method of inducing efficiency gains in the healthcare market. The NHO has operated completely independently in such a market environment, competing with the private sector, and not relying on government funding. However, there is a general reluctance to allow public hospitals, including the independent administrative agencies, to strengthen or enter into businesses that compete with the private sector for managerial advantages, as this would put pressure on the private sector businesses.

The analysis of the 15 years of management performance in this paper provides a basis for determining if public hospitals, which are expected to serve as infrastructure for managing healthcare crises, are financially sustainable after their conversion into independent administrative agencies that are required to have the same financial independence as the private sector while maintaining their current roles. The medical fees are set uniformly in Japan by the government according to the quality and the difficulty of the treatment, and the aggregate medical profit can be viewed as a measure of hospital management. The NHO, similar to the national government, has a common set of salaries according to the job type and age, which makes the comparison with the labor costs a good indicator to benchmark a hospital's performance [20]. Furthermore, given the staffing and the functional requirements that are linked to the 'medical fee schedule', as described above, the costs that can realistically be managed by the healthcare providers are limited to how many personnel are added from the minimum number that is determined in the system, and to what extent the facilities are renovated or the medical equipment is replaced. On the revenue side, the real issue is the balance of provision, i.e., what medical specialties of doctors are employed and what type of medical care is provided. Thus, the managers in Japan only have control over the growth of the labor costs, the amount of investment, and the number of patients, which are closely linked to the corresponding sales. Therefore, the RMP, the RIP and the OPP are effective and simple for the assessment of hospital management in the NHO, in terms of the balance among the medical income, the labor costs, and the medical functions that are associated with the equipment.

The RIP shows the ratio of the indirect costs (investment) to the labor costs, and, thus, indicates the balance between the capital and the labor costs that are required in order to provide medical functions. For example, the new capital expenditure in the third period was on a downward trend, as evidenced by the growth rate of the capital expenditure (Table 3, Figure 4). However, this value was higher in the third period than in the first period, when the capital investment was also limited, due to the impact of capital investment that was made in the second period. On the other hand, the capital expenditure in the PLS is depreciation, which does not increase rapidly unless new buildings are constructed, and shows a downward trend over time. Therefore, if the labor costs continue to rise, the RIP will fall. With the exception of group 3, the RIP in the third period was higher than that in the first period in all of the years, and this was a factor in the deterioration of management. The year 2009, when significant investment resumed, was the year in which the government was replaced by the opposition. Thus, it is undeniable that the political pressure on the previous government in healthcare policy had an impact. In fact, the capital investment has been rapid since FY 2009 (Figure 4). This may have been an investment that made it impossible to maintain the replacement cycle of capital investment, which is clearly evident from the investment situation in the third period. When such unplanned investments are made, they include wasteful investments with a bias, such as that due to political pressure. Of course, the political influence is unavoidable when an independent administrative body operates under the approval and the direction of the administration. However, it may also be a turning point where the very strong political influence has made it difficult to maintain managerial independence. Despite the investment being lower than in the second period, the third period resulted in a negative FCF in cash flow, which did not generate the resources to repay the debt (Table 3).

Group 3 had stable management throughout the first two periods, and for this reason, it appeared that the group 3 hospitals were likely to be stable businesses, unless major capital investments were made (Figure 5c). However, in FY 2016, group 3 posted its only loss in 15 years. The reason for the deficit was the low growth rate of medical revenue, as shown by the decline in the RMP, and the increased growth rate of the personnel-related expenses of 7.2% and 2.8% between FY 2015 and FY 2016, respectively, which could not be covered (Table 3).

There was also an increase in the cost of materials in the acute care hospitals, particularly in groups 2 and 3 (Table 3). This may be due to the introduction of high-priced drugs in recent years. However, while the use of high-cost materials led to an increase in the medical revenue, it did not necessarily translate into medical profit. This was evident in the OPP of groups 2 and 3 in FY 2015 (Figure 5b,c). Furthermore, the large increase in the labor costs in 2015 was due to the fact that, although 50% of the labor insurance premiums are paid from the state treasury in the private sector, this was not applied to the NHO, and the subsequent policy changes increased the labor insurance premiums [18]. Although the growth rate of the personnel-related costs is presented for a single year, it is closely linked to the subsequent hospital management, and its impact over the medium- to long-term was seen for all of the RMP, RIP, and OPP indicators. This large increase in the labor costs in 2015 was not necessary for medical treatment, but purely due to political factors. These increases in labor costs, which have nothing to do with the medical practice and do not generate so-called medical income, naturally had a significant impact on the hospital management. This was a factor that caused most of the hospitals to suffer downward pressure on their management in the third phase.

Regarding the third period, during which the NHO had the worst business conditions, the revisions of the medical fees in FY 2014, FY 2016, and FY 2018 were +0.82%, +0.56%, and +0.63% for medical treatment, and −0.05%, −0.11%, and −0.09% for materials, respectively. These data at least indicate a positive revision for medical treatment. According to the 2021 white paper on small and medium enterprises in Japan, the BER (%) of small enterprises (with a capitalization of less than USD 0.09 million) is 90.9% (FY2018), which means that they are less resilient to crises [26]. In the NHO, only groups 1–4 in the first period had a BER that was below 0.9 (BER (%): 90%). In all of the other periods, the BER was above 0.9, and in the third period, it was almost 1 (Figure 7). The capital of the NHO was about USD 1.8 billion in 2020. In other words, the hospital management by independent administrative agencies in Japan is worse than the BER of a small company and is very vulnerable to a crisis.

The labor costs in the NHO have increased by an average of 3.3–3.4% in each period (Table 3). This is partly due to the increase in the number of staff, but also largely due to the pay structure of the organization. While the hospital director is empowered to increase or decrease the number of staff with the approval of the HQ, it is currently impossible for the NHO to make major changes to the staff salary structure, partly because it has taken over the national system. This analysis suggests that, under the current reimbursement system, even the natural increase in labor costs cannot be covered if strict public management continues after the transformation to an independent agency. In other words, if the public hospitals were legally (or in case implicitly) obliged to take on a public role after this transformation, they would be difficult to maintain and manage under the current reimbursement system. Of course, the long-term management of hospitals is possible if the official price of the medical care (reimbursement), which is revised every two years in Japan, is revised positively and can cover the higher labor costs in order to meet the political demands that are specially imposed on the public hospitals and are determined by a salary structure that is influenced by the national system. However, about 70% of the hospitals in Japan are private hospitals, which are free from policy objectives. The official prices are to be the same for all hospitals everywhere, and the official prices do not vary specifically by the public or the private sector. Therefore, a public pricing system is established with the main focus on the management of the private hospitals. This may be partly due to the historical setting of the medical fees in Japan by the Central Social Insurance Medical Council (CSIMC), which mainly operates through consultations between the private hospital owners and the insurers [1,27,28]. In fact, the representatives of the public hospitals are still not on the committee [29]. These hospitals were originally funded by public money and did not have to make a profit on the medical fees alone. However, this problem has arisen in recent years, as the public hospitals have had to generate income through the medical fees without changing their role or the cost structure after becoming independent administrative agencies.

The hospitals that are providing chronic care have increased their staffing levels in order to improve their earnings and to obtain higher levels of remuneration. In the reimbursement system in Japan, the basic fee is determined by the number of nurses that are assigned to a ward. Although this has improved the quality of care and the working environment, it has not led to a significant increase in the number of inpatients and, because of the nature of the patient population, it is unlikely to lead to a significant increase in remuneration. Thus, in order to improve management in the current situation, it is important for the acute hospitals to have an RMP above 0.25 so that the number of hospitals that are in surplus is greater than those that are in deficit. The BEP was also lower than 1 (Figure 8), which means that the RMP should be at least 0.25. For the chronic care hospitals (groups 4 to 6), the number of surplus hospitals is greater than the number of deficit hospitals when the RMP exceeds 0.21 and the BEP is also below 1 (Figure 9). This situation can be achieved by attracting more new patients or/and by reducing the labor costs in order to increase the RMP and by limiting the investment in order to reduce the RIP. In the NHO, functional restraint to the extent that is permitted by the legal system and a reduction in hospital beds have been pursued in the past. However, the OPP decreased to 0.001 in the third period. In addition, continuous negative FCF despite the reduction in the capital expenditure would create a shortage of facilities and financial inflexibility in a situation such as the COVID-19 pandemic that occurred in FY 2020.

If the independent administrative agencies are to become fully economically independent, the government should not impose special institutional restrictions in order to meet the political and administrative requirements. In order tobe more competitive in the market, it is essential to weaken the special political controls that are currently in operation and to create a freer structure that is aimed at a profit-making system with private management. However, this will make it more difficult to prepare for infectious diseases and disasters, which can put downward pressure on the business. This has also been pointed out as an explanation for the decline in the research power of national university medical departments, as a result of the change to an independent administrative agency. University hospitals now have to compete in the general healthcare market, which requires a concentration of management resources on the profitable areas (i.e., the medical treatment), rather than research [30]. In the event of a catastrophe or a pandemic, such as COVID-19, this could create a number of obstacles to a national or local government-led response. If the national government were to completely relinquish their ability to manage the situation, they would also lose the opportunity to have a free hand in the provision of healthcare, which is required by policy. In order to avoid such a situation, a higher public price for healthcare may be needed, including private hospitals, in order to allow for uncertainty in the normal course of events or a rapid provision of the necessary facilities in the event of a pandemic or a disaster. The same problem arises in local regions. Local government hospitals are required to respond to local health crises, similarly to the NHO; however, in order to decouple the local government hospitals from the local government finances, these hospitals are being converted into local independent administrative agencies. The results of this study suggest that the same problems might occur in municipal hospitals if they were to become independent administrative agencies, as is the case with the NHO.

Although the NHO provides a broad range of healthcare functions that are a microcosm of the Japanese healthcare delivery system, the study has the limitation that it cannot be adapted for the evaluation of efficiency in organizations that are more competitively managed when they are viewed on a hospital-by-hospital basis. The evaluation criteria are based on the personnel costs; however, if the safety and the functionality of the hospitals can be adjusted, comparisons can be made in terms of how well they are maintained and how much income they generate in relation to the personnel costs. On the other hand, as comparable treatment outcome data have not been taken in Japan, it is still difficult to conduct an efficiency assessment of costs based on outcomes.

5. Conclusions

The transformation of national hospitals and sanatoriums into independent administrative corporations was partly evaluated in this study as an improvement in profitability. However, in the third period of the study, there was an increasing tendency towards deficits. In particular, controlling the investment did not increase the profits and the FCF was negative for five years. This situation raises doubts about the long-term sustainability of independent management. Our results suggest that further organizational reforms are needed in order to sustain the country's infrastructure in the long term. This is particularly important for health crisis management in areas such as infectious diseases, where continued investment is difficult. At the same time, it is important to evaluate and discuss the future of public hospitals, including the question of whether they should become independent administrative agencies.

Supplementary Materials: The following supporting information can be downloaded at: https://www.mdpi.com/article/10.3390/healthcare10102084/s1, Table S1: Governance structures of health organizations (detailed); Table S2: Final review of the medium-term management plan (detailed).

Author Contributions: Conceptualization, Y.N. (Yoshiaki Nakagawa); Data curation, Y.N. (Yoshiaki Nakagawa); Formal analysis, Y.N. (Yoshiaki Nakagawa), K.I., and Y.N. (Yoshinobu Nakagawa); Funding acquisition, Y.K.; Investigation, Y.N. (Yoshiaki Nakagawa); Methodology, Y.N. (Yoshiaki Nakagawa); Resources, Y.N. (Yoshiaki Nakagawa) and Y.K.; Supervision, Y.K. and Y.N. (Yoshinobu Nakagawa); Visualization, Y.N. (Yoshiaki Nakagawa), K.I., and Y.N. (Yoshinobu Nakagawa); Writing—original draft, Y.N. (Yoshiaki Nakagawa) and K.I.; Writing—review and editing, Y.K. and Y.N. (Yoshinobu Nakagawa). All authors have read and agreed to the published version of the manuscript.

Funding: This research was partly supported by a Grant-in-Aid for Scientific Research (S) from the Japan Society for the Promotion of Science (grant number 21H05001). The funding source had no involvement in study design; in collection, analysis, and interpretation of data; in writing of the report; or in the decision to submit the paper for publication.

Institutional Review Board Statement: Not applicable.

Informed Consent Statement: Not applicable.

Data Availability Statement: All data in the study will be made available upon reasonable request to the corresponding author.

Conflicts of Interest: The authors declare no conflict of interest.

References

1. Ikegami, N.; Campbell, J.C. Health care reform in Japan: The virtues of muddling through. *Health Aff.* **1999**, *18*, 56–75. [CrossRef] [PubMed]
2. Ikegami, N.; Yoo, B.; Hashimoto, H.; Matsumoto, M.; Ogata, H.; Babazono, A.; Watanabe, R.; Shibuya, K.; Yang, B.M.; Reich, M.R.; et al. Japan: Universal Health Care at 50 Years 2: Japanese universal health coverage: Evolution, achievements, and challenges. *Lancet* **2011**, *378*, 1106–1115. [CrossRef]
3. Huntington, D. Public Hospital Governance in the Asia Pacific Region–Drivers of Change. In *Public Hospital Governance in Asia and the Pacific*; Huntington, D., Hort, K., Eds.; World Health Organization Regional Office for the Western Pacific: Manila, Philippines, 2015; pp. 2–25.
4. Nakagawa, Y.; Ito, M.; Nakagawa, Y. Analysis of financial status and personnel investment of National Hospital Organization (NHO) in Japan. *J. Jpn. Soc. Health Care Manag.* **2018**, *19*, 109–114.
5. Tagawa, Y.; Tsugawa, Y.; Ikegami, N. National Hospital Reform in Japan: Results and Challenges. In *Universal Health Coverage for Inclusive and Sustainable Development: Lessons from Japan*; Ikegami, N., Ed.; World Bank Group: Washington, DC, USA, 2014; pp. 149–162.
6. Act on the National Hospital Organization, Independent Administrative Agency. 2002. Available online: https://elaws.e-gov.go.jp/document?law_unique_id=414AC0000000191_20150801_000000000000000 (accessed on 18 October 2022).
7. Results of the Final Evaluation of the Performance of the Independent Administrative Agencies National Hospital Agency in Relation to its Mid-Term Objectives.–1st Period. Available online: https://nho.hosp.go.jp/files/000027938.pdf (accessed on 3 October 2022).
8. Results of the Final Evaluation of the Performance of the Independent Administrative Agencies National Hospital Agency in Relation to Its Mid-Term Objectives.–2nd Period. Available online: https://nho.hosp.go.jp/files/000034104.pdf (accessed on 3 October 2022).
9. Results of the Final Evaluation of the Performance of the Independent Administrative Agencies National Hospital Agency in Relation to Its Mid-Term Objectives.–3rd Period. Available online: https://nho.hosp.go.jp/files/000115005.pdf (accessed on 3 October 2022).
10. Nakanishi, W. Independent administrative institutions (dokuritsu gyosei hojin): Passage of revised and maintenance Acts. *Law Res.* **2014**, *357*, 3–22.
11. Furukawa, S. Independent administrative institutions (dokuritsu gyosei hojin): Institutional design and political process. *J. Public Policy Stud.* **2001**, *1*, 166–178.

12. Uchiyama, Y. Policy Diffusion and political institutions: Comparing administrative reforms in Japan and the United Kingdom. *J. Public Policy Stud.* **2005**, *5*, 119–129.
13. Shibata, Y. National Hospital Special Accounting. In *Heisei Fiscal History: 1989–2000*; Hayashi, K., Ishi, H., Horiuchi, A., Eds.; Ministry of Finance, Policy Research Institute: Tokyo, Japan, 2012; Volume 3, pp. 206–212.
14. Outline of the National Hospital Special Account Scheme. Available online: https://www.mhlw.go.jp/wp/yosan/other/zaimu0307/dl/1-3.pdf (accessed on 24 May 2022).
15. National Hospital Special Accounting. Available online: https://www.mhlw.go.jp/wp/yosan/other/syocho02/dl/6.pdf (accessed on 24 May 2022).
16. Report on the Inspection of Accounts for 2003. Available online: https://report.jbaudit.go.jp/org/h15/2003-h15-1325-0.htm (accessed on 24 May 2022).
17. Nakagawa, Y.; Takemura, T.; Yoshihara, H.; Nakagawa, Y. Financial analysis at the National Hospital Organization's hospitals-introducing new financial management indicators based on personnel cost. *J. Jpn. Soc. Health Care Manag.* **2010**, *11*, 15–23.
18. Report on the Inspection of the Financial Statements for the Financial Year 2017. pp. 928–948. Available online: https://report.jbaudit.go.jp/org/pdf/H29kensahoukoku.pdf (accessed on 24 May 2022).
19. National Hospital Organization-Financial Statements. Available online: https://nho.hosp.go.jp/disclosure/disclosure_zaimu.html (accessed on 24 May 2022).
20. Nakagawa, Y.; Yoshihara, H.; Nakagawa, Y. A new cost accounting model and new indicators for hospital management based on personnel cost. In *Management Engineering for Effective Healthcare Delivery: Principles and Applications*; Pierce, S., Alexander, K., Eds.; IGI Global: Hershey, PA, USA, 2011; pp. 419–434.
21. Nakagawa, Y.; Yoshihara, H.; Nakagawa, Y. New indicators based on personnel cost for management efficiency in a hospital. *J. Med. Syst.* **2011**, *35*, 625–637. [CrossRef]
22. Kakinaka, M.; Kato, R. Regulated medical fee schedule of the Japanese health care system. *Int. J. Health Care Financ. Econ.* **2013**, *13*, 301–317. [CrossRef] [PubMed]
23. Ikegami, N. Controlling Health Expenditures by Revisions to the Fee Schedule in Japan. In *Universal Health Coverage for Inclusive and Sustainable Development: Lessons from Japan*; Ikegami, N., Ed.; World Bank Group: Washington, DC, USA, 2014; pp. 69–100.
24. World Health Statistics 2022: Monitoring Health for the SDGs, Sustainable Development Goals. Available online: https://apps.who.int/iris/rest/bitstreams/1435584/retrieve (accessed on 3 October 2022).
25. Health at a Glance 2021. Available online: https://www.oecd-ilibrary.org/deliver/ae3016b9-en.pdf?itemId=%2Fcontent%2Fpublication%2Fae3016b9-en&mimeType=pdf (accessed on 3 October 2022).
26. The Small and Medium Enterprise Agency. *Part 2: The Ability to Overcome the Crisis-Chapter 1: The Financial Basis of Small and Medium-Sized Enterprises and Management Strategies in the Face of the Impact of Infectious Diseases. 2021 White Paper on Small and Medium Enterprises in Japan*; The Small and Medium Enterprise Agency, Ed.; The Small and Medium Enterprise Agency: Tokyo, Japan, 2021; pp. II-6–II-7.
27. Campbell, J.C.; Takagi, Y. The political economy of the fee schedule in Japan. In *Universal Health Coverage for Inclusive and Sustainable Development: Lessons from Japan*; Ikegami, N., Ed.; World Bank Group: Washington, DC, USA, 2014; pp. 101–118.
28. Social Insurance Medical Council Act. 1950. Available online: https://www.japaneselawtranslation.go.jp/en/laws/view/3266/en (accessed on 25 September 2022).
29. List of members of the Central Social Insurance Medical Council. Available online: https://www.mhlw.go.jp/content/12404000/000851671.pdf (accessed on 24 May 2022).
30. Yuta, K. Impact of university reform on research performance aggregated and disaggregated across research fields: A case study of the partial privatization of Japanese national universities. *Jpn. Econ. Rev.* **2021**, *6*, 1–27. Available online: https://link.springer.com/article/10.1007/s42973-021-00074-y (accessed on 24 May 2022).

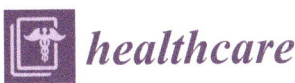

Article

Investigation of Mental and Physical Health of Nurses Associated with Errors in Clinical Practice

Despoina Pappa [1,*], Ioannis Koutelekos [1], Eleni Evangelou [1], Evangelos Dousis [1], Georgia Gerogianni [1], Evdokia Misouridou [1], Afroditi Zartaloudi [1], Nikoletta Margari [1], Georgia Toulia [1], Polyxeni Mangoulia [2], Eftychia Ferentinou [1], Anna Giga [1] and Chrysoula Dafogianni [1]

[1] Department of Nursing, University of West Attica, 12243 Athens, Greece
[2] Department of Nursing, Evangelismos General Hospital, 10676 Athens, Greece
* Correspondence: dpappa@uniwa.gr; Tel.: +30-6908894588

Citation: Pappa, D.; Koutelekos, I.; Evangelou, E.; Dousis, E.; Gerogianni, G.; Misouridou, E.; Zartaloudi, A.; Margari, N.; Toulia, G.; Mangoulia, P.; et al. Investigation of Mental and Physical Health of Nurses Associated with Errors in Clinical Practice. *Healthcare* 2022, 10, 1803. https://doi.org/10.3390/healthcare10091803

Academic Editor: Daniele Giansanti

Received: 4 September 2022
Accepted: 16 September 2022
Published: 19 September 2022

Publisher's Note: MDPI stays neutral with regard to jurisdictional claims in published maps and institutional affiliations.

Copyright: © 2022 by the authors. Licensee MDPI, Basel, Switzerland. This article is an open access article distributed under the terms and conditions of the Creative Commons Attribution (CC BY) license (https://creativecommons.org/licenses/by/4.0/).

Abstract: Background: Errors are common among all healthcare settings. The safety of patients is linked directly with nursing errors because nurses stand by them more often than any other healthcare professional. The role of mental and physical health of nurses is of great interest for a good and efficient job performance, but also for maintaining good patient care delivery. This study aimed to investigate the association between nurses' general health and making errors during clinical practice. Methods: A total of 364 nurses completed a specially designed questionnaire anonymously and voluntarily. The sample consisted of nurses with all educational degrees. The questionnaire included demographic data and questions about general health issues, resilience status and nurses' possible experience with errors within a hospital. Results: 65,8% of the participants stated that at least one error had happened at their workplace, and 49,4% of them reported that the error was caused by them. Somatic symptoms were found to have a positive correlation with making errors ($p < 0.001$). However, the other aspects of general health, which were anxiety/insomnia, social dysfunction and severe depression, had no statistical significance with adverse events. The most common type of error reported (65,5%) was a medication adverse event. Resilience level was found to be statistically significant ($p < 0.001$) when correlated with all aspects of general health (anxiety/insomnia, severe depression, somatic symptoms), but not with social dysfunction. Conclusion: Nurses are affected by their somatic symptoms in their daily clinical practice, making them vulnerable to making errors that compromise patient safety. A high resilience level could help them cope with unfavorable situations and prevent them from doing harm to a patient or themselves.

Keywords: mental health; physical health; resilience; nurses; errors

1. Introduction

The incidence of errors is high worldwide [1–3], with reports indicating that 1 out of 10 patients is affected during their hospitalization [4–6]. Furthermore, for a percentage of approximately 7%[5], these mistakes have irreversible consequences. The World Alliance for Patient Safety adds that 10% of hospitalized patients in developed countries experience an adverse event annually. At the same time, there is increasing concern about reversible deaths because of in-hospital errors [7].

A nursing error involves an unintended "accident" made by a nurse that adversely affects—or could adversely affected—the safety and quality of care of a patient [8]. According to the Nurses Ethical Codes [9], nurses have an important role in safeguarding the integrity of patients, as they spend more time with them than any other healthcare professional. Therefore, most errors are more likely to be made by the nursing staff within a hospital. In a large research study where more than 43,000 nurses participated [10,11], the essential magnitude of the problem was shown, as the factors of burnout, understaffing, non-observance of duties and insufficient nursing support contributed dramatically to the improper delivery of health care. The most common errors within a hospital are infections, falls, pressure ulcers, medication errors, documentation errors and equipment injuries [12].

Nurses are particularly affected by the workplace. Stress and constant association with patients who are dying or suffering directly affect their mental health. Shift work that affects the circadian rhythm [13] as well as workload have been extensively studied in terms of their impact on the physical condition of nurses [14–21]. The hospital's largest workforce, which works under a shift system, has been shown to have a higher rate of cardiovascular diseases, diabetes, dementia, sleep and weight disorders, obesity and more [13,22]. Olds& Clarke [23] reported that for every hour of work, the possibility of the wrong drug or the wrong dose increases by 2%. Along with prolonged burnout and a less than optimal state of well-being in nurses, the quality of care provided is inadvertently affected [24,25]. The management of psychological and physical stress, as well as the adoption of good health practices, are issues of major importance for nurses in terms of the effective performance of their duties, since they are the ones that directly affect the quality-of-care provision [14,21]. This study aimed to investigate the association between nurses' general health and making errors during clinical practice.

2. Materials and Methods

2.1. Participants

The study participants consisted of nurses with all educational degrees, such as university nurses, nurses from technological institutions and assistant nurses of secondary education. The population of the present study was working at general hospitals.

2.2. Data Collection

The present study was a cross-sectional study performed through completion of an anonymous and voluntary questionnaire from November 2019 to November 2020. The research was approved by the Ethics Committee of the University of West Attica and the scientific councils of all the hospitals involved. Due to restrictive measures for the worldwide pandemic from hospitals' policies within the total study period, it was necessary to create a different way to distribute and collect questionnaires, so an electronic form of the tool was developed too.

2.3. Instruments

The research tool consisted of four sections: 1. The demographic data: questions concerning the demographic and occupational status of the participants, such as gender, age, marital and educational status, working section (inpatient nurse/outpatient nurse/operating nurse/oncology nurse/other) and duration of work under a specific unit, 2. The General Health Questionnaire (GHQ-28) [26], which describes a 4-factor structure (somatic symptoms, anxiety/insomnia, social dysfunction and depression), 3. The Taxonomy of Error, Root Cause Analysis and Practice-responsibility (TERCAP) [27], which is designed to collect nursing practice breakdown data from boards of nursing. It describes a set of categories that is based on notions of good nursing practice, such as Safe Medication Administration, Documentation, Surveillance, Prevention, Intervention, Clinical Reasoning, Interpretation of Orders and Professional Responsibility, and 4. The Brief Resilience Scale (BRS) [28], which is a 5-point Likert scale about six specific statements of daily life routine.

2.4. Data Analysis

In this study, quantitative variables were initially tested for normality using the Kolmogorov–Smirnov criterion. The same variables were expressed as mean (SD = Standard Deviation) or median (interquantile range), absolute and relative frequencies. Student's t-tests were computed for the comparison of mean values. Multiple linear regression analysis was used with the dependentGHQ-28 scores. The regression equation included terms for participants' demographics, work-related characteristics and the occurrence of an error during their work. Adjusted regression coefficients (β) with standard errors (SE) were computed from the results of the linear regression analyses. In this study, the *p*-values were two-tailed. Statistical significance was set at $p < 0.05$. The analysis was accomplished using SPSS-version 22.0 statistical software.

3. Results

Demographic Characteristics

In this study, 364 nurses were included. Their demographics and occupational characteristics are presented in Table 1. Most of the participants were women (87.3%), were aged from 22 to 35 years (43.6%), were married or living with their partner (50%) and had children (45.6%). Moreover, 48% of the sample had a university degree, 10.2% were specialized, 50.5% had a monthly income of EUR 500–1000, 12.1% had a second job and almost all (94.7%) were Greek native speakers. The median number of years of working experience in their present hospital was 9 years (IQR: 1–15 years). The mean resilience score was 20.4 (SD = 4.2).

Table 1. Participants' characteristics.

	N (%)
Gender	
Men	46 (12.7)
Women	318 (87.3)
Age	
22–35	159 (43.6)
36–45	132 (36.2)
46+	73 (20.2)
Married/Living with partner	182 (50)
Children	166 (45.6)
Educational level	
High school/secondary education	36 (9.9)
Two-year college graduate	27 (7.4)
University alumni	175 (48)
MSc/PhD holder	126 (34.7)
Specialized	37 (10.2)
Monthly income	
EUR 500–EUR 1000	184 (50.5)
EUR 1001– EUR 1500	170 (46.7)
EUR 1501– EUR 2000	9 (2.5)
EUR 2001 and above	1 (0.3)
Second job	44 (12.1)
Greek native speaker	345 (94.7)
Years of experience in present hospital, median (IQR)	9 (1–15)
Total number of beds in use in your unit, median (IQR)	12 (7–20.5)
Total number of beds in your unit, median (IQR)	14.5 (9–30)
Brief Resilience Score, mean (SD)	20.4 (4.2)

Almost 7 out of 10 participants (65.8%) had experienced an error in their job. More specifically, 49.4% of the participants stated that they had caused an adverse event themselves, and 73.2% that someone else had caused it. The most frequent places that errors occurred were the room of the patient (29.2%) and the Intensive Care Unit (ICU) (24.3%). Most of the errors were made on male patients (65.1%), and in 32.1% of the cases, there was a complication in the patient's health after the error. The error involved some kind of intention or criminal behavior in only 6.7% of the cases, and the error involved a drug error in 65.5% of the cases.

Participants' scores on the GHQ-28 subscales, as well as their total scores, are presented in Table 2. Somatic symptoms' scores were found to differ significantly between participants who had experienced an error in their work and those who had not ($p = 0.030$). More specifically, participants who had experienced an error in their work had significantly greater somatic symptoms. All the other GHQ-28 subscales, as well as total score, were similar in both participants' groups.

Table 2. GHQ-28 subscales by total sample, and by having an error occur in the workplace.

	Total Sample		During Your Professional Career, Has Any Error Ever Occurred in Your Workplace?				
			No (N = 124; 34.1%)		Yes (N = 240; 65.9%)		
	Mean	SD	Mean	SD	Mean	SD	p Student's t-Test
Somatic symptoms	7.67	4.64	6.93	4.48	8.06	4.68	**0.030**
Anxiety/insomnia	7.48	5.15	6.93	5.30	7.77	5.07	0.147
Social dysfunction	8.31	3.66	8.11	4.13	8.42	3.39	0.435
Severe depression	2.23	3.54	2.10	3.69	2.30	3.46	0.617
Total GHQ-28 score	25.78	12.64	24.18	11.53	26.58	13.11	0.094

The difference on the somatic symptoms scale between participants who had experienced an error in their work and those who had not remained significant after adjusting for all other demographical and occupational characteristics (Table 3).

Table 3. Multiple linear regression results with somatic symptoms and anxiety/insomnia subscales as dependent variables.

	Somatic Symptoms			Anxiety/Insomnia		
	β +	SE ++	p	β +	SE ++	p
Gender						
Men						
Women	1.22	0.80	0.130	0.34	0.80	0.670
Age						
22–35						
36–45	−1.39	0.71	**0.050**	−2.56	0.73	**<0.001**
46+	−0.99	1.12	0.375	−3.46	1.15	**0.003**
Married/Living with partner						
No						
Yes	0.44	0.69	0.525	−0.28	0.70	0.688
Children						
No						
Yes	0.56	0.76	0.456	1.78	0.78	**0.022**
Educational level						
High school graduate/Two-year college graduate						
University alumni	−0.95	0.78	0.226	−0.65	0.81	0.423
MSc/PhD holder	0.36	0.82	0.664	1.13	0.85	0.185
Specialized						
No						
Yes	0.50	0.93	0.595	−0.36	0.96	0.709
Monthly income						
EUR 500-EUR 1000						
EUR 1001 and above	−0.13	0.60	0.824	−0.38	0.61	0.540
Second job						
No						
Yes	1.43	0.75	0.057	1.21	0.77	0.118
Greek native speaker						
No						
Yes	1.02	1.59	0.522	0.56	1.64	0.732

Table 3. Cont.

	Somatic Symptoms			Anxiety/Insomnia		
	β [+]	SE [++]	p	β [+]	SE [++]	p
Years of experience in present hospital	−0.01	0.05	0.879	0.05	0.05	0.256
Total number of beds in use in your unit	−0.003	0.019	0.873	−0.001	0.020	0.953
Total number of beds in your unit	0.001	0.014	0.935	0.002	0.014	0.893
Brief Resilience Score	−0.39	0.06	**<0.001**	−0.61	0.06	**<0.001**
During your professional career, has any error ever occurred in your workplace?						
No						
Yes	1.05	0.54	**0.050**	0.42	0.55	0.449

[+] Regression coefficient; [++] Standard Error.

In addition, participants who were 36–45 years old had fewer somatic symptoms compared ($p = 0.050$) to those who were 22–35 years old, and participants who had greater resilience also had fewer somatic symptoms. Furthermore, participants with children had more anxiety/insomnia symptoms. On the other hand, participants who were 36–45 years old ($p < 0.001$) or more than 46 years old ($p = 0.003$) had fewer anxiety/insomnia symptoms compared to participants who were 22–35 years old. Participants who had greater resilience were found to experience fewer anxiety/insomnia symptoms.

Social dysfunction was not associated with any of the demographical and occupational characteristics (Table 4). On the contrary, participants with greater resilience were significantly associated with less severe depression symptoms ($p < 0.001$).

Table 4. Multiple linear regression results with social dysfunction and severe depression subscales as dependent variables.

	Social Dysfunction			Severe Depression		
	β [+]	SE [++]	p	β [+]	SE [++]	p
Gender						
Men						
Women	0.32	0.65	0.624	0.56	0.60	0.349
Age						
22–35						
36–45	−1.04	0.59	0.080	−0.53	0.54	0.325
46+	−1.11	0.94	0.236	−1.66	0.86	0.054
Married/Living with partner						
No						
Yes	0.70	0.57	0.225	0.07	0.53	0.889
Children						
No						
Yes	−0.42	0.63	0.508	0.45	0.58	0.439
Educational level						
High school graduate/Two-year college graduate						
University alumni	−0.89	0.65	0.173	−0.68	0.60	0.257
MSc/PhD holder	−0.94	0.69	0.170	0.13	0.63	0.842
Specialized						
No						
Yes	0.54	0.78	0.487	−0.07	0.72	0.922

Table 4. Cont.

	Social Dysfunction			Severe Depression		
	β +	SE ++	p	β +	SE ++	p
Monthly income						
EUR 500–EUR 1000						
EUR 1001 and above	−0.70	0.50	0.164	−0.72	0.46	0.119
Second job						
No						
Yes	−0.48	0.63	0.444	0.09	0.58	0.879
Greek native speaker						
No						
Yes	−1.65	1.34	0.217	0.48	1.22	0.698
Years of experience in present hospital	0.03	0.04	0.498	0.05	0.04	0.130
Total number of beds in use in your unit	0.008	0.016	0.606	−0.019	0.015	0.197
Total number of beds in your unit	0.005	0.012	0.641	0.013	0.011	0.223
Brief Resilience Score	−0.06	0.05	0.255	−0.25	0.05	**<0.001**
During your professional career, has any error ever occurred in your workplace?						
No						
Yes	0.20	0.45	0.657	0.42	0.41	0.305

+ Regression coefficient; ++ Standard Error.

Participants who were 36–45 years old ($p = 0.003$) or more than 46 years old had better total GHQ-28 total scores compared to participants who were 22–35 years old ($p = 0.013$) (Table 5). Greater resilience of participants was significantly associated with better total GHQ scores ($p < 0.001$).

Table 5. Multiple linear regression results with total GHQ-28 score as a dependent variable.

	Total Score GHQ-28		
	β +	SE ++	p
Gender			
Men			
Women	3.49	2.09	0.095
Age			
22–35			
36–45	−5.49	1.85	**0.003**
46+	−7.24	2.91	**0.013**
Married/Living with partner			
No			
Yes	1.11	1.79	0.535
Children			
No			
Yes	2.31	1.97	0.241
Educational level			
High school graduate/Two-year college graduate			
University alumni	−3.56	2.06	0.085
MSc/PhD holder	0.35	2.15	0.873
Specialized			
No			
Yes	0.56	2.43	0.818

Table 5. Cont.

	Total Score GHQ-28		
	β [+]	SE [++]	p
Monthly income			
EUR 500–EUR 1000			
EUR 1001 and above	−1.77	1.56	0.256
Second job			
No			
Yes	2.42	1.96	0.216
Greek native speaker			
No			
Yes	0.35	4.15	0.934
Years of experience in present hospital	0.13	0.12	0.293
Total number of beds in use of your unit	−0.014	0.050	0.779
Total number of beds of your unit	0.022	0.036	0.546
Brief Resilience Score	−1.28	0.16	**<0.001**
During your professional career, has any error ever occurred in your workplace?			
No			
Yes	2.34	1.40	0.097

[+] Regression coefficient; [++] Standard Error.

4. Discussion

This study aimed to examine the relationship between nurses' physical and mental health status, resilience and occurrence of errors during daily job practice. A significant correlation was found between physical symptoms and occurrence of adverse events for nurses who participated in the research. Similar results were found by Arimura et al. [29], who indicated that there was a statistical significance between poor physical health and errors.

This study also showed that one third of the nurses reported that they were making errors mostly on day or evening shifts. Similarly, Gold et al. [30] found in their study that nurses working on rotating shifts and occasionally at night mentioned more medication errors due to insufficient sleep management.

Additionally, in the present study, one third of the participants referred to errors made while changing shifts (patient hand-offs). These results are congruent with those of Drach-Zahavy and Hadid [31], who examined handover communication between nurses and the types of errors happening at shift change. More specifically, inaccurate drug dosage and missing documentation were found to be the top errors reported at that time.

The present study also found that errors were significantly correlated with physical fatigue and anxiety. Similarly, West et al. [32], who investigated in-hospital errors associated with fatigue, anxiety and insomnia, found relevant findings, since nurses' fatigue was provoked by heavy workload. When the workload was consistent, fatigue and burnout were regarded as chronic. In this study, also, eight out of ten nurses stated that the workload of nursing staff negatively affected the occurrence of their reported error. According to Al-Kandari and Thomas [33], adverse events had a significant correlation with workload, resulting mostly in medication delays or omissions.

The findings of this study indicate that patients' wards and ICUs are the most risky departments for an adverse event to happen. It is of great importance to mention that several studies [34,35] have investigated the occurrence rate of nursing errors within hospital units. In ICUs, the seriousness of patients' medical conditions makes nursing practice more specialized, focused, demanding and exhausting. A recent study by Melnyk et al. [36]

examined the association between errors and nurses' mental and physical health. Their results indicated that when nurses were in poor mental and physical health, reporting an error was much more statistically significant. However, according to "Project to collect medical near miss/adverse events information", [37] nurses make errors 0.56 times more often in outpatient departments. Similarly, in Melnyk's study [36], it was found that nurses in poor physical and mental health presented with 26% higher likelihood of making errors and 71% higher possibility of having an adverse event. They also stated that depression had a significant association with errors.

The present study also showed that the association of nurses' general health with level of resilience had a positive impact on somatic symptoms, anxiety/insomnia and severe depression. So, when nurses were more resilient, they presented fewer physical symptoms. This finding was congruent with those of Koen et al. [38], who examined the prevalence of resilience in professional nurses, stating that low levels of mental discomfort were presented by resilient nurses. However, Koen et al. [38] indicated that although half of the nurses were flourishing with regards to their general health, the other half were not. So, they might need special support for social well-being and job satisfaction. It is important to recognize the actual needs of health professionals on time.

5. Limitations

A part of this study was conducted during the first wave of the COVID-19 pandemic. Due to the restrictive measures on hospital access, electronic questionnaires were distributed to nursing staff after their agreement. This situation had the impact of eliminating direct communication with the personnel and further explanation of the study purpose and necessity. There was phone contact with the head nurses to obtain information about the proper execution of the procedure.

6. Conclusions

Nurses were affected mostly by their physical health in making errors in their daily practice. Fatigue, headaches, sickness tendency and exhaustion were the main descriptions for poor physical status in nurses in this study. A significant association was reported between nursing errors and somatic symptoms. Although several researchers associated errors with poor mental health, this study revealed no such connection. However, a prolonged stay of physical symptoms could lead to disrupted mental status, correlating errors with mental health in that way. Resilience might be a useful capacity to be obtained and developed in the nursing population, as it was shown that the more resilient a nurse was, the less somatic symptoms they had. This study would be necessary to continue due to the increased need for errors examination.

Author Contributions: Conceptualization, D.P. and C.D.; supervision, C.D.; methodology, D.P. and C.D.; analysis, D.P. and I.K.; data curation, D.P., C.D., G.G. and A.Z.; writing—original draft preparation, D.P., C.D., G.G., E.E. and P.M.; investigation and resources, N.M. and G.T.; visualization and writing—review and editing, D.P., E.D., E.M., E.F. and A.G. All authors have read and agreed to the published version of the manuscript.

Funding: This research received no external funding.

Institutional Review Board Statement: The present study was approved by the Ethics Committee, University of West Attica.

Informed Consent Statement: Informed consent was obtained from all study participants for the survey.

Data Availability Statement: All the data generated during this study are included in this published article.

Conflicts of Interest: The authors declare no conflict of interest.

References

1. Garrouste-Orgeas, M.; Philippart, F.; Bruel, C.; Max, A.; Lau, N.; Misset, B. Overview of medical errors and adverse events. *Ann. Intensiv. Care* **2012**, *2*, 2. [CrossRef] [PubMed]
2. Crigger, N.J. Always Having to Say You're Sorry: An ethical response to making mistakes in professional practice. *Nurs. Ethic* **2004**, *11*, 568–576. [CrossRef] [PubMed]
3. Hashemi, F.; Nikbakht Nasrabadi, A.; Asghari, F. Nurses perceived worries from error disclosure: A qualitative study. *Iran. J. Nurs. Res.* **2011**, *20*, 30–43.
4. Schwappach, D.L.; Boluarte, T.A. The emotional impact of medical error involvement on physicians: A call for leadership and organisational accountability. *Swiss Med. Wkly.* **2009**, *139*, 9–15.
5. De Vries, E.N.; Ramrattan, M.A.; Smorenburg, S.M.; Gouma, D.J.; Boermeester, M.A. The incidence and nature of in-hospital adverse events: A systematic review. *BMJ Qual. Saf.* **2008**, *17*, 216–223. [CrossRef] [PubMed]
6. Valiee, S.; Peyrovi, H.; Nasrabadi, A.N. Critical care nurses' perception of nursing error and its causes: A qualitative study. *Contemp. Nurse* **2014**, *46*, 206–213. [CrossRef] [PubMed]
7. World Health Organization. *World Alliance for Patient Safety: Forward Programme*; WHO: Geneva, Switzerland, 2004.
8. Johnstone, M.-J.; Kanitsaki, O. The ethics and practical importance of defining, distinguishing and disclosing nursing errors: A discussion paper. *Int. J. Nurs. Stud.* **2006**, *43*, 367–376. [CrossRef]
9. Washington State Nurses' Association. *Medical Errors and Patient Safety*; Paper; WSNA Board of Directors: Tukwila, WA, USA, 2005.
10. Aiken, L.H.; Clarke, S.; Sloane, D.M. Hospital staffing, organization, and quality of care: Cross-national findings. *Int. J. Qual. Health Care* **2002**, *14*, 5–14. [CrossRef]
11. Aiken, L.H.; Clarke, S.; Sloane, D.M.; Sochalski, J.A.; Busse, R.; Clarke, H.; Giovannetti, P.; Hunt, J.; Rafferty, A.M.; Shamian, J. Nurses' Reports on Hospital Care in Five Countries. *Health Aff.* **2001**, *20*, 43–53. [CrossRef]
12. Delamont, A. How to avoid the top seven nursing errors. *Nurs. Made Incred. Easy* **2013**, *11*, 8–10. [CrossRef]
13. Shim, J.Y.; Seo, N.S.; Kim, M.A.; Park, J.S. Influence of Job Stress, Sleep Quality and Fatigue on Work Engagement in Shift Nurses. *Korean J. Stress Res.* **2019**, *27*, 344–352. [CrossRef]
14. Jørgensen, J.T.; Karlsen, S.; Stayner, L.; Andersen, J.; Andersen, Z.J. Shift work and overall and cause-specific mortality in the Danish nurse cohort. *Scand. J. Work Environ. Health* **2017**, *43*, 117–126. [CrossRef] [PubMed]
15. Vetter, C.; Devore, E.E.; Wegrzyn, L.R.; Massa, J.; Speizer, F.E.; Kawachi, I.; Rosner, B.; Stampfer, M.J.; Schernhammer, E. Association Between Rotating Night Shift Work and Risk of Coronary Heart Disease Among Women. *JAMA* **2016**, *315*, 1726–1734. [CrossRef]
16. Wang, Y.; Gu, F.; Deng, M.; Guo, L.; Lu, C.; Zhou, C.; Chen, S.; Xu, Y. Rotating shift work and menstrual characteristics in a cohort of Chinese nurses. *BMC Women's Health* **2016**, *16*, 24. [CrossRef] [PubMed]
17. Fujishiro, K.; Hibert, E.L.; Schernhammer, E.; Rich-Edwards, J.W. Shift work, job strain and changes in the body mass index among women: A prospective study. *Occup. Environ. Med.* **2016**, *74*, 410–416. [CrossRef] [PubMed]
18. Lee, G.-J.; Kim, K.; Kim, S.Y.; Kim, J.-H.; Suh, C.; Son, B.-C.; Lee, C.-K.; Choi, J. Effects of shift work on abdominal obesity among 20–39-year-old female nurses: A 5-year retrospective longitudinal study. *Ann. Occup. Environ. Med.* **2016**, *28*, 69. [CrossRef] [PubMed]
19. Vedaa, Ø.; Mørland, E.; Larsen, M.; Harris, A.; Erevik, E.; Sivertsen, B.; Bjorvatn, B.; Waage, S.; Pallesen, S. Sleep Detriments Associated with Quick Returns in Rotating Shift Work. *J. Occup. Environ. Med.* **2017**, *59*, 522–527. [CrossRef]
20. Scott, L.D.; Arslanian-Engoren, C.; Engoren, M.C. Association of Sleep and Fatigue with Decision Regret Among Critical Care Nurses. *Am. J. Crit. Care* **2014**, *23*, 13–23. [CrossRef]
21. Arslanian-Engoren, C.; Scott, L.D. Clinical decision regret among critical care nurses: A qualitative analysis. *Heart Lung* **2014**, *43*, 416–419. [CrossRef]
22. Barger, L.K.; Rajaratnam, S.; Wang, W.; O'Brien, C.S.; Sullivan, J.P.; Qadri, S.; Lockley, S.W.; Czeisler, C.A. Common Sleep Disorders Increase Risk of Motor Vehicle Crashes and Adverse Health Outcomes in Firefighters. *J. Clin. Sleep Med.* **2015**, *11*, 233–240. [CrossRef]
23. Olds, D.M.; Clarke, S.P. The effect of work hours on adverse events and errors in health care. *J. Saf. Res.* **2010**, *41*, 153–162. [CrossRef] [PubMed]
24. Hall, L.H.; Johnson, J.; Watt, I.; Tsipa, A.; O'Connor, D.B. Healthcare Staff Wellbeing, Burnout, and Patient Safety: A Systematic Review. *PLoS ONE* **2016**, *11*, e0159015. [CrossRef] [PubMed]
25. Makary, A.M.; Daniel, M. Medical error—the third leading cause of death in the US. *BMJ* **2016**, *353*, i2139. [CrossRef] [PubMed]
26. Goldberg, D.P.; Hillier, V.F. A scaled version of the General Health Questionnaire. *Psychol. Med.* **1979**, *9*, 139–145. [CrossRef]
27. Benner, P.; Malloch, K.; Sheets, V.; Bitz, K.; Emrich, L.; Thomas, M.B.; Bowen, K.; Scott, K.; Patterson, L.; Schwed, K.; et al. TERCAP: Creating a national database on nursing errors. *Harv. Health Policy Rev.* **2006**, *7*, 48–63.
28. Smith, B.W.; Dalen, J.; Wiggins, K.; Tooley, E.; Christopher, P.; Bernard, J. The brief resilience scale: Assessing the ability to bounce back. *Int. J. Behav. Med.* **2008**, *15*, 194–200. [CrossRef]
29. Arimura, M.; Imai, M.; Okawa, M.; Fujimura, T.; Yamada, N. Sleep, Mental Health Status, and Medical Errors among Hospital Nurses in Japan. *Ind. Health* **2010**, *48*, 811–817. [CrossRef]

30. Gold, D.R.; Rogacz, S.; Bock, N.; Tosteson, T.D.; Baum, T.M.; Speizer, F.E.; Czeisler, C.A. Rotating shift work, sleep, and accidents related to sleepiness in hospital nurses. *Am. J. Public Health* **1992**, *82*, 1011–1014. [CrossRef]
31. Drach-Zahavy, A.; Hadid, N. Nursing handovers as resilient points of care: Linking handover strategies to treatment errors in the patient care in the following shift. *J. Adv. Nurs.* **2015**, *71*, 1135–1145. [CrossRef]
32. West, C.P.; Tan, A.D.; Habermann, T.M.; Sloan, J.A.; Shanafelt, T.D. Association of Resident Fatigue and Distress with Perceived Medical Errors. *JAMA* **2009**, *302*, 1294–1300. [CrossRef]
33. Al-Kandari, F.; Thomas, D. Perceived adverse patient outcomes correlated to nurses' workload in medical and surgical wards of selected hospitals in Kuwait. *J. Clin. Nurs.* **2009**, *18*, 581–590. [CrossRef] [PubMed]
34. Moyen, E.; Camiré, E.; Stelfox, H.T. Clinical review: Medication errors in critical care. *Crit. Care* **2008**, *12*, 208. [CrossRef] [PubMed]
35. Kane-Gill, S.; Weber, R.J. Principles and Practices of Medication Safety in the ICU. *Crit. Care Clin.* **2006**, *22*, 273–290. [CrossRef] [PubMed]
36. Melnyk, B.M.; Orsolini, L.; Tan, A.; Arslanian-Engoren, C.; Melkus, G.D.; Dunbar-Jacob, J.; Rice, V.H.; Millan, A.; Dunbar, S.B.; Braun, L.T.; et al. A National Study Links Nurses' Physical and Mental Health to Medical Errors and Perceived Worksite Wellness. *J. Occup. Environ. Med.* **2018**, *60*, 126–131. [CrossRef]
37. Project to Collect Medical Near-Miss/Adverse Events Information 2010 Annual Report. Available online: http://www.med-safe.jp/pdf/report_21.pdf (accessed on 3 March 2022).
38. Koen, M.P.; Van Eeden, C.; Wissing, M.P. The prevalence of resilience in a group of professional nurses. *Health SA Gesondheid* **2011**, *16*, 11. [CrossRef]

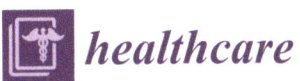

Article

Perceptions, Knowledge and Attitudes among Young Adults about Prevention of HPV Infection and Immunization

Maria Sidiropoulou [1], Georgia Gerogianni [2,*], Freideriki Eleni Kourti [3], Despoina Pappa [2], Afroditi Zartaloudi [2], Ioannis Koutelekos [2], Evangelos Dousis [2], Nikoletta Margari [2], Polyxeni Mangoulia [4], Eftychia Ferentinou [2], Anna Giga [2], Michail Zografakis-Sfakianakis [5] and Chrysoula Dafogianni [1,2]

[1] School of Social Sciences, Hellenic Open University, 26335 Patra, Greece
[2] Department of Nursing, University of West Attica, 12243 Athens, Greece
[3] School of Medicine, National and Kapodistrian University of Athens, 10679 Athens, Greece
[4] Department of Nursing, National and Kapodistrian University of Athens, 10679 Athens, Greece
[5] Department of Nursing, Hellenic Mediterranean University, 72100 Crete, Greece
* Correspondence: ggerogiani@uniwa.gr

Abstract: Introduction: Human papilloma virus (HPV) is one of the most common sexually transmitted infections and is widely known as the main causative agent for cervical cancer. The aim of this study was to investigate the perceptions, knowledge and attitudes of young Greek adults concerning prevention of HPV infection and HPV immunization. Material and Methods: This constitutes a cross-sectional online survey. A convenience sample of young Greek adults (n = 883) residing in Greece, aged 17 to more than 35 years was surveyed from December 2020 to March 2021. Two validated questionnaires were used to collect data. Results: Participants demonstrated moderate knowledge about HPV infection and vaccination, with a mean knowledge score of 53.26 (SD ± 20.65) and 38.92 (SD ± 17.58), respectively. Cronbach's alpha value was 0.77 and 0.80. Female participants were better informed than males. Approximately 52.3% of respondents had been vaccinated and 65.5% were willing to get vaccinated in the future. Vaccination rate was significantly associated with gender (OR = 11.99; 99% CI = 6.59–21.84), knowledge about the HPV vaccine (OR = 1.04; 99% CI = 1.03–1.04) and age (OR = 0.07; 99% CI = 0.03–0.15). Reasons for vaccine refusal were insufficient information (36.8%) and fear of side effects (19%). Correlates of positive vaccination intention were knowledge about HPV (OR = 1.02; 99% CI = 1.01–1.02). Conclusions: The findings suggest that the Greek government's continuing HPV promotion efforts and education on the risks of HPV infection among young people are likely to increase vaccination acceptance among this group.

Keywords: HPV vaccine; human papilloma virus; attitudes; cervical cancer; prevention; knowledge; perception

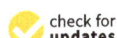

Citation: Sidiropoulou, M.; Gerogianni, G.; Kourti, F.E.; Pappa, D.; Zartaloudi, A.; Koutelekos, I.; Dousis, E.; Margari, N.; Mangoulia, P.; Ferentinou, E.; et al. Perceptions, Knowledge and Attitudes among Young Adults about Prevention of HPV Infection and Immunization. Healthcare 2022, 10, 1721. https://doi.org/10.3390/healthcare10091721

Academic Editor: Marco Dettori

Received: 23 July 2022
Accepted: 5 September 2022
Published: 8 September 2022

Publisher's Note: MDPI stays neutral with regard to jurisdictional claims in published maps and institutional affiliations.

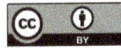

Copyright: © 2022 by the authors. Licensee MDPI, Basel, Switzerland. This article is an open access article distributed under the terms and conditions of the Creative Commons Attribution (CC BY) license (https://creativecommons.org/licenses/by/4.0/).

1. Introduction

Human papilloma virus (HPV) is one of the most common sexually transmitted infections, with an estimated 80% of people being infected with HPV in their lifetime [1]. HPV is widely known as the main causative agent for cervical cancer. Multiple HPV types are capable of infecting the anogenital tract, although only the high-risk types of HPV are oncogenic. The two most common are HPV-16 and -18, which, between them, are detected in 60–78% of cervical carcinomas and 72–94% of adenocarcinomas [2]. In Greece, HPV prevalence ranges between 5.2 and 6.7% and in Europe between 3.7 and 3.9% [3]. About 5–10% of all infected women develop persistent infection, which may progress to premalignant and malignant conditions [4]. The potential exists, however, to prevent the majority of these cancers through increased awareness programs leading to higher HPV vaccine uptake.

There are today three licensed prophylactic vaccines against HPV, exhibiting an excellent safety and immunogenicity profile. The quadrivalent vaccine (targeting HPV types 6,

11, 16 and 18) was first licensed in 2006, the bivalent vaccine (targeting HPV types 16 and 18) in 2007, and the 9-valent vaccine (targeting HPV types 6, 11, 16, 18, 31, 33, 45, 52 and 58) in 2014 [5]. By March 2017, globally, 71 countries had introduced the HPV vaccine into their national immunization program for girls and 11 countries also for boys. The World Health Organization (WHO) recommends the vaccination of young girls 9–13 years old, i.e., before the onset of sexual activity [4].

In Greece, since the introduction date in 2008, all vaccines have been fully financed by the national authorities and are offered to females 11–18 years old and to young men and women 18–26 years old who belong to special risk groups, according to the Greek National Immunization Programme (NIP) [6]. However, a number of Greek studies indicate low vaccination rates [7–9]. This low level of coverage has been attributed to the fact that HPV vaccination is considered the responsibility of the parents, there being as yet no national school-based program [10].

In order to achieve high vaccination coverage, it is necessary to obtain an overview of the knowledge about and attitude toward HPV vaccination in the general population. Previous studies have revealed that despite the high prevalence of HPV, there are misconceptions or else a lack of awareness about HPV even among otherwise well-informed people while, by contrast, there is evidence that vaccination uptake is increased when the targeted population is well-informed about the risks and benefits [11–13]. Thus, the present study aimed at assessing the extent of knowledge about, awareness of, and attitude toward HPV and its vaccine in a Greek population of young adults. We hypothesized that young adults who were considered vaccine-eligible (aged 25 years or younger) would have higher awareness and knowledge of HPV and HPV vaccination compared to older ages (i.e., somewhat older than 35 years). Similarly, we hypothesized that parameters such as the parents' educational background, presymptomatic screening, and safe sexual behavior would influence vaccination acceptance among participants.

Aim

The aim of this study was to investigate the perceptions, knowledge, and attitudes of young Greek adults concerning the prevention of HPV infection and HPV immunization.

2. Methods
2.1. Study Design

This study is based on a cross-sectional online survey.

2.2. Sample

A convenience sample was used to implement the present study. The study sample consisted of young Greek adults aged 17 to more than 35 years, living in Athens and urban areas. Participants who did not consent to participate in the study and those outside the study age range (under 17 years and over 40 years) were excluded. A total of 883 out of 926 people participated in the study. The inclusion criteria for participants were to be students attending medical schools and other higher education institutions and health professionals and be able to speak, read, and write in Greek. Exclusion criteria were inadequate language skills and age under 17 years.

2.3. Data Collection

The data collection was carried out through the completion of two anonymous questionnaires, after receiving informed consent from each participant. The questionnaires were converted into an online file via an electronic questionnaire creation platform and then posted in an electronic communication environment. Research data were collected from December 2020 to March 2021. Participation was voluntary and anonymity was assured. At the beginning of the research study, participants were asked to study the consent text, and only if they agreed would they complete the other sections. There was another consent question at the end of the questionnaire and answers were recorded only if the participants consented.

Before collecting data, we obtained approval by the Research Committee of the Hellenic Open University.

The research tools which evaluated the participants' perceptions, knowledge, and attitudes concerning the prevention of HPV infection and HPV immunization were as follows:

A structured questionnaire indicated by Dafermou et al. [14] which included 67 questions and had five sub-dimensions, namely: demographic variables, knowledge of HPV, knowledge of the HPV vaccine, presymptomatic screening, and sexual behavior. The question items were open-ended and closed-ended, of which 10 items were addressed to female participants and the remainder were the same for both genders. This questionnaire had high reliability in Greek population [14].

A questionnaire indicated by Agorastos et al. [15] which included questions about personal history, knowledge about natural history and cervical-cancer prevention, HPV infection, its role in cervical malignancy, and the attitude of women toward HPV vaccination for themselves and their children. The above research tools were licensed with authorized permission for usage from the scientific authors. In addition, socio-demographic characteristics of the participants were collected.

2.4. Data Analysis

The Statistical Package for Social Sciences version 22.0 was used to perform the statistical analysis. Mean values and standard deviations (SD) were used to describe the quantitative variables. Absolute (N) and relative (%) frequencies were used to describe the qualitative variables. Pearson's χ^2 test or Fisher's exact test was used to compare ratios where necessary. Student's *t*-test was used to compare quantitative variables between two groups. Parametric dispersion analysis (ANOVA) was used to compare quantitative variables between more than two groups. To identify a type-I error due to multiple comparisons, Bonferroni correction was used, according to which the significance level was set at 0.05/k (k = number of comparisons). Linear regression analysis was used to find independent factors related to the knowledge scores, from which dependence coefficients (b) and their standard errors (standard errors = SE) were derived. In order to find independent factors related to vaccination and vaccination intention, a logistic regression analysis was performed, and the odds ratio (OR) was derived with 99% confidence intervals (99% DE). The internal reliability of the knowledge questionnaire was tested using Cronbach's alpha coefficient. The significance levels were bilateral, and the statistical significance was set at 0.01.

3. Results

3.1. Participants' Demographic Information

In total, 926 people participated in the survey, of whom 883 consented to participate; the response rate being 95.5% (Table 1). The mean age of the participants was 25.5 years (SD ± 8; range 17 to more than 35 years) and the majority (86.4%) (*n* = 763) were women. A total of 62.5% (*n* = 552) were students in higher education and 23.4% were full-time employees. Inhabitants of urban areas accounted for 73.5% of the study population and the remaining 24.6% lived in the capital city of Athens. In total, 863 participants (97.7%) were ethnic Greek. A total of 48.8% of respondents were unmarried, while 32.5% were in a relationship. In addition, 56.4% (*n* = 498) had a sibling and 46.5% had at least one parent with a higher-education qualification. Finally, 22.9% of the participants had a monthly family income of over EUR 2000.

3.2. Sexual Behavior and Screening

Most participants (81.1%) stated that they take precautions during sexual intercourse (Table 2). Males indicated a significantly higher rate of safe sexual behavior (90.8%), compared to females (80.3%) (*p* = 0.006). About 16.5% of respondents (*n* = 146) reported that they had been infected by HPV in the past, while male participants had a significantly lower HPV incidence rate compared to women (13.3% vs. 17%) ($p < 0.001$). The highest HPV infection rate according to age was found in the 26–35 age group (31.1%) ($p < 0.001$).

Table 1. Sociodemographic characteristics of participants.

		n	Valid %
Gender (n = 883)	Female	763	86.4
	Male	120	13.6
Age	Mean in years	883	25.5 (SD ± 8.0)
	Range in years	883	17–40
Ethnicity	Greek	863	97.7
	Albanian	12	1.4
	Other [a]	8	0.9
Profession	Full-time employee	207	23.4
	Part-time employee	35	4.0
	Unemployed	42	4.8
	Student	552	62.5
	Household	7	0.8
	Do not know	6	0.5
	Student and Employee	34	3.9
Residence	Athens	217	24.6
	Urban area	649	73.5
	Foreign country	17	1.9
Marital status	Single	431	48.8
	Married	154	17.4
	Divorced	11	1.2
	In a relationship	287	32.5
Siblings	None	110	12.5
	One	498	56.4
	Two	183	20.7
	Three	62	7.0
	More	30	3.4
Parents' Education	Primary education	138	15.6
	Secondary education	361	40.9
	Higher education	302	34.2
	Master's	82	9.3
Monthly family income	EUR 500–1000	187	21.2
	EUR 1001–1500	155	17.6
	EUR 1501–2000	161	18.2
	Over EUR 2000	202	22.9
	Do not know	178	20.2

SD: standard deviation, [a] Other ethnicities were, in descending order: Cypriot (5), Bulgarian (1), Hungarian (1), Romanian (1).

Approximately 57.2% of female participants (n = 431) had visited a gynecologist at least once in the past year. The frequency of visits to the gynecologist was found to be highest in the age group 26–35 years old (72.9%) and the lowest in the age group under 25 years old (22.0%) ($p < 0.001$). The majority (98.8%) knew about the Pap test, having been informed mainly by their family and the doctor (72.8 and 59.8%, respectively). It was found that, as participants' age increased, the information rate via the gynecologist increased, while information via the Internet decreased ($p < 0.001$). Nearly 66.2% of the female population regularly had a Pap test, of whom 79.8% did it once a year, while 24% had been infected with HPV at some point in their lives. The Pap test rate differed significantly between the three age groups, with the lowest rate being in the age group of 25 years and under (50.4%) and the highest among women over 35 years (97.1%) ($p < 0.001$). Moreover, the rate of HPV infection among women who had cervical screening differed significantly between the age groups, with the lowest being in the group under 25 years of age (16.4%) and the highest in the 26–35 age group (29.9%, $p < 0.001$). The main reasons for not being screened were not being sexually active (62.5%), followed by the absence of symptoms (20.3%).

Table 2. Sexual behavior and screening among participants.

	Total n (%)	Men n (%)	Women n (%)	p Pearson's χ^2 Test *	≤25 n (%)	Age 26–35 n (%)	>35 n (%)	p Pearson's χ^2 Test
Variables								
Sexual Behavior								
Precaution during sexual intercourse								
Yes	722 (81.8)	109 (90.8)	613 (80.3)		510 (86.9)	135 (76.3)	77 (64.7)	
No		11 (9.2)	150 (19.7)	0.006	77 (13.1)	42 (23.7)	42 (35.3)	0.310
HPV infection								
Yes	146 (16.5)	16 (13.3)	130 (17.0)		57 (9.7)	55 (31.1)	34 (28.6)	
No		104 (86.7)	633 (83.0)	<0.001	530 (90.3)	122 (68.9)	85 (71.4)	<0.001
Individual history of women								
Annual gynecology visit								
None			116 (15.0)		113 (22.0)	0 (0.0)	3 (2.9)	
Once			437 (57.2)		249 (49.8)	116 (72.9)	72 (69.9)	
6 months			142 (18.8)		102 (20.7)	26 (16.8)	13 (12.6)	<0.001
Every 2 years			50 (6.6)		28 (5.7)	11 (7.1)	11 (10.7)	
>3 years			18 (2.4)		9 (1.8)	5 (3.2)	4 (3.9)	
Knowledge about cervical screening								
Yes			754 (98.8)		492 (98.2)	155 (100.0)	103 (100.0)	0.109 [a]
No			9 (1.8)		9 (1.8)	0 (0.0)	0 (0.0)	
Information sources								
Family			549 (72.8)		377 (76.6)	116 (74.8)	52 (50.5)	<0.001
Friends			183 (24.3)		123 (25.0)	36 (23.2)	22 (21.4)	0.703
Television			102 (13.5)		66 (13.4)	16 (10.3)	19 (18.4)	0.173
Gynecologist			451 (59.8)		260 (25.8)	106 (68.4)	83 (80.6)	<0.001
Pediatrician			62 (8.2)		46 (9.3)	13 (8.4)	2 (1.9)	0.043
Press			54 (7.2)		26 (5.9)	14 (9.0)	9 (8.7)	0.301
Internet			293 (38.9)		212 (43.1)	51 (32.9)	28 (27.2)	0.003
School			195 (25.9)		139 (28.3)	33 (21.3)	22 (21.4)	0.120
Personal cervical screening								
Yes			502 (66.2)		252 (50.4)	150 (96.8)	100 (97.1)	<0.001
No			256 (33.8)		248 (49.6)	5 (3.2)	3 (2.9)	
Frequency of cervical screening								
Once a year			398 (79.8)		20 (80)	121 (81.2)	76 (76.8)	
Every 6 months			34 (6.6)		23 (8.8)	9 (6.0)	2 (2.0)	
Every 2 years			53 (10.4)		26 (10.0)	14 (9.4)	13 (13.1)	0.011
>3 years			17 (3.2)		3 (1.2)	6 (3.4)	8 (8.1)	
Reasons for not screening								
Ignorance			18 (7.0)		18 (7.3)	0 (0.0)	0 (0.0)	1.000 [a]
Absence of sexual intercourse			160 (62.5)		154 (62.1)	4 (80.0)	2 (66.7)	0.847 [a]
Absence of symptoms			52 (20.3)		51 (20.6)	1 (20.0)	0 (0.0)	1.000 [a]
Fear of the result			10 (3.9)		9 (3.6)	0 (0.0)	1 (33.3)	0.125 [a]
Difficult access			19 (7.4)		19 (7.7)	0 (0.0)	0 (0.0)	1.000 [a]
Financial reasons			34 (13.3)		33 (13.3)	1 (20.0)	0 (0.0)	0.686 [a]
Positive PAP Test for HPV [b]								
Yes			145 (24.0)		71 (16.4)	46 (29.9)	28 (27.5)	
No			543 (76.0)		361 (83.6)	108 (70.1)	74 (72.5)	<0.001

* Pearson's χ^2 test < 0.01, [a] Fisher's exact test, [b] Concerns women who had cervical screening.

3.3. HPV Awareness

The majority of the study population was aware of HPV (90%) (Table 3). The mean HPV knowledge score was 53.26 out of 100 (SD ± 20.65). The internal consistency of the knowledge item regarding HPV evaluated by Cronbach's alpha, was 0.77. Bivariate correlates of positive HPV awareness included the following: female sex ($p = 0.001$), employed ($p = 0.001$), married ($p = 0.006$), living in Athens ($p = 0.001$) and having previously been infected with HPV ($p < 0.001$). Moreover, there were significant differences in overall mean knowledge scores among the three age groups and the frequency of gynecologist visits. Participants who were 26–35 years old were more likely to report that they had heard of HPV, compared to those under 25 years ($p = 0.001$). Female participants who had cervical screening, visited the doctor regularly, and knew about the Pap test and HPV-DNA test had a higher score, indicating more knowledge regarding HPV ($p < 0.001$). In the multivariable model, the following factors were positively associated with HPV awareness: female sex ($p = 0.007$; referent = male sex), residence in the region of Athens ($p = 0.002$; referent = urban area) and positive HPV infection ($p < 0.001$; referent = negative infection). Parents' educational level and safe sexual behavior were not associated with HPV awareness.

Table 3. Awareness of HPV and HPV vaccination among participants.

	Mean Knowledge Score % (SD)				Aware of HPV ($n = 801; 90.7\%$)			Aware of HPV Vaccination ($n = 782; 88.6\%$)		
	HPV 53.26 (20.65)	p Student's t-Test *	HPV Vaccination 38.92 (17.58)	p Student's t-Test	β [a]	SE [b]	p ** Value	β	SE	p Value
Variables										
Age										
≤25	51.83 (21.10)		38.59 (17.59)		(Referent)			(Referent)		
26–35	58.19 (18.67)		42.42 (16.33)		0.28	2.39	0.908	0.86	2.06	0.677
>35	53.00 (20.26)	0.001	35.37 (18.55)	0.002	−4.13	2.73	0.131	−5.98	2.36	0.011
Sex										
Male	47.32 (26.09)		32.92 (20.22)		(Referent)			(Referent)		
Female	54.19 (19.52)	0.001	39.87 (16.95)	<0.001	5.45	2.01	0.007	6.43	1.73	<0.001
Occupation										
Students	51.35 (21.30)		38.15 (17.42)		(Referent)			(Referent)		
Employed	57.08 (18.68)		40.40 (17.42)		4.40	2.32	0.058	2.52	2.00	0.209
Unemployed	57.29 (18.47)	<0.001	41.00 (18.54)	0.170	5.68	3.24	0.080	3.55	2.80	0.204
Residence										
Urban area	51.68 (21.29)		38.02 (17.77)		(Referent)			(Referent)		
Athens	57.41 (18.17)		41.20 (16.54)		4.92	1.59	0.002	3.03	1.37	0.027
Foreign country	60.50 (17.52)	0.001	44.12 (20.44)	0.033	6.18	5.06	0.222	5.27	4.36	0.227
Marital status										
Single	51.35 (21.54)		37.38 (17.88)		(Referent)			(Referent)		
Married	55.17 (19.56)	0.006	40.47 (17.15)	0.009	2.80	1.47	0.058	2.87	1.27	0.024
HPV infection										
No	51.60 (21.12)		38.41 (17.87)		(Referent)			(Referent)		
Yes	61.64 (15.67)	<0.001	41.50 (15.86)	0.050	8.47	1.90	<0.001	2.39	1.63	0.144
Data for women only:										
Annual gynecology visit										
None	47.60 (19.13)		35.76 (16.63)							
Once	55.55 (18.62)		41.25 (16.52)							
6 months	53.67 (19.73)		39.60 (16.17)							
Over 2–3 years	58.82 (23.03)	<0.001	41.18 (20.05)	0.020						

Table 3. Cont.

		Mean Knowledge Score % (SD)				Aware of HPV (n = 801; 90.7%)	Aware of HPV Vaccination (n = 782; 88.6%)
	Personal cervical screening						
Yes		57.53 (18.63)		41.71 (17.01)			
No		47.56 (19.68)	<0.001	36.42 (16.27)	<0.001		
	Knowledge about HPV–DNA Test						
Yes		64.66 (16.58)		47.44 (15.53)			
No		45.52 (17.53)	<0.001	33.84 (15.25)	<0.001		
	Knowledge about cervical screening						
Yes		54.40 (19.38)		40.03 (16.92)			
No		30.95 (23.15)	<0.001	28.79 (13.64)	0.047		

SD: standard deviation, [a] dependency factor, [b] standard factor error, * $p < 0.01$, ** P Student's t-test < 0.01.

3.4. HPV Vaccination Awareness

Similarly, most respondents (88.6%) were aware of HPV vaccination. The mean HPV vaccine knowledge score was 38.92 out of 100 (SD ± 17.58). Internal consistency regarding the HPV-vaccine-knowledge item was 0.80. The most common information resources reported concerning the vaccine were the gynecologist (50.6%), followed by the Internet (43.6%) and the family (39.9%). Bivariate correlations of positive HPV vaccine awareness included the following: female sex ($p < 0.001$), married ($p = 0.009$), and women who had cervical screening and knew about the HPV-DNA test ($p < 0.001$). Participants 26–35 years old were better informed about the HPV vaccine than those over 35 years ($p = 0.002$). In the multivariable model, the factor of female sex was positively associated with vaccine knowledge ($p < 0.001$; referent = male sex). Occupation, residence, parents' educational level, sexual behavior and HPV prevalence were not associated with HPV vaccine awareness.

3.5. Vaccination Uptake

Of the participants, almost 52.3% ($n = 462$) had already been vaccinated. Approximately 50.3% did not know which vaccine type they had received, while 60.9% had received all three HPV injections. Of those who had refused, a total of 36.8% reported lack of information as the main reason, followed by the fear of side effects (19%) and not being sexually active (15%).

Bivariate correlates of HPV vaccination included the following: female sex, students, age up to 25 years, and HPV and HPV vaccination knowledge ($p < 0.001$) (Table 4). Vaccination uptake was lower among participants over 35 years ($p < 0.001$). Vaccinated participants knew significantly more about HPV and the vaccination ($p < 0.001$). In the logistic regression model, age, sex and the HPV-vaccine-knowledge score were positively associated with HPV acceptance. The results showed that the factors associated with higher vaccination rate in the entire sample were vaccinated participants being up to 25 years (OR = 0.07; 99% CI = 0.03–0.15; referent = participants up to 35 years), being female (OR = 11.99; 99% CI = 6.59–21.84; referent = male sex) and knowing better about the vaccine (OR = 1.04; 99% CI = 1.03–1.06). Screening factors for women, residence, marital status, parents' educational background, sexual behavior and HPV infection were not associated with vaccination uptake, as had been hypothesized.

3.6. Vaccination Intention

Among the non-vaccinated respondents, 67.5% ($n = 284$) indicated that they would like to receive the vaccine if they were to decide in the future. According to bivariate correlation, the following factors significantly contributed to the participant's vaccination intention: age, occupation, safe sexual behavior and greater knowledge about HPV (Table 5). The results showed that as age increases, the vaccination-intention rate decreases ($p < 0.002$).

Students as well as those who take precautions during sexual intercourse had a significantly higher intention rate ($p = 0.005$). Moreover, participants who intended to get vaccinated knew better about HPV, compared to those who had no such intention ($p = 0.001$). Multiple logistic regression was performed to assess predictors of intention. The results indicated that the more participants knew about HPV, the more likely they were to have the intention to be vaccinated (OR = 1.22; 99% CI = 1.01–1.03). Screening for women, sex, the vaccine knowledge score and previous HPV infection did not appear to influence participants' intention to be vaccinated.

Table 4. Multivariable logistic regression analysis for factors associated with vaccination uptake.

		Vaccinated			Logistic Regression OR (99% CI) [a]		
		Yes n (%)	No n (%)	p Pearson's χ^2 Test *	OR	CI	p ** Value
Variables							
Age							
≤25		346 (58.9)	241 (41.1)			(Referent)	
26–35		103 (58.2)	74 (41.8)	<0.001	0.95	0.54–1.66	0.859
>35		13 (10.9)	106 (89.1)		0.07	0.03–0.15	<0.001
Sex							
Male		12 (12.5)	105 (87.5)	<0.001		(Referent)	
Female		447 (58.6)	316 (41.4)		11.99	6.59–21.84	<0.001
Ethnicity							
Other		12 (60.0)	8 (40.0)	0.487		(Referent)	
Greek		450 (52.1)	413 (47.9)		1.15	0.4–3.35	0.794
Occupation							
Students		334 (57.0)	252 (43.0)			(Referent)	
Employed		101 (41.7)	141 (58.3)	<0.001	0.82	0.47–1.44	0.483
Unemployed		25 (51.0)	24 (49.0)		0.86	0.39–1.87	0.701
Residence							
Urban area		347 (53.5)	302 (46.5)			(Referent)	
Athens		105 (48.4)	112 (51.6)	0.372	0.69	0.48–1.01	0.054
Foreign country		10 (58.8)	7 (41.2)		1.77	0.5–6.19	0.373
		Marital status					
Single		230 (52.0)	212 (48.0)	0.845		(Referent)	
Married		232 (52.6)	209 (47.4)		1.09	0.77–1.53	0.623
		Educational level of parents					
Primary		27 (40.9)	39 (59.1)				
Secondary		153 (52.2)	140 (47.8)	0.050	0.94	0.76–1.16	0.547
Higher		212 (51.6)	199 (48.8)				
Master's		70 (61.90)	43 (38.1)				
		Safe sexual behavior					
No		72 (44.7)	89 (55.3)	0.033		(Referent)	
Yes		390 (54.0)	332 (46.0)		1.42	0.92–2.19	0.118
		HPV infection					
No		393 (53.3)	344 (46.7)	0.180		(Referent)	
Yes		69 (47.3)	77 (52.7)		0.92	0.58–1.44	0.703
Mean HPV knowledge (SD)		56.4 (18.7)	49.9 (22.1)	<0.001 [b]	1	0.99–1.01	0.584
Mean HPV vaccine knowledge (SD)		43.9 (15.2)	33.4 (18.4)	<0.001 [b]	1.04	1.03–1.06	<0.001

* Pearson's χ^2 test < 0.01, ** $p < 0.01$, [a] odds ratio (99% confidence interval), [b] Student's t-test,.

Table 5. Multivariable logistic regression analysis for factors associated with vaccination intention.

	Intention to Vaccinate			Logistic Regression OR (99% CI) [a]		
	Yes n (%)	No n (%)	p Pearson's χ^2 Test *	OR	CI	p ** Value
Variables						
Age						
≤25	179 (74.3)	62 (25.7)		(Referent)		
26–35	46 (62.2)	28 (37.8)	0.002	0.68	0.3–1.57	0.368
>35	59 (55.7)	47 (44.3)		0.58	0.26–1.29	0.180
Sex						
Male	73 (69.5)	32 (30.5)	0.602	(Referent)		
Female	211 (66.8)	105 (32.2)		0.97	0.57–1.64	0.899
Ethnicity						
Other	7 (87.5)	1 (12.5)	0.447 [b]	(Referent)		
Greek	277 (67.1)	136 (32.9)		0.3	0.04–2.61	0.278
Occupation						
Students	186 (73.8)	66 (26.2)		(Referent)		
Employed	83 (58.9)	58 (41.1)	0.002	0.73	0.34–1.59	0.432
Unemployed	12 (50.0)	12 (50.0)		0.45	0.17–1.24	0.124
Residence						
Urban area	201 (66.6)	101 (33.4)		(Referent)		
Athens	79 (70.5)	33 (29.5)	0.587 [b]	1	0.6–1.67	0.991
Foreign country	4 (57.1)	3 (42.9)		0.65	0.12–3.42	0.610
Marital status						
Single	153 (72.2)	59 (27.8)	0.038	(Referent)		
Married	131 (62.7)	78 (37.3)		0.92	0.55–1.52	0.739
Educational level of parents						
Primary	24 (61.5)	15 (38.5)				
Secondary	91 (65.0)	49 ()35.0)	0.652	0.96	0.72–1.29	0.799
Higher	139 (69.8)	60 (30.2)				
Master's	30 (36.8)	13 (30.2)				
Safe sexual behavior						
No	49 (55.1)	40 (44.9)	0.005	(Referent)		
Yes	235 (70.8)	97 (29.2)		1.76	1.01–3.07	0.046
HPV infection						
No	229 (66.6)	115 (33.4)	0.411	(Referent)		
Yes	55 (71.4)	22 (28.6)		1.49	0.81–2.74	0.203
Mean HPV knowledge (SD)	52.2 (21.9)	44.9 (21.8)	0.001 [c]	1.02	1.01–1.03	**0.004**
Mean HPV Vaccine knowledge (SD)	34.5 (18.6)	31.2 (17.8)	0.080 [c]	1	0.98–1.01	0.651

* Pearson's χ^2 test < 0.01, ** p < 0.01, [a] odds ratio (99% confidence interval), [b] Fisher's exact test, [c] Student's t-test.

3.7. Attitudes toward Vaccination

Among the total sample, 59.5% were willing to copay for the vaccine if it was not offered for free, while 26.2% indicated that they would pay only the participation rate in cost. The great majority (96.0%) stated that young people should be informed about the association between HPV with sexual behavior and cervical cancer before being vaccinated. Approximately 57.2% of participants believed that vaccination is beneficial for people who have already been infected by a specific HPV type, by offering protection from other HPV types.

4. Discussion

This study aimed to investigate the perceptions, knowledge, and attitudes of young Greek adults concerning the prevention of HPV infection and HPV immunization. The study results were encouraging, as they showed a favorable attitude toward vaccination and a moderate knowledge score for HPV and the vaccine. More than half of the study population had been vaccinated and about two out of three of the non-vaccinated were willing to receive the vaccine in the future.

The research findings revealed the moderate knowledge level of participants about HPV. Although the majority was aware of HPV, fewer than half knew of the possible transmission modes and only a quarter of the overall sample about the HPV–cancer association. To our knowledge, few similar studies on young adults have been conducted in Greece. One study on Greek students 15–18 years old observed limited knowledge about HPV [16], while another study on Greek females 17–24 years old found that 69.7% of them reported adequate knowledge about HPV [17]. On the other hand, a low knowledge level was also observed in several previous studies from other countries. A study in Romania revealed that 69.2% of women had heard about HPV, but their knowledge was minimal and incomplete [18]. Similarly, a study in China indicated that the participants had a poor understanding of HPV transmission [19]. Marek et al. [20] found that only 17% of Hungarian adolescents knew about HPV, while other studies reported a higher level of knowledge in this age group [21,22]. These findings suggest that, on the whole, participants did not have sufficient perceptions about HPV. Thus, there is an urgent need to raise public awareness about and increase education on the risks of HPV infection. In our study, as in other studies [23,24], female gender and marital status were found to be significantly related to knowledge level, as women and married participants proved to be more aware of HPV. This is possibly because, since females are more concerned about cervical cancer, they are better informed about HPV, and married people are more concerned about the perceived risk of HPV infection for themselves or for their daughter since they take most of the responsibility for their children's healthcare. Furthermore, participants living in urban areas had a lower level of HPV knowledge, probably due to the fact that people living in large capital cities have greater access to health information sources. Varela and Saridi [25] showed similar results in their study. It was observed that people with a history of HPV know better about the transmission of HPV and the methods of protection. Focusing on age, the older age group proved to be more aware of HPV issues than the younger group. This is possibly due to the lack of information among the latter group as to HPV infection risks. Similar studies conducted in Nigerian and Canadian populations are in agreement with these findings [26,27].

Vaccination-related knowledge was at a lower level than HPV knowledge. More than three-quarters of respondents stated that they were aware of the HPV vaccine, but only one-third answered all the vaccine questions correctly. Similarly, a previous Greek study by Vaidakis et al. [28] found that less than half of the sample knew about the HPV vaccination. An international review of surveys on young people aged up to 26 years reported poor knowledge and misconceptions about HPV and its vaccine [29]. Furthermore, a meta-analysis of studies on European adolescents revealed a poor understanding of basic HPV vaccine knowledge [30]. Women were more knowledgeable about vaccination compared to men. These results are consistent with other previous studies, which showed that most females of the study population aged 18–26 years were more aware of the vaccine [31–33]. Women are probably more concerned about cervical cancer and want to be fully informed on prevention methods. Moreover, males have lower access to related information than women, who have more opportunities to acquire such information from healthcare professionals though cervical screening and routine gynecological visits. The younger participants received significantly lower scores than the older age groups, similarly to findings in previous research [34]. This is possibly explained by older people having attended more courses on sex education, knowing someone who has been diagnosed with HPV or experiencing infection themselves. Screening among female participants was positively associated with vaccine knowledge, as it was revealed that women who did not undergo Pap tests regularly had a lower knowledge level. Similar studies accord with these results [35,36]. This might be explained by the fact that HPV is statistically the main causative agent of cervical cancer, and it is detected in women only through presymptomatic screening. This accounts for HPV vaccination programs being targeted mostly at the female population [37].

Despite the relatively high level of awareness of HPV, only half of participants had been vaccinated. This rate is, nevertheless, well above the estimated national vaccination coverage of 9%. These results correspond to those of previous Greek research, which demonstrated above-average vaccination coverage [6,38,39]. Furthermore, consistent with the literature, our study results showed that young participants (<25 years old) and women were more likely to have been vaccinated [40–42]. This is probably due to the Greek vaccination program, which is targeted at young girls (12–18 years). Moreover, participants who were knowledgeable about HPV had higher acceptance of HPV vaccination. Evidence varies across countries as to whether knowledge impacts vaccination uptake. Some studies report a positive correlation [43,44], while others reported no correlation [45,46].

The study findings shed light on the need for the provision of more information on HPV, given that the main reason reported for vaccination reluctance was insufficient information, followed by fear of side effects. This can partly be attributed to misinformation spread by the Internet and the media, which leads to misconception about the safety and efficacy of the HPV vaccine. In fact, many international studies have determined that inadequate information about the vaccine and safety issues are common among both parents and adolescents [47–49].

Vaccination intention among non-vaccinated participants proved to be high, with more than half of participants stating that they were willing to be vaccinated in the future. Intention rate was higher among young participants, given that this age group (20–24 years old) are at the highest risk for contracting HPV, while older participants were less positive about vaccination, probably due to the perception of their low risk of HPV infection and being in a monogamous relationship. Moreover, people who followed safe sexual behavior were found to have a higher intention rate, the latter surely reflecting their awareness of and sensitivity to preventive measures. Xiao [50] demonstrated that sexual history is an important factor in predicting general behavior toward vaccination. Finally, participants who were knowledgeable about HPV were more likely to receive the vaccine in the future, this observation being in-line with other studies [14,51].

Regarding the source of information and trust, respondents stated that the gynecologist along with the Internet and family provided most of their information and were the most trusted. However, as mentioned, given that the Internet does not always provide accurate information, this finding suggests that governments must consider taking steps so that the Internet becomes part of a communication strategy that will promote the dissemination on the Web of reliable, scientifically evaluated information to young people and to the population at large. Meanwhile, healthcare providers can play a pivotal role in promoting vaccination, by cooperating with schools in providing health education to adolescents.

With respect to screening, two out of three female participants regularly had a Pap test, the majority of whom were over 35 years old. This is likely explained by the inclusion in the questionnaire of older women (over 35), who appear to have greater awareness of health issues and to routinely apply preventive behaviors. This finding is in-line with other Greek studies [52,53]. Participants aged 26–35 years old and especially women in this age group were more likely to be infected by HPV. This is probably due to the fact that these age groups take fewer sexual precautions, because they consider themselves to be at low infection risk. Moreover, women are more likely to be diagnosed with HPV through their routine gynecologist visits.

Limitations

One limitation of the current study is its Web-based nature. Online surveys may have advantages related to the high speed and low cost of data collection. However, they may be biased by limited and selective participation, as certain populations with no access are unable to participate. Furthermore, using a convenience sample means that the sample is not representative of the general population so that there is the risk of bias. In terms of external validity, a larger sample size including more male participants as well as inhabitants of capital cities would render more valid results. One strength of the study is that the results may be used in the implementation of future research as well as in awareness campaigns concerning HPV prevention.

5. Conclusions

The aim of the present study was to investigate young Greek adults' awareness of and attitudes toward HPV vaccination. In conclusion, the participants' general attitude proved positive, as about half had been vaccinated and more than half were willing to receive the vaccine in the future. Vaccination uptake was significantly associated with knowledge of HPV and its vaccine, as well as other factors. The knowledge level was moderate and related to sex, residence, and previous HPV infection. The main vaccination barrier was inadequate information. Consequently, more educational programs are needed to raise awareness regarding HPV and the vaccination. These programs should be targeted both at health professionals and the general public. Future research studies need to collect and use data from a representative sample of the Greek population to provide a more in-depth evaluation of the views and predictors influencing HPV vaccination uptake in Greece.

Author Contributions: Conceptualization, M.S. Methodology and writing—original draft, G.G. Writing—review and editing; methodology, F.E.K. Data curation and software, I.K. and E.D. Validation and formal analysis, N.M. and P.M. Investigation and resources, A.Z. Visualization and writing—review and editing, M.Z.-S. Investigation and visualization, D.P., E.F. and A.G. Writing—original draft and data curation, C.D. All authors have read and agreed to the published version of the manuscript.

Funding: This research received no external funding.

Institutional Review Board Statement: The present study was conducted according to the guidelines of the Declaration of Helsinki, and approved by the Research Committee of Hellenic Open University.

Informed Consent Statement: Informed consent was obtained from all subjects involved in the study.

Data Availability Statement: The data presented in this study are available on request from the corresponding author. The data are not publicly available due to privacy reasons.

Conflicts of Interest: All authors declare no conflict of interest in this paper.

References

1. Chesson, H.W.; Dunne, E.F.; Hariri, S.; Markowitz, L.E. The estimated lifetime probability of acquiring human papillomavirus in the United States. *Sex. Transm. Dis.* **2014**, *41*, 660–664. [CrossRef] [PubMed]
2. Hopkins, T.G.; Wood, N. Female human papillomavirus (HPV) vaccination: Global uptake and the impact of attitudes. *Vaccine* **2013**, *31*, 1673–1679. [CrossRef] [PubMed]
3. Bruni, L.; Albero, G.; Serrano, B.; Mena, M.; Gómez, D.; Muñoz, J.; Bosch, F.X.; de Sanjosé, S. *Human Papillomavirus and Related Diseases in the World*; Summary Report; ICO/IARC Information Centre on HPV and Cancer (HPV Information Centre): Lyon, France, 2021.
4. WHO. *Human Papillomavirus Vaccines: Who Position Paper, May 2017*; Weekly Epidemiological Report; WHO: Geneva, Switzerland, 2017.
5. Taebi, M.; Riazi, H.; Keshavarz, Z.; Afrakhteh, M. Knowledge and attitude toward human papillomavirus and HPV vaccination in Iranian population: A systematic review. *Asian Pac. J. Cancer Prev. APJCP* **2019**, *20*, 1945–1949. [CrossRef] [PubMed]
6. Jelastopulu, E.; Fafliora, E.; Plota, A.; Babalis, V.; Bartsokas, C.; Poulas, K.; Plotas, P. Knowledge, behaviours and attitudes regarding HPV infection and its prevention in female students in West Greece. *Eur. Rev. Med. Pharmacol. Sci.* **2016**, *20*, 2622–2629.
7. Kanellopoulou, A.; Giannakopoulos, I.; Fouzas, S.; Papachatzi, E.; Nasikas, S.; Papakonstantinopoulou, A.; Gkentzi, D. Vaccination coverage among school children in Western Greece from 2016 to 2019. *Hum. Vaccines Immunother.* **2021**, *17*, 4535–4541. [CrossRef]

8. Xenaki, D.; Plotas, P.; Michail, G.; Poulas, K.; Jelastopulu, E. Knowledge, behaviours and attitudes for human papillomavirus (HPV) prevention among educators and health professionals in Greece. *Eur. Rev. Med. Pharmacol. Sci.* **2020**, *24*, 7745–7752. [CrossRef]
9. Valasoulis, G.; Pouliakis, A.; Michail, G.; Kottaridi, C.; Spathis, A.; Kyrgiou, M.; Daponte, A. Alterations of HPV-Related Biomarkers after Prophylactic HPV Vaccination. A Prospective Pilot Observational Study in Greek Women. *Cancers* **2020**, *12*, 1164. [CrossRef]
10. Paraskevaidis, E.; Athanasiou, A.; Paraskevaidi, M.; Bilirakis, E.; Galazios, G.; Kontomanolis, E.; Kyrgiou, M. Cervical pathology following HPV vaccination in Greece: A 10-year HeCPA observational cohort study. *Vivo* **2020**, *34*, 1445–1449. [CrossRef]
11. Suzuki, Y.; Sukegawa, A.; Ueda, Y.; Sekine, M.; Enomoto, T.; Miyagi, E. Effect of a Brief Web-Based Educational Intervention on Willingness to Consider Human Papillomavirus Vaccination for Children in Japan: Randomized Controlled Trial. *J. Med. Internet Res.* **2021**, *23*, e28355. [CrossRef]
12. Zhang, X.; Liu, C.R.; Wang, Z.Z.; Ren, Z.F.; Feng, X.X.; Ma, W.; Li, J. Effect of a school-based educational intervention on HPV and HPV vaccine knowledge and willingness to be vaccinated among Chinese adolescents: A multi-center intervention follow-up study. *Vaccine* **2020**, *38*, 3665–3670. [CrossRef]
13. Dixon, B.E.; Zimet, G.D.; Xiao, S.; Tu, W.; Lindsay, B.; Church, A.; Downs, S.M. An educational intervention to improve HPV vaccination: A cluster randomized trial. *Pediatrics* **2019**, *143*, e20181457. [CrossRef] [PubMed]
14. Dafermou, H.M.; Tsoumakas, K.; Pavlopoulou, I. Human papillomavirus vaccines. Knowledge and compliance of health science students. *Arch. Greek Med.* **2015**, *32*, 202–209.
15. Agorastos, T.; Chatzistamatiou, K.; Zafrakas, M.; Siamanta, V.; Katsamagkas, T.; Constantinidis, T.C.; Lampropoulos, A.F. Epidemiology of HPV infection and current status of cervical cancer prevention in Greece. *Eur. J. Cancer Prev.* **2014**, *23*, 425–431. [CrossRef] [PubMed]
16. Anagnostou, P.A.; Aletras, V.H.; Niakas, D.A. Human papillomavirus knowledge and vaccine acceptability among adolescents in a Greek region. *Public Health* **2017**, *152*, 145–152. [CrossRef] [PubMed]
17. Michail, G.; Smaili, M.; Vozikis, A.; Jelastopulu, E.; Adonakis, G.; Poulas, K. Female students receiving post-secondary education in Greece: The results of a collaborative human papillomavirus knowledge survey. *Public Health* **2014**, *128*, 1099–1105. [CrossRef]
18. Grigore, M.; Teleman, S.I.; Pristavu, A.; Matei, M. Awareness and knowledge about HPV and HPV vaccine among Romanian women. *J. Cancer Educ.* **2018**, *33*, 154–159. [CrossRef]
19. Deng, C.; Chen, X.; Liu, Y. Human papillomavirus vaccination: Coverage rate, knowledge, acceptance, and associated factors in college students in mainland China. *Hum. Vaccines Immunother.* **2021**, *17*, 828–835. [CrossRef]
20. Marek, E.; Dergez, T.; Rebek-Nagy, G.; Kricskovics, A.; Kovacs, K.; Bozsa, S.; Gocze, P. Adolescents' awareness of HPV infections and attitudes towards HPV vaccination 3 years following the introduction of the HPV vaccine in Hungary. *Vaccine* **2011**, *29*, 8591–8598. [CrossRef]
21. Preston, S.M.; Darrow, W.W. Are men being left behind (or catching up)? Differences in HPV awareness, knowledge, and attitudes between diverse college men and women. *Am. J. Men's Health* **2019**, *13*, 1–12. [CrossRef]
22. Navarro-Illana, P.; Diez-Domingo, J.; Navarro-Illana, E.; Tuells, J.; Alemán, S.; Puig-Barberá, J. Knowledge and attitudes of Spanish adolescent girls towards human papillomavirus infection: Where to intervene to improve vaccination coverage. *BMC Public Health* **2014**, *14*, 490. [CrossRef]
23. Holcomb, B.; Bailey, J.M.; Crawford, K.; Ruffin, M.T. Adults' knowledge and behaviors related to human papillomavirus infection. *J. Am. Board Fam. Pract.* **2004**, *17*, 26–31. [CrossRef] [PubMed]
24. Marlow, L.A.; Zimet, G.D.; McCaffery, K.J.; Ostini, R.; Waller, J. Knowledge of human papillomavirus (HPV) and HPV vaccination: An international comparison. *Vaccine* **2013**, *31*, 763–769. [CrossRef] [PubMed]
25. Varela, P.; Saridi, M. Factors related to the attitudes and knowledge of parents about the vaccination of adolescents against the human wart virus (HPV). *Hell. J. Nurs. Sci.* **2014**, *7*, 24–32.
26. Makwe, C.C.; Anorlu, R.I.; Odeyemi, K.A. Human papillomavirus (HPV) infection and vaccines: Knowledge, attitude and perception among female students at the University of Lagos, Lagos, Nigeria. *J. Epidemiol. Glob. Health* **2012**, *2*, 199–206. [CrossRef]
27. Dell, D.; Chen, H.; Ahmad, F.; Stewart, D. Knowledge about human papillomavirus among adolescents. *J. Low. Genit. Tract Dis.* **2001**, *5*, 115–116. [CrossRef]
28. Vaidakis, D.; Moustaki, I.; Zervas, I.; Barbouni, A.; Merakou, K.; Chrysi, M.S.; Panoskaltsis, T. Knowledge of Greek adolescents on human papilloma virus (HPV) and vaccination: A national epidemiologic study. *Medicine* **2017**, *96*, e5287. [CrossRef] [PubMed]
29. Hendry, M.; Lewis, R.; Clements, A.; Damery, S.; Wilkinson, C. "HPV? Never heard of it!": A systematic review of girls' and parents' information needs, views and preferences about human papillomavirus vaccination. *Vaccine* **2013**, *31*, 5152–5167. [CrossRef] [PubMed]
30. Patel, H.; Jeve, Y.B.; Sherman, S.M.; Moss, E.L. Knowledge of human papillomavirus and the human papillomavirus vaccine in European adolescents: A systematic review. *Sex. Transm. Infect.* **2016**, *92*, 474–479. [CrossRef]
31. Thompson, E.L.; Wheldon, C.W.; Rosen, B.L.; Maness, S.B.; Kasting, M.L.; Massey, P.M. Awareness and knowledge of HPV and HPV vaccination among adults ages 27–45 years. *Vaccine* **2020**, *38*, 3143–3148. [CrossRef]
32. Oh, J.K.; Lim, M.K.; Yun, E.H.; Lee, E.H.; Shin, H.R. Awareness of and attitude towards human papillomavirus infection and vaccination for cervical cancer prevention among adult males and females in Korea: A nationwide interview survey. *Vaccine* **2010**, *28*, 1854–1860. [CrossRef]

33. Jain, N.; Euler, G.L.; Shefer, A.; Lu, P.; Yankey, D.; Markowitz, L. Human papillomavirus (HPV) awareness and vaccination initiation among women in the United States, National Immunization Survey—Adult 2007. *Prev. Med.* **2009**, *48*, 426–431. [CrossRef] [PubMed]
34. Garcini, L.M.; Murray, K.E.; Barnack-Tavlaris, J.L.; Zhou, A.Q.; Malcarne, V.L.; Klonoff, E.A. Awareness and knowledge of human papillomavirus (HPV) among ethnically diverse women varying in generation status. *J. Immigr. Minority Health* **2015**, *17*, 29–36. [CrossRef] [PubMed]
35. Williams, W.W.; Lu, P.J.; Saraiya, M.; Yankey, D.; Dorell, C.; Rodriguez, J.L.; Kepka, D.; Markowitz, L.E. Factors associated with human papillomavirus vaccination among young adult women in the United States. *Vaccine* **2013**, *31*, 2937–2946. [CrossRef]
36. Dinas, K.; Nasioutziki, M.; Arvanitidou, O.; Mavromatidis, G.; Loufopoulos, P.; Pantazis, K.; Dovas, D.; Danilidis, A.; Tsampazis, N.; Zepiridis, L.; et al. Awareness of human papillomavirus infection, testing and vaccination in midwives and midwifery students in Greece. *J. Obstet. Gynaecol.* **2009**, *29*, 542–546. [CrossRef]
37. Shaikh, M.H.; Bortnik, V.; McMillan, N.A.; Idris, A. cGAS-STING responses are dampened in high-risk HPV type 16 positive head and neck squamous cell carcinoma cells. *Microb. Pathog.* **2019**, *132*, 162–165. [CrossRef]
38. Papagiannis, D.; Rachiotis, G.; Symvoulakis, E.K.; Daponte, A.; Grivea, I.N.; Syrogiannopoulos, G.A.; Hadjichristodoulou, C. Vaccination against human papillomavirus among 865 female students from the health professions in central Greece: A questionnaire-based cross-sectional study. *J. Multidiscip. Healthc.* **2013**, *6*, 435–439. [CrossRef]
39. Donadiki, E.M.; Jiménez-García, R.; Hernández-Barrera, V.; Carrasco-Garrido, P.; de Andrés, A.L.; Velonakis, E.G. Human papillomavirus vaccination coverage among Greek higher education female students and predictors of vaccine uptake. *Vaccine* **2012**, *30*, 6967–6970. [CrossRef]
40. Swiecki-Sikora, A.L.; Henry, K.A.; Kepka, D. HPV Vaccination Coverage Among US Teens Across the Rural-Urban Continuum. *J. Rural Health* **2019**, *35*, 506–517. [CrossRef]
41. Adjei Boakye, E.; Lew, D.; Muthukrishnan, M.; Tobi, B.B.; Rohde, R.L.; Varvares, M.A.; Osazuwa-Peters, N. Correlates of human papillomavirus (HPV) vaccination initiation and completion among 18–26 year old in the United States. *Hum. Vaccines Immunother.* **2018**, *14*, 2016–2024. [CrossRef]
42. Lewis, R.M.; Markowitz, L.E. Human papillomavirus vaccination coverage among females and males, National Health and Nutrition Examination Survey, United States, 2007–2016. *Vaccine* **2018**, *36*, 2567–2573. [CrossRef]
43. Natipagon-Shah, B.; Lee, E.; Lee, S.Y. Knowledge, Beliefs, and Practices Among US College Students Concerning Papillomavirus Vaccination. *J. Community Health* **2021**, *46*, 380–388. [CrossRef]
44. Nickel, B.; Dodd, R.H.; Turner, R.M.; Waller, J.; Marlow, L.; Zimet, G.; Ostini, R.; McCaffery, K. Factors associated with the human papillomavirus (HPV) vaccination across three countries following vaccination introduction. *Prev. Med. Rep.* **2017**, *8*, 169–176. [CrossRef] [PubMed]
45. Fishman, J.; Taylor, L.; Kooker, P.; Frank, I. Parent and adolescent knowledge of HPV and subsequent vaccination. *Pediatrics* **2014**, *134*, e1049–e1056. [CrossRef] [PubMed]
46. Lenselink, C.H.; Schmeink, C.E.; Melchers, W.J.G.; Massuger, L.F.A.G.; Hendriks, J.C.M.; Van Hamont, D.; Bekkers, R.L.M. Young adults and acceptance of the human papillomavirus vaccine. *Public Health* **2008**, *122*, 1295–1301. [CrossRef]
47. Cataldi, J.R.; O'Leary, S.T.; Markowitz, L.E.; Allison, M.A.; Crane, L.A.; Hurley, L.P.; Kempe, A. Changes in Strength of Recommendation and Perceived Barriers to Human Papillomavirus Vaccination: Longitudinal Analysis of Primary Care Physicians, 2008–2018. *J. Pediatrics* **2021**, *234*, 149–157. [CrossRef]
48. Thompson, E.L.; Rosen, B.L.; Vamos, C.A.; Kadono, M.; Daley, E.M. Human Papillomavirus Vaccination: What Are the Reasons for Nonvaccination among US Adolescents? *J. Adolesc. Health* **2017**, *61*, 288–293. [CrossRef]
49. Mammas, I.N.; Theodoridou, M.; Koutsaftiki, C.; Bertsias, G.; Sourvinos, G.; Spandidos, D.A. Vaccination against Human Papillomavirus in relation to Financial Crisis: The "Evaluation and Education of Greek Female Adolescents on Human Papillomaviruses' Prevention Strategies" ELEFTHERIA Study. *J. Pediatric Adolesc. Gynecol.* **2016**, *29*, 362–366. [CrossRef] [PubMed]
50. Xiao, X. Follow the heart or the mind? Examining cognitive and affective attitude on HPV vaccination intention. *Atl. J. Commun.* **2019**, *29*, 93–105. [CrossRef]
51. Zimet, G.D.; Weiss, T.W.; Rosenthal, S.L.; Good, M.B.; Vichnin, M.D. Reasons for non-vaccination against HPV and future vaccination intentions among 19–26-year-old women. *BMC Women's Health* **2010**, *10*, 27. [CrossRef]
52. Vakfari, A.; Gavana, M.; Giannakopoulos, S.; Smyrnakis, E.; Benos, A. Participation rates in cervical cancer screening: Experience in rural Northern Greece. *Hippokratia* **2011**, *15*, 346–352.
53. Simou, E.; Maniadakis, N.; Pallis, A.; Foundoulakis, E.; Kourlaba, G. Factors Associated with the Use of Pap Smear Testing in Greece. *J. Women's Health* **2010**, *19*, 1577–1585. [CrossRef] [PubMed]

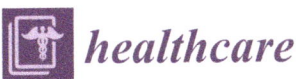

Review

Basics of Sustainable Diets and Tools for Assessing Dietary Sustainability: A Primer for Researchers and Policy Actors

Ioanna Alexandropoulou [1,*], Dimitrios G. Goulis [2], Theodora Merou [3], Tonia Vassilakou [4], Dimitrios P. Bogdanos [5] and Maria G. Grammatikopoulou [5,*]

1. Department of Nutritional Sciences & Dietetics, Faculty of Health Sciences, International Hellenic University, Alexander Campus, GR-57400 Thessaloniki, Greece
2. Unit of Reproductive Endocrinology, 1st Department of Obstetrics and Gynecology, Medical School, Aristotle University of Thessaloniki, 76 Agiou Pavlou Street, GR-56429 Thessaloniki, Greece
3. Department of Forest and Natural Environment Sciences, International Hellenic University, GR-66100 Drama, Greece
4. Department of Public Health Policy, School of Public Health, University of West Attica, 196 Alexandras Avenue, GR-11521 Athens, Greece
5. Department of Rheumatology and Clinical Immunology, Faculty of Medicine, School of Health Sciences, University of Thessaly, Biopolis, GR-41110 Larissa, Greece
* Correspondence: ialexand@med.duth.gr (I.A.); mariagram@auth.gr (M.G.G.)

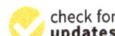

Citation: Alexandropoulou, I.; Goulis, D.G.; Merou, T.; Vassilakou, T.; Bogdanos, D.P.; Grammatikopoulou, M.G. Basics of Sustainable Diets and Tools for Assessing Dietary Sustainability: A Primer for Researchers and Policy Actors. *Healthcare* 2022, 10, 1668. https://doi.org/10.3390/healthcare10091668

Academic Editors: Sofia Koukouli and Areti Stavropoulou

Received: 11 July 2022
Accepted: 30 August 2022
Published: 31 August 2022

Publisher's Note: MDPI stays neutral with regard to jurisdictional claims in published maps and institutional affiliations.

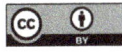

Copyright: © 2022 by the authors. Licensee MDPI, Basel, Switzerland. This article is an open access article distributed under the terms and conditions of the Creative Commons Attribution (CC BY) license (https://creativecommons.org/licenses/by/4.0/).

Abstract: Climate change can have economic consequences, affecting the nutritional intake of populations and increasing food insecurity, as it negatively affects diet quality parameters. One way to mitigate these consequences is to change the way we produce and consume our food. A healthy and sustainable diet aims to promote and achieve the physical, mental, and social well-being of the populations at all life stages, while protecting and safeguarding the resources of the planet and preserving biodiversity. Over the past few years, several indexes have been developed to evaluate dietary sustainability, most of them based on the EAT-*Lancet* reference diet. The present review explains the problems that arise in human nutrition as a result of climate change and presents currently available diet sustainability indexes and their applications and limitations, in an effort to aid researchers and policy actors in identifying aspects that need improvement in the development of relevant indexes. Overall, great heterogeneity exists among the indicators included in the available indexes and their methodology. Furthermore, many indexes do not adequately account for the diets' environmental impact, whereas others fall short in the economic impact domain, or the ethical aspects of sustainability. The present review reveals that the design of one environmentally friendly diet that is appropriate for all cultures, populations, patients, and geographic locations is a difficult task. For this, the development of sustainable and healthy diet recommendations that are region-specific and culturally specific, and simultaneously encompass all aspects of sustainability, is required.

Keywords: environment; plant-based diet; resilience; one health; ecological footprint; water footprint; greenhouse gas; land occupation; sustainable diet index; Sustainable-HEalthy-Diet (SHED) index; food packaging; business as usual

1. Introduction

Despite the numerous technological advantages and the evolution of science, the agricultural and fishery sectors still fail to fulfill the dietary needs of the global population [1]. In addition, climate change has economic consequences and increases the threat of food insecurity, as it negatively affects agricultural and livestock production, and also fisheries [2–4]. With regard to human nutrition, climate change impacts food quality parameters, including protein, micronutrients, and vitamin content, mainly in basic crops [5]. For proteins in particular, the projected estimated reduction in some basic grains, such as rice and barley, can have an important impact on population health [5,6]. On the other end of the spectrum, human nutrition also impacts climate change by increasing greenhouse gas emissions (GHGe, including methane, CO_2, and N_2O), overconsumption of water resources, and extensive land use [7]. It was found that one-quarter of GHGe are released due to agricultural activity, with animal husbandry accounting for the largest percentage [8]. In addition, studies revealed that dietary patterns with high animal food content are releasing greater GHGe. The increase in GHGe, mainly due to human activity, leads to an increase in the planet's temperature, resulting in the observed climate change and the effects it brings [9].

Counterbalancing the results of climate change on our diet requires changing the way we produce and consume food. The development of sustainable food standards is a key objective of the United Nations (UN), aiming to achieve the Sustainable Development Goals (SDGs) [10]. Although we currently lack a unanimous definition of what a sustainable diet is, according to the Food and Agriculture Organization (FAO) (Figure 1) [11], it aims to achieve and maintain the physical, mental, and social health and well-being of the populations at all life stages, while protecting and safeguarding the resources of the planet and preserving the biodiversity [12]. In this context, a sustainable diet is also an accessible one, ensuring equity while based on fair trade principles, encompassing eco-friendly, local, and seasonal foods that are covering the nutritional needs of the people, limiting food insecurity [11].

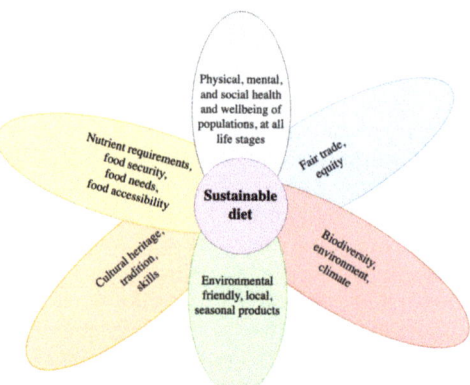

Figure 1. Components of sustainable diets according to the FAO [11].

Since the EAT-*Lancet* Commission on healthy diets from sustainable food systems was published [7], consumers' concerns for the critical role of food systems were heightened, propelling research interest in achieving and quantifying a sustainable diet. Clearly, a single agenda integrating global health and environmental sustainability would not be adequate in achieving the SDGs. Hence, various tools and indexes have been designed and proposed, aiming to assess dietary sustainability using different components and food groups. A variety of indicators can be used to evaluate the impact of certain food groups on the environment, with GHGe being the most used in research [13]. Other indicators include pesticides, land and blue water use, biodiversity, and eutrophication (i.e., the increase in the supply rate of organic matter to an ecosystem) [14].

There is a need to recognize the impact of human nutrition on the environment and how changes in the way we eat will contribute to a more sustainable environment. There is also a need to measure how sustainable the population's diet is and calculate its environmental impact. Thus, it is necessary to describe the current indexes, their advantages and disadvantages, and how to use them, in order to aid researchers and policy actors in identifying aspects that need improvement in the development of novel indexes.

For this reason, the aims of the present review are (a) to understand the problems that arise in human nutrition due to climate change and present sustainable food systems as one of solutions to the problem, and (b) to showcase the existing indexes/tools for evaluating sustainable nutrition, as well as the advantages and disadvantages that each one displays.

2. Nutrition and Climate Change

Climate change poses a threat to food security, mainly due to its negative impacts on agricultural productivity. In the past few decades, research has also focused on how climate change affects main crops' quality parameters [2,5]. Recent studies suggest that the change in the climate will lead to modifications in the nutrient content of basic staple foods consumed in our daily diet, including rice, barley, flour, legumes, etc. [15–17]. In some cases, these modifications concern reductions in the content of basic nutrients, such as proteins, but with regard to the micronutrient content of foods, including iron (Fe) and zinc (Zn) levels. The content of staple crops with respect to these micronutrients is an important determinant in estimating the dietary intake of micronutrients in a population [15,16]. Nutrient deficiencies involving Fe and Zn constitute major global public health issues, particularly in areas where people base their dietary intake on these crops, such as women and children residing in sub-Saharan Africa [14]. The main parameters of climate change affecting food nutrient composition include the increasing ambient temperature, followed by drought and the subsequent increases in atmospheric CO_2 concentration.

2.1. Effects of Drought

Drought reduces the concentration of nutrients in plants such as legumes, cereals, and grasses. In particular, it affects the cultivation of beans and *Hordeum vulgare* (barley), *Zeamays* (Zea), and ryegrass [15]. Common beans are the most important legumes supporting food security and human nutrition globally. In particular, they provide almost 15% of daily calories and 36% of daily protein in many African and South American countries [18]. For smallholder farmers in sub-Saharan Africa, beans are an important crop and a key nutritional component in the diets of poor rural communities. Inevitably, such small farming communities are more vulnerable to the negative effects of climate change [19,20]. For common beans, it is not known whether drought-related crop reductions will also lead to changes in nutritional quality under future drought scenarios [21]. A modeling study investigating the impact of changes in heat and rainfall frequency in southeastern Africa [15] predicted that by the year 2050, common beans will become unsuitable for cultivation in the vast majority of the current bean-growing areas. Thus, the transfer and relocation of crops to new areas should be performed with careful selection of suitable varieties for each new geographical area [15].

Drought also reduces approximately 50% the nitrogen (N) and phosphorus (P) concentration in the susceptible barley and Zea plants and in the drought-resistant *Andropogon gerardii* (big bluestem). This is due to the decrease in the level of nutrient uptake proteins or transporters in plant roots, such as the NRT1 protein for the uptake of nitrate (NO_3), the ammonium transporter 1 (AMT1) for ammonium (NH_4), and the PHT1 transporter for P [17]. The negative effects of drought have also been detected on the mRNA levels of nutrient uptake proteins, including the Zn transporter in maize, the silicon (Si) transporter in rice, and the NO_3 and sulfate (SO_4) transporters in grapes [22]. In parallel, heat stress also induces negative effects on the antioxidant enzyme content of *Zea mays* [23]. In contrast, up-regulation of the NRT1, AMT1, and PHT1 proteins per unit of total root protein during drought was observed in a recent study, associated with increases in the mRNA levels of these proteins in maize [24]. However, since nutrient uptake proteins can be post-transcriptionally regulated, it is important to assess the levels of these components in order to understand how exposure to drought affects their expression and uptake rate [25].

2.2. Increase in CO_2 Concentration

Over the next 30–80 years, the rate of increase in atmospheric CO_2 is likely to exceed 550 ppm. According to the literature, increased levels of CO_2 in the atmosphere will affect plant growth and suppress Zn, Fe, and protein levels in staple crops. In a recent study conducted by Smith and Myers [16], 41 cultivars of six food crops were grown over 10 years on three continents to determine the effect of elevated CO_2 levels on their quality. The results revealed reduced levels of Fe and Zn in all crops. In another study, protein levels were also decreased in grains, but legumes were not as affected, probably due to the general ability of legumes to extract and assimilate more N than other grains under increased CO_2 exposure in order to maintain the C:N ratio (25). The levels of some vitamins have been reported to change. For example, Zhu and associates [5] found that in rice, the level of vitamin E increased, while other vitamins (vitamins B_1, B_2, B_5, and B_9) were reduced.

Another research group [26] studied the effects of increased CO_2 on plant growth in greenhouses, or indoors. The results revealed that in artificial environments, the changes, particularly the increase in CO_2, can negatively affect the concentration of nutrients in some plants [26]. C3 plants, such as rice and wheat, have less energy-efficient photosynthesis compared to C4 plants, such as maize [24]. This is due to the different photosynthesis mechanism in these plants. In C3 plants, the first product of photosynthesis is a sugar with three carbon atoms, while C4 plants produce sugar with four carbon atoms. C4s are very efficient at using CO_2 and thus lose less water [27]. If a C3 plant grows in an environment abundant in CO_2, then it will produce more carbohydrates, but it will concurrently reduce its concentration of other elements, including vitamins of the B complex. In particular, if wheat is grown in a CO_2 concentration exceeding 546 ppm, then it will have approximately 6–13% less protein, 4–7% less Zn, and 5–8% less Fe [28].

In field experiments grown under elevated CO_2 conditions, Meden and associates [6] observed a reduction in the protein content of rice, barley, potato, and wheat, ranging from 6.5% to 14%. The negative effect of high ambient CO_2 concentration on the Zn, Fe, and protein content of plants was also shown in experiments involving different rice varieties in China and Japan [5]. In the same study, the effects on the levels of B vitamins were also investigated and it was observed that the reduction in the nutrient content of rice was even greater, ranging between 13% and 30%, with the greatest reduction in folic acid concentrations. On the other hand, an increase in vitamin E (α-tocopherol) levels was also observed [5].

2.3. Effects on Human Health

As already mentioned, increases in atmospheric CO_2 content induce significant reductions in the protein content of plants such as rice, potatoes, wheat, and barley. Therefore, populations that depend on these plants to meet their dietary protein goals are expected to experience a reduction in their protein intake, exceeding 5% [6]. According to Medek [6], it has been estimated that by the year 2050, approximately 150 million people may be at risk of protein deficiency as a consequence of increased ambient CO_2. Zhu and associates [5] used a food balance sheet developed by the FAO and gross domestic product (GDP) to estimate the risk of nutritional deficiencies for the 10 largest rice-consuming countries. Their results indicated that shortfalls were larger for countries with the lowest GDP [5]. Another study suggested that the countries at greater risk include Tajikistan, Bangladesh, Burundi, Liberia, the Occupied Palestinian Territories, Iraq, and Afghanistan, while in India, an additional 5% of the population is estimated to be at risk of developing protein deficiency due to the changes in rice content [6].

According to Bennett's law, an increased income can provide alternative food sources for energy, and consequently protein, including meat, fish, and dairy, whereas low income is associated with more carbohydrate intake and reduced protein sources [29]. Therefore, in economically developed countries such as South Korea and Japan, the reduced protein in rice is not expected to alter the dietary intake of the populations. In contrast, in developing countries such as Guinea and Madagascar, dependence on rice persists. Hence, poorer countries are bound to be more affected by this nutritional deficit [5]. These predicted results are based on the Intergovernmental Panel on Climate Change's climatic scenarios, which estimate that CO_2 concentrations will reach 570 μmol mole^{-1} by the end of the century [30].

Based on these observations, Smith and Myers [31] estimated the public health implications of the deficiency of dietary B-complex vitamins in rice as a result of climate change. They also tried to quantify the risk of developing neural tube defects in babies born from mothers suffering from folate deficiency. Their results showed an increased risk for folate, thiamine, and riboflavin deficiencies in an additional 132, 67, and 40 million people, respectively. They used a statistical model in which the data came from estimates of nutrient stocks and corresponding requirements at a national level [31].

In parts of the world with a great prevalence of food insecurity, the reduced nutritional value of cheap and easily accessible diet seeds exacerbates the problem. It is estimated that 1.4 billion women and children under the age of five living in countries with high rates of anemia will lose an additional 4% of their dietary Fe intake. Iron deficiency can lead to stunted growth and reduced mental and physical abilities. In countries where manual labor is the main type of work, this can have a negative effect on income, and therefore further limit access to adequate and nutritious food [16]. Moreover, nutrient depletion projections suggest that by the year 2050, an additional 175 million people worldwide will be Zn-deficient [16]. As a result, geographic areas exhibiting less diet diversity such as India, sub-Saharan Africa, and parts of South Asia will be more affected by changes in the nutrient levels of staple crops [16].

2.4. Impact of Human Nutrition on Climate Change

Food is a basic human right and a healthy diet can contribute to our health and well-being. Distinct types of foods differ, not only in terms of their nutrient content, but also in the amount of land, water, energy, and GHGe required to produce them (ecological footprint) [32]. Today, the complex and global food production and distribution system is created to meet our ever-increasing nutritional needs, in terms of both quantity and taste. Nowadays, it is possible, for example, to fish in the Atlantic Ocean and consume the products within a few days on the European continent, as well as to supply European products all over the world.

Nonetheless, for many scientists, the food sector is considered an important effector of environmental change. It has been estimated that 30% of the GHGe are food-derived, while 70% of the drinking water is used for food production globally. The extensive use of land for crops has altered natural ecosystems, leading to the extinction of several species [7]. The rate of extinction and reduction in species population is greater than that of the Holocene era and is estimated at 1 species/million species/year. The amount in kilograms of insects decreased by 75% in the past three decades, while that of domestic birds decreased by 30% in one and a half decades [7]. Results from food life cycle assessment (LCA) studies reveal that the environmental impacts of food production are higher for animal products, and even greater for ruminants [33].

Total food demand is expected to increase by 70% by the year 2050, with a shift to animal-based foods including seafood, the consumption of which is expected to increase by 80%. It is believed that the global demand for beef may increase by 95% [9]. A consequence of the ever-higher consumption of animal products, and especially meat, is the increase in GHGe, which may reach 80% by the year 2050. The long-term overconsumption of meat can also affect the availability and prices of other food products [9]. This increasing consumption is mainly located in the urban areas of emerging economies in Asia, such as India and China [34]. In the U.S. and Europe, a decrease in beef consumption per capita was noticed since the 1970s, mainly due to public health concerns and rise in ready-to-go foods that give more alternatives. Projections indicate that beef consumption/capita on the European continent is expected to remain almost steady. Nevertheless, the consumed amount/person/day of animal products remains higher among high-income countries compared to low-income ones [9,35].

2.5. Sustainable Diets

The change in the way we produce and consume food is a key goal for the UN in order to achieve the SDGs. There are four SDGs for sustainable food systems and healthy eating standards: (a) SDG 2 aims to stop hunger, accomplish food security, enhance nutrition, and encourage sustainable agriculture; (b) SDG 3 aims to ensure healthy living and supporting well-being for everyone at any age; (c) SDG 12 aims to establish sustainability in producing and wasting systems; and (d) SDG 13 addresses the need for immediate actions to combat the effects of climate change [10].

The concept of a sustainable diet has been around for several years and links the environmental impact of our food choices. It includes meeting nutritional requirements with diets having a low environmental impact and respecting the biodiversity and cultural heritage of each region, and at the same time, it covers the parameters of accessibility and affordability. Studies have shown that these diets can reduce GHGe via the reduction in the intake of animal foods and their replacement with plant foods [36]. According to the FAO [11], a sustainable and healthy diet should take into account several factors. The most important of them are environmental (climate change, loss of biodiversity, land use, air and water pollution), food security issues (access to it, availability, stability of production), nutritional adequacy (enrichment with all necessary macro- and micro-nutrients), people's socio-economic background, culture, and animal welfare issues [11].

These diets should be designed to be specific to each distinct environment, and therefore, there is no ideal dietary pattern for all. Our knowledge is growing about healthier eating habits with a lower environmental impact, but we should also include the socio-economic dimensions of sustainability in this context. We already know that the nutritional needs differ between sexes and age groups, but this is also happening between countries. There are different energy and dietary requirements for macro- and micronutrients between low- and high-income countries [37].

In addition, a review comparing the results of several studies relating different dietary patterns to the produced GHGe and the land use required for the production of the diets revealed that the least GHGe and land use requirements were observed in vegetarian and other "healthy" diets. Nevertheless, the substitution of red meat with poultry may induce a lower impact on global warming [38]. However, there is the risk that reducing animal foods will lead to a subsequent reduction in protein intake, so ideally, they should be replaced by alternative protein sources. In this context, researchers also focused on identifying alternative sources of protein with a smaller environmental footprint. MacDiarmid and Whybrow [36] reviewed relevant studies investigating (a) the use of already existing protein-rich plant foods, such as legumes; (b) alternative animal sources, such as edible insects; and (c) the development of novel foods, including lab-grown meat. Studies based on the LCA revealed that insect-based products had a lower environmental impact, including lower GHGe and land use, compared to animal products [39]. In contrast, in the case of lab-grown meat, the lower environmental impact compared to animal products is dependent on the production unit. Further studies are required to clarify the suitability of alternative protein sources [40].

The aforementioned issues associated with climate change and the projection trends indicate that the time for action and changing the food system is now. The lack of specific scientific targets for what a healthy and sustainable diet constitutes was apparent [7], leading to the development of specific expert groups aiming to solve the problem.

3. The EAT-*Lancet* Reference Diet

The EAT-*Lancet* Commission on Food, Planet, Health brought together 37 renowned scientists to evaluate if the future population can be fed on a healthy diet within planetary boundaries [41]. The Commission proposed the first targets for the consumption of a sustainable diet and the environmental boundaries regarding food production in order to meet the SDGs [42]. These targets formed the eponymous reference diet based on the universal diet that theoretically promotes human and environmental health simultaneously, under the "one health" principle [7]. It is based on eight food groups: whole grains, tubers and starchy vegetables (potatoes and cassava), vegetables, fruits, dairy foods, protein sources (meat, eggs, fish, legumes, nuts), added fats, and added sugars. The diet is mainly plant-based, with whole grains, vegetables, fruits, nuts, and legumes comprising the majority of the consumed foods. Meat and dairy are also included in the diet, but their target consumption is significantly less than that of plant-products and they are consumed periodically. The EAT-*Lancet* diet was disseminated in nine languages and funded by the Wellcome Trust and the EAT forum, a Norwegian-based independent non-profit organization founded by the Stordalen Foundation, the Wellcome Trust, and the Stockholm Resilience Centre [41].

3.1. Methodological Limitations of the EAT-Lancet Reference Diet

Despite its novelty, the EAT-*Lancet* reference diet has several methodological limitations. The suggested consumption thresholds for each food group were based mainly on epidemiological data (cohort and cross-sectional studies), with few meta-analyses (one published in 2007). No grading system was employed to rate evidence quality and produce valid recommendations for the selected thresholds. The Commission's experts made recommendations based on selected data published during the previous decades. For instance, the results of the "Seven countries study" [43], a landmark cross-sectional study initiated in 1958, investigating the relationship between diet and disease, has numerous methodological flaws, and due to its design, cannot provide evidence for the development of informed decisions [44,45], despite being innovative at its time. In the EAT-*Lancet* report, this specific reference is used to introduce the notion that lower meat intake is associated with reduced cardiovascular risk. As Trijsburg noted [13], the EAT-*Lancet* authors based their recommendations on previously published systematic reviews, meta-analyses, and pooled analyses of primary data, added as a supplementary material to the report, without developing a new systematic product to answer each research question. According to Zagmutt [46], the report failed to use systematic methods for the selection of the health impacts of foods and their corresponding risk ratios (RRs), despite the fact that these were crucial to their findings and the proposed diet. The report resembles a narrative review more than a systematic report driving recommendations.

Additionally, the report makes inconsistent use of the scientific literature for associations between food groups and diseases, without any methodology to grade the evidence [47]. Subsequently, attempts to replicate the U.S. mortality calculations proposed by the EAT-*Lancet* report [48] revealed flaws in the methods and assumptions used to estimate the avoided mortalities, calling into question the global conclusions of the Commission. The arbitrary associations of foods with diseases bring to light the concerns raised over nutrition epidemiology [49,50]. For instance, with regard to meat intake, recent state-of-the-art meta-analyses from expert scientists have revealed that the actual magnitude of association between red and processed meat intake and all-cause mortality and adverse cardiometabolic outcomes is very small, but on the other hand, the existing evidence is of low certainty [51]. Similar results were also apparent with regard to cancer mortality and incidence, where the certainty of evidence using the Grading of Recommendations Assessment, Development, and Evaluation (GRADE) [52] approach was low to very low [53]. An akin meta-analysis examining meat intake and cancer outcomes also revealed that low- or very-low-certainty evidence suggests that the adoption of diets with less red/processed meat may induce very small reductions in adverse cancer outcomes [54].

Meta-analyses are performed to gather primary evidence and pool data in order to guide decision making in science, including nutrition and medicine [55]. When old meta-analyses are used to inform decisions, more recent studies are not included, while in parallel, the methodological quality of the meta-analyses is not always up-to-date. For this reason, for each recommendation regarding clinical decisions, either in nutrition or in medicine, the conduction of a systematic review and/or meta-analysis is required to provide up-to-date information for the examined hypothesis, including the most recent evidence. As a result, all clinical practice guidelines and nutrition recommendations must be developed under this methodology, which has been described in detail in the AGREE consortium [56]. In the EAT-*Lancet* report, neither the GRADE [52] nor the AGREE [56] were used to produce evidence tables and guide recommendations regarding dietary targets, although they are considered as the standard in the development of clinical recommendations [55]. Moreover, given that nutrition recommendations have already been criticized deeply for not meeting scientific standards [57–60], it is important to safeguard sustainable nutrition from this saga. Critical evaluation of the process used to synthesize the evidence when making recommendations for clinical practice (as in the EAT-*Lancet* report) enables users to assess the trustworthiness of these recommendations [61]. Health professionals are increasingly dependent on valid recommendations in everyday clinical practice since they do not always have the time to keep up with the medical literature, and for providing evidence-based practice [61,62]. According to Lunny and associates [61], high-quality systematic review products are required for the identification and pooling of the best available up-to-date evidence in order to inform clinical recommendations. The use of non-systematic methods, as seen in the EAT-*Lancet* report [7], may greatly compromise the validity and reliability of the evidence used to inform the formulation of recommendations—let alone global nutritional policy recommendations—and ultimately leads to over- or under-estimation of the treatment effect estimates and potentially untrustworthy and misleading recommendations [61,63].

According to Kaiser [64], the EAT-*Lancet* report [7] acts as a "brokerage between science and policy"; that is, it failed to meet transparency and replicability standards, providing great statistical uncertainty [48]. For some scientists [65], the narrow manner in describing the measures to tackle broken food systems and lack of health is also questionable. For example, anthropologists [65] noted the ill-suited association between premature death as the main residual of unhealthy dietary choices. Furthermore, they pointed out that the term "healthy diets" was repeated approximately 100 times in the report text. For a solution to be evidence-based, it must be transparent, replicable, and supported by the proper quantification of its impact [46]. Nevertheless, this does not appear to be the case for the report [46], despite the fact that the authors claim to use "the best available evidence" [7].

Apart from methodological limitations, the EAT-*Lancet* reference diet also entails economic limitations and raises concerns regarding the efficacy of the diet to provide nutritional adequacy and the suitability of the diet for specific patient populations.

3.2. Economic Limitations of the EAT-Lancet Reference Diet

Low basic income constitutes a major health constraint [66], associated with increased food insecurity [67]. Economic analyses of the reference diet have revealed that the cost of the diet exceeded the household/capita income of at least 1.58 billion people worldwide, making it unaffordable [68–70]. Based on 2011 commodities prices, it was calculated that the most affordable version of the EAT–*Lancet* diet cost a global median of USD 2.84 daily (IQR 2.41–3.16), which may be a small fraction of the average income in developed countries, but still, it is an unaffordable amount for poor populations of the world [68]. In rural India, people are currently spending an average of USD 1.00/person/day for their diets and the cost of the EAT-*Lancet* diets ranges between USD 3.00 and 5.00/person/day [71]. Not surprisingly, the higher costs of the reference diet are attributed mainly to fresh fruits and vegetables [68]. Moreover, the cost of the benchmarking diet ranged between 3% and 73% of the national income in several low-income and middle-income countries [69].

Interestingly, although the Commission included high-ranking officials of the World Health Organization (WHO) and FAO, the WHO rushed to drop its sponsorship of the EAT-*Lancet* Commission [72] and withdraw endorsement [73], citing concerns regarding the economic impact of the reference diet on poor, livestock-producing countries. There were concerns that the widespread adoption of the diet could risk jobs and traditional diets linked to cultural heritage [73]. It is believed however, that this move by the WHO to withdraw endorsement was propelled by political interests and motivation. According to Drewnowski [69], the FAO description of sustainable diets is based on four pillars: health, society, economics, and the environment; nevertheless, the suggested reference diet falls short on the social and economic aspects of the definition. Other scientists [46] argued that, at the moment, the reference diet appears to promote a solution favoring high-income countries, without providing solutions for major global health issues, including maternal and child malnutrition.

3.3. Nutritional Adequacy of the EAT-Lancet Diet

According to a relevant press release of the UN Italian Representation [74], due to its restrictive manner regarding several food groups, adopting the reference diet might be nutritionally deficient and even dangerous for human health in the long run, particularly for populations with enhanced dietary requirements. Furthermore, the nutritional inadequacy of the diet might enhance the need for dietary supplements or food fortification, which in turn may inflate the cost of the diet. Of note, in this situation, given that the carbon footprint of dietary supplements has never been assessed, the final result of balancing nutrient needs through supplements might, in fact, counterbalance the postulated environmental benefits of the reference diet.

3.4. Restriction of Animal-Sourced Foods

Many independent researchers revealed flaws in the analyses behind the EAT-*Lancet* report [46,48,75]. Great concern was also raised regarding the restrictive nature of the reference diet for animal food sources [47]. This restrictive manner concerning animal foods seems to disregard recent meta-analyses published in top journals exonerating the association between meat intake and health [51,54]. Furthermore, as Thorkildsen and Reksnesit [47] pointed out, the report does not consider regional and national differences in the available natural resources. Sustainable production for one country is not always sustainable somewhere else in the world [47], and meat production seems to fall within this category. The report also raised concerns regarding the economic future of countries involved in cattle farming, including Ethiopia and other developing countries. The absolute or relative elimination of foods of animal origin would ultimately end cattle farming and all related activities [74], ending the viability of all the cattle farming companies situated in these countries. However, according to the UN Italian Representation [74], in the EAT-*Lancet* report [7], meat products were "arbitrarily regarded as unhealthy".

Subsequently, two new members were recently appointed to the EAT-*Lancet* Commission, a Zambian agricultural nutritionist and the General Director's Representative to Ethiopia at the International Livestock Research Institute, aiming to add heterogeneity to the pool of Commission members and provide advice on this issue [76].

3.5. Application of the Reference Diet to Specific Patient Populations

An additional important limitation involves the adoption of the diet by patients with diseases limiting the intake of vegetables and fruits, such as irritable bowel syndrome or inflammatory bowel disease. For these patients, achieving health while following the EAT-*Lancet* diet is unrealistic. Moreover, those with drug-resistant epilepsy following a ketogenic diet are unlikely to adhere to the proposed sustainable dietary regime. According to the WHO, "a standard diet for the whole planet, regardless of the age, sex, metabolism, general state of health and eating habits of each person, has no scientific justification at all" [74].

4. Indexes Assessing Dietary Sustainability Based on the EAT-*Lancet* Reference Diet

The publication of the EAT-*Lancet* report [7] initiated the need to "quantify" the sustainability of diets. This resulted in the development of several indexes, many based on the EAT-*Lancet* report [7] and others developed *de novo* (Table 1). In order to fulfill all sustainability criteria, these indexes must also account for the economic, environmental, fair trade, cultural heritage, and population health aspects of sustainability, as previously detailed in Figure 1.

Table 1. Indexes assessing dietary sustainability.

Index Name	Origin	Main Domains of the Index	Components	Dietary Intake Domains (Foods and Food Groups)	Environmental Impact	Based on the EAT-Lancet Reference Diet [7]	Score Range
EAT-Lancet diet score [77]	U.K.	Dietary intake	14 food items, each providing a score of 0 or 1.	Whole grains, tubers, starchy vegetables (potatoes and cassava), vegetables, fruits, dairy foods, protein sources (meat, eggs, fish, legumes, nuts), added fats, added sugars.	Not accounted for	Yes	0–14
WISH [13]	Global (The Netherlands, Italy, Brazil, USA)	Dietary intake	13 components, each scored between 0 and 10.	Whole grains, vegetables, fruits, dairy foods, red meat, fish, eggs, chicken/poultry, legumes, nuts, unsaturated fats, saturated fats, added sugars.	GHGe, land use, eutrophication, acidification, scarcity weighted water	Yes	0–130
PHDI [78]	Brazil	Dietary intake	16 food items, each providing a maximum score of 10 or 5 and a minimum of 0.	Nuts and peanuts, legumes, fruits, total vegetables, whole grains, eggs, fish and seafood, tubers and potatoes, dairy, vegetable oils, dark green vegetables/total vegetable ratio, red and orange/total vegetable ratio, red meats, chicken and substitutes, animal fats, added sugars.	Not accounted for	Yes	0–150
SHED Index [79]	Israel	Healthy eating (overall dietary consumption), drinking habits (intake of sweetened beverages and bottled water), sustainable eating (plant-based), socio-cultural aspects (organic foods, food consumerism), intake of ultra-processed and plant-based foods, environmental aspects (food waste, domestic waste streams)	30 items, each with a different weight to the score.	The healthy eating domain includes consumption frequency questions regarding meat products, plant-based foods, fruit/vegetable variety, preference for plant-based over animal products, drinking water preference, low-salt products, ultra-processed products, low-sugar foods, sweetened beverages, sweets, salt intake, recycle food scraps with a composter, preferring foods made in the country.	Accounted for, although it does not quantify GHGe	Yes, and the MDS	0–100
IDSS [80]	Mexico	Dietary intake	13 food items, each providing a binary score of 0 or 1.	Whole-grain foods, tubers and starchy vegetables, vegetables, fruits, milk and by-products, beef/pork, chicken and other birds, eggs, fish and seafood, legumes/soybeans/tree nuts, saturated fats, unsaturated oils, added sugars.	Not accounted for	Yes	0–13
HSDI [81]	Australia	NR	NR	NR	NR	No	NR
SDI [82]	France	Environmental, nutritional, economic, and socio-cultural aspects of the diet	4 components, providing a score of 1–5.	A nutritional sub-index reflects the adequacy between energy intake and needs. The PANDiet is included as a sub-index, assessing the adequacy in nutrient intake based on the French recommendations for 24 nutrients.	Accounted for	No	4–20

GHGe, greenhouse gas emissions; HSDI, Healthy and Sustainable Diet Index [81]; IDSS, Indice de dietasaludable y sostenible [80]; MDS, Mediterranean diet score [83]; PANDiet, probability of adequate nutrient intake [84]; PHDI, Planetary Health Diet Index [78]; SDI, sustainable diet index; SHED, Sustainable-HEalthy-Diet [79]; U.K., United Kingdom; USA, United States of America; WISH, World Index for Sustainability and Health [13].

4.1. The EAT-Lancet Diet Score

The EAT-*Lancet* diet score [77] was the first by-product of the EAT-*Lancet* report. It is based on 14 food items according to the eight food groups suggested in the reference diet. The suggested energy intake is 2500 kcal/day, as in the reference diet. For each food group, a threshold intake of dry, raw weight is recommended; consumptions below each threshold add one point to the index score (i.e., above the minimum intake or below the maximum intake). Any intake not meeting the threshold of a specific food group receives a score of 0, based on a binary scoring system [77]. With regard to whole grains, roots, and tubers in particular, recommendations were increased to ensure reaching a daily energy intake of 2500 kcal; thus, the suggested intakes were not based on disease prevention or environmental impact suggestions [13].

The use of the reference diet showed beneficial associations with ischemic heart disease and diabetes in the U.K. European Prospective Investigation into Cancer and Nutrition (EPIC)-Oxford cohort [77]. However, an analysis using the U.S. Department of Agriculture (USDA) food database showed that the maximum score can be achieved by consuming a small apple, approximately 200 g of tomatoes, 28 g of nuts, 10 g of extra-fiber all-bran cereals, and nothing else whatsoever each day [80]. For this reason, it has been argued that the results of the score "have no relevance" to the EAT-*Lancet* report [80]; the Commission has not commented on the subject, nor has it endorsed the score.

Cacau et al. [78] spotted several limitations regarding the score. Using reference values in grams does not allow for assessing individual adherence, irrespective of the total energy intake of the participants. For example, the 2500 kcal/d diet cannot apply to infants, young children, or athletes. Furthermore, it does not include intermediate intake and interchangeable group values [78]. An additional bottleneck is that the score does not account for sustainability's environmental and economic aspects.

Finally, since it is based on the EAT-*Lancet* report, it also carries all the previously mentioned limitations of the reference diet.

4.2. The World Index for Sustainability and Health (WISH)

The WISH was designed with the aim to monitor the healthiness and environmental sustainability of the diet of a population [13], based on the EAT-*Lancet* recommendations [7]. However, the authors omitted tubers and starchy vegetables from the scoring, arguing that neither the WHO nor the Global Burden of Disease (GBD) included them in their recommendations. With the removal of the tubers and starchy vegetables food group, the WISH consists of 13 foods and food groups. Its scoring is based on a gradual system according to the classification of each food group as neutral, protective, or negative for human and planet health, without requiring food composition tables or LCA data, as the authors considered that these data are unavailable for different countries [13]. Food groups considered as more protective had a greater consumption recommendation, whereas those deemed as more harmful for human health and the environment were suggested to be consumed in smaller amounts. Moreover, scores are assigned assuming a linear relationship between the component and the health outcomes, with protective food groups providing greater scores with increased consumption and negative food groups providing lower scores when consumed in greater amounts. Additionally, food groups are also divided in three categories based on their environmental impact (low, medium, and high environmental impact food groups).

The index was validated in a small sample of 396 urban Vietnamese men and women using duplicate 24 h dietary recalls [13]. The initial analysis revealed that the score could differentiate between the healthiness and environmental sustainability of the Vietnamese diet.

The index uses reference values in grams, not allowing for the assessment of individual adherence regardless of the total energy intake of the diet [78]. Moreover, it fails to include all intermediate values and interchangeable groups proposed in the EAT-*Lancet* report [78], meaning that for each food group, meeting the threshold or not, is the only parameter affecting the score received, in a binary manner. When half the amount of foods is consumed, no intermediate score can be provided. A total of four distinct sub-scores are added for the calculation of the total WISH, namely, (i) the healthy sub-score, evaluating how healthy the diet is (sum of the eight protective and two neutral food groups), (ii) the less healthy sub-score assessing how unhealthy a diet is (sum of the three "unhealthy" food groups), (iii) the low environmental impact sub-score (sum of the six low environmental impact food groups), and (iv) the high environmental impact sub-score (sum of the three high and four moderate environmental impact food groups) [13]. As a result, one individual may score high in the healthy sub-score but low in the low environmental impact sub-score, indicating a healthy diet for humans, but unhealthy for the planet. Similarly to the EAT-*Lancet* diet score, it inevitably carries all the limitations of the respective reference diet. Finally, although developed as a world index for measuring dietary sustainability, it has only been validated in a Vietnamese sample.

4.3. The Planetary Health Diet Index (PHDI)

The PHDI [78] is based on 16 components with proportional scoring, considering the EAT-*Lancet* food groups as energy intake ratios. The components include nuts and peanuts, legumes, fruits, total vegetables, whole grains, eggs, fish and seafood, tubers and potatoes, dairy, vegetable oils, dark green vegetables-to-total vegetable ratio, red and orange to total vegetable ratio, red meats, chicken and substitutes, animal fats, and added sugars. A daily intake of 2500 kcal was set with different intakes from 16 distinct food groups, expressed in two manners, as g/day and as kcal/day [78], according to the EAT-*Lancet* reference diet [7]. The energy contribution of all intake tiers and midpoints proposed for each food group were calculated to the reference diet of 2500 kcal/d. Each component was weighted based on adequacy, moderation, and optimum intake ratio, based on whether intake values suggest a greater or lower adherence to the reference diet assumptions, according to the system indicated by the Dutch Healthy Eating Index (HEI) group [85]. Concerning the scoring system, each of the 16 components of the PHDI provides a maximum of 10 or 5 points, with the total score ranging from 0 to 150 points.

The ELSA-Brasil multicenter cohort validated the index (N = 15,105 men and women aged 35–74 years) [78]. The construct validity and reliability of the index were performed based on the methodology proposed for the HEI [86], according to the relevant Brazilian-revised tool [87]. The internal reliability was evaluated using Cronbach's α, which had a value of 0.51. For the construct validity, three separate sets of examinations were performed. In the first, linear regression models adjusted for sex and age were used to assess correlations between the PHDI score with selected nutrients. In the second set of examinations, it was assessed whether the PHDI could assess adherence to EAT-*Lancet* recommendations, irrespective of the amount of energy consumed in the diet. In the third, a principal component analysis (PCA) was performed to investigate whether the PHDI had more than one factor explaining the variability of the data. Finally, the degree that the PHDI could discriminate between groups with known differences in the quality of their diets was also evaluated [86]. The results of the construct validity revealed that the PHDI showed a positive correlation with the intake of carbohydrates; PUFA; vegetable proteins; dietary fiber; vitamins A, C, E, and K; folate and thiamine; and several elements, including Fe, K, Zn, Se, Mg, and Cu [78]. Moreover, the PHDI was negatively associated with total and saturated fat, animal protein, cholesterol, MUFA, etc. No association was observed between the index and total protein intake, total energy, Calcium, or Na consumption [78]. The PCA revealed a variety of factors that explain the variability in the PHDI, although none of the 16 components were deemed responsible for a significant proportion of the observed covariance in the data [78].

In parallel, GHGe was calculated to adjust for the ecological aspect of the sustainable diet definition. For this, the "Environmental Footprints of Food and Culinary Preparations Consumed in Brazil" database was used to estimate the carbon footprint of each consumption data, based on the FFQ [88]. Nevertheless, the GHGe was only used to "validate" the index and is not used in the calculation of the score, which is only based on the quantity of the consumed food groups and the respective caloric densities, without any specific weighing according to the GHGe.

A cohort analysis revealed that Brazilians with greater PHDI scores (greater adherence to the EAT-*Lancet* diet) were 24% less likely to be overweight/obese [89]. Moreover, findings from the National Dietary Survey 2017–2018 revealed that the average PHDI score of the Brazilian population reached 45.9 points (95% CI 45.6–46.1), indicating extremely low adherence [90].

An important limitation of the index is that it does not account for the environmental and economic aspects of sustainability.

4.4. The Sustainable-HEalthy-Diet (SHED) Index

The SHED Index [79] was based on the EAT-*Lancet* reference diet and the Mediterranean Diet Score (MDS) [83]. It is based on 30 components, namely, healthy eating, dietary consumption, intake of sweetened beverages and bottled water, intake of ultra-processed food and plant-based foods, purchase of organic food, and food consumerism, including food waste and domestic waste streams [79]. In the final index, dietary intake is not accounted for, but sustainable dietary habits are evaluated through several questions (Table 1). The methodology behind the development of the SHED was innovative since it includes a variety of sustainable diet components, without relying solely on dietary intake cutoffs.

The Delphi method was applied to define the exact questions to be included in the questionnaire, with overall agreement on most issues. The participating experts had nutrition, public health, risk-assessment, environmental science, methodology, agriculture, and consumer behavior backgrounds, although no information regarding the number of experts was reported. According to the authors, organic farming was one of the issues not reaching a unanimous expert agreement, in light of the limited agricultural land per person in Israel, thus excluding this particular question [79]. Another issue of concern involved fresh food packaging—given that Israel has a warm climate, and fruits and vegetables are either sold in bulk, or packaged servings. Concerning this issue, the panel agreed not to include information regarding food packaging due to the lack of conclusiveness regarding the benefits and harms between health and the environment [79]. Two questions were assessed on a visual analog scale (VAS) of 100%, namely, compliance with recycling waste and packaging and the proportion of plant-based food in the diet. Regarding dietary intake, a semi-quantitative FFQ [91] with 115 food items, each with nine frequency options, was used to validate food consumption questions. Finally, a PCA was performed to evaluate the loading of each component in the algorithm.

A total of 348 Israeli men and women aged 20–45 years completed the questionnaire. Greater intake of animal protein intake was associated with a lower SHED Index, whereas more recycling efforts were associated with a higher score. As expected, MDS and SHED were highly correlated [79]. Furthermore, the SHED Index was consistent with the EAT-*Lancet* reference diet. No other studies have applied the SHED index to date.

According to the authors, an important limitation of the questionnaire is that it assesses various sustainable diet dimensions without quantifying GHGe, the main metric for evaluating environmental burden [79]. Another limitation is that dietary intake is not calculated or directly accounted for in the index; rather, sustainable dietary habits are evaluated. Furthermore, the index can assess the sustainability of nutritional choices without considering individual economic constraints, falling short of this specific aspect of the sustainable diet definition [11].

4.5. Indice de Dieta Saludable y Sostenible (IDSS)

The Mexican IDSS [80] was developed according to the EAT-*Lancet* reference diet. It is constructed of 13 food groups, including whole-grain foods, tubers and starchy vegetables, vegetables, fruits, milk and by-products, beef or pork, chicken and other birds, eggs, fish and seafood, legumes/soybeans/tree nuts, saturated fats, unsaturated oils, and added sugars. PCA was used to assess the loading of each component. The scoring is categorized in ≤ 5, 6, 7, 8, or ≥ 9 total points.

The index was validated in a sample of Mexican adults (N = 11,506) from the National Health and Nutrition Survey 2018–2019. The results revealed that men with higher scores demonstrated a lower prevalence of obesity, although the association between IDSS and obesity was not significant in women [80].

5. Other Indexes Assessing Dietary Sustainability, Developed Independently of the EAT-*Lancet* Reference Diet

5.1. The Healthy and Sustainable Diet Index (HSDI)

The HSDI [81] was the first reported effort to devise an index assessing dietary sustainability. The proposed methodology suggested its validation in a sample of 247 Australian young adults, aged between 18 and 30 years, participants of the Connecting Health and Technology study. According to the published protocol, 4 days of food and beverage images would be analyzed from a mobile food record (mFR) application. The mFR would calculate servings of eggs, red meat, dairy, fish and poultry, fruit and vegetables (including seasonality), ultra-processed energy-dense nutrient-poor foods and beverages, individually packaged foods, and plate waste [81]. This would result in the development of a prediction model for the HSDI. However, despite its novelty, the final product was never published.

5.2. The Sustainable Diet Index (SDI)

The SDI was designed to assess dietary sustainability, incorporating individual multi-dimensional indicators of sustainability [82], based on the FAO's definition of sustainable diets [11]. It includes seven indicators categorized into four standardized domains, representing the diet's environmental, nutritional, economic, and socio-cultural aspects.

An annual organic, previously validated, semi-quantitative 264-item FFQ [92] was used to collect data regarding the dietary intake of participants. The reported consumption and the probability of adequate nutrient intake (PANDiet) [84] were calculated for each participant, assessing dietary adequacy. Apart from nutrient adequacy, an additional sub-index was developed, assessing the adequacy of energy intake to meet energy needs.

Concerning the environmental impact, a specifically developed database of environmental indicators of raw agricultural products was used, assessing three indicators: GHGe, primary energy consumption, and land occupation. A partial score was calculated for each food product. The total dietary and environmental impact was estimated by multiplying the score by the quantity of food consumed, accounting for the agricultural production methods in each case.

The share of organic food in the diet was included in the index (biodiversity preservation), and the individual daily monetary cost of each diet was computed by multiplying the quantity of consumed goods by their price. Furthermore, an index was developed, evaluating the diversity of purchase places other than supermarkets and an additional one assessing the intake of ready-made products.

Each of the four domains (environmental, nutritional, economic, and socio-cultural aspects of the diet) receives a score between 1 and 5; thus, the total score can range from 4 to 20, with greater scores indicative of more sustainable diets.

The index was validated in a sample of 29,388 participants in the Nutri Net-Santé cohort study [82]. The results revealed that participants exhibiting a high SDI were concordant with the proposed sustainable diets in the literature.

As the authors noted [82], selecting a 1–5 rating scheme in each domain has an important effect on the index development. The authors opted for five categories, one for each sustainable diet indicator, aiming to discriminate participants without having many categories. Additionally, equal weights were given to the four sub-indexes, reflecting the absence of hierarchy in the FAO's sustainable diet definition [11]. Additionally, the authors expressed their interest in expanding the index in the future, aiming to include water footprint, fair trade, or crop treatment frequency indexes [82]. Last, but not least, since the index is based on the French recommendations for dietary intake, adaptation of the score and extrapolation outside France are not warranted.

Publication of the SDI gave the idea for cultural adaptations of the index in other countries. In this context, a Malaysian SDI was proposed and is currently being developed [81].

6. Conclusions

Despite the various tools and indexes developed to assess dietary sustainability, a gold standard is still missing. This is because the sustainable diet option is yet novel, requiring further research to understand the concept and reach a consensus on its aspects. Furthermore, most of the indexes are based on the EAT-*Lancet* reference diet, which has raised concerns regarding its limitations. After all, indexes developed using an a priori method tend to inherit various methodological limits [93]. However, no other alternative reference diets have been developed, and this indicates that research should be shifted towards new prototype diets before the development of more indexes. Undoubtedly, the EAT-*Lancet* report was the first attempt to solve a difficult problem and it was not within the scope of the present review to offer criticism without aiming to improve the development of future reference diets and upgrade the science of nutrition. Version 2.0 of the EAT-*Lancet* report is expected to be published in the year 2024, acknowledging that a consensus regarding the global targets is still missing [42]. Clearly, a takeaway point from the present review is that the design of one diet that is appropriate for all cultures, populations, patients, and geographic locations—that is environmentally friendly at the same time—is a difficult, if not impossible task.

For this, the development of sustainable and healthy diet recommendations that are region-specific and culturally specific, while at the same time, encompass all aspects of sustainability, is required. Researchers argue that increasing population adherence to the existing government dietary guidelines in each country would be a more realistic approach to improving the health and environmental impact of the consumed diets [94]. According to Springmann [95] and Kovacs [96], however, the current food-based dietary guidelines are incompatible with climate change, freshwater, land use, and nitrogen targets, and this should be corrected. As a result, the FAO and several individual researchers have pledged the incorporation of sustainability in the national and global dietary guidelines [95,97,98]. According to the Intergovernmental Panel on Climate Change, every country needs to evaluate how land and natural resources can be used for food production in the most sustainable manner, and consider socio-economic, natural site-specific, and cultural particularities of each geographic area before making suggestions for a sustainable diet policy [99].

The principles of sustainable healthy diets are set to provide flexible roadmaps for policy actors [100]. On the other hand, for a sustainable and healthy diet to be quantified, the dimensions selected for each index require meticulous assessment by relevant indicators [101]. According to Eme [102], and as demonstrated in the present review, the evidence basis for selecting specific and robust indicators for sustainable diet indexes is frequently weak, fragmented, and arbitrary. Furthermore, great heterogeneity is apparent among the included indicators and their weight on population health [100]. Many indexes do not adequately account for the diets' environmental impact, whereas others fall short in the economic impact domain. In parallel, consideration of the water footprint is missing from most indexes.

Last, but not least, the ethical aspect of the sustainable diet is under-examined in the currently available indexes. Fair trade is only accounted for in the SHED index, but the remaining authors have failed to incorporate this component in their sustainability scores. Environmental ethics are linked to food choice morality, and meeting social standards can often be more costly than meeting nutrient requirements [69,103].

In summary, it appears that the methodology behind the development of indexes to assess dietary sustainability is demanding, requiring the consideration of several sustainability aspects. Furthermore, the need for reliable, evidence-based prototype diets is also a demanding task, in order to ensure the trust of the public and the scientific community.

Author Contributions: Conceptualization, I.A. and M.G.G.; methodology, D.P.B., D.G.G. and M.G.G.; investigation, I.A., M.G.G., T.V. and T.M.; resources, D.P.B. and T.M.; data curation, I.A. and M.G.G.; writing—original draft preparation, M.G.G. and I.A.; writing—review and editing, T.V., D.G.G., T.M. and D.P.B.; supervision, D.P.B.; project administration, D.P.B. All authors have read and agreed to the published version of the manuscript.

Funding: This research received no external funding.

Institutional Review Board Statement: Not applicable.

Informed Consent Statement: Not applicable.

Data Availability Statement: Not applicable.

Conflicts of Interest: The authors declare no conflict of interest.

References

1. Vassilakou, T.; Grammatikopoulou, M.G.; Gkiouras, K.; Lampropoulou, M.A.; Pepa, A.; Katsaridis, S.; Alexandropoulou, I.; Bobora, D.; Bati, Z.; Vamvakis, A.; et al. *Practical Sustainable Nutrition Guide for Young People: Shifting Our Dietary Habits from Animal, to Plant-Based Foods*; WWF World Wild Fund: Athens, Greece, 2022.
2. DaMatta, F.M.; Grandis, A.; Arenque, B.C.; Buckeridge, M.S. Impacts of climate changes on crop physiology and food quality. *Food Res. Int.* **2010**, *43*, 1814–1823. [CrossRef]
3. Escarcha, J.F.; Lassa, J.A.; Zander, K.K. Livestock Under Climate Change: A Systematic Review of Impacts and Adaptation. *Climate* **2018**, *6*, 54. [CrossRef]
4. Brander, K. Impacts of climate change on fisheries. *J. Mar. Syst.* **2010**, *79*, 389–402. [CrossRef]
5. Zhu, C.; Kobayashi, K.; Loladze, I.; Zhu, J.; Jiang, Q.; Xu, X.; Liu, G.; Seneweera, S.; Ebi, K.L.; Drewnowski, A.; et al. Carbon dioxide (CO_2) levels this century will alter the protein, micronutrients, and vitamin content of rice grains with potential health consequences for the poorest rice-dependent countries. *Sci. Adv.* **2018**, *4*, eaaq1012. [CrossRef]
6. Medek, D.E.; Schwartz, J.; Myers, S.S. Estimated Effects of Future Atmospheric CO_2 Concentrations on Protein Intake and the Risk of Protein Deficiency by Country and Region. *Environ. Health Perspect.* **2017**, *125*, 087002. [CrossRef] [PubMed]
7. Willett, W.; Rockström, J.; Loken, B.; Springmann, M.; Lang, T.; Vermeulen, S.; Garnett, T.; Tilman, D.; DeClerck, F.; Wood, A.; et al. Food in the Anthropocene: The EAT–Lancet Commission on healthy diets from sustainable food systems. *Lancet* **2019**, *393*, 447–492. [CrossRef]
8. Grossi, G.; Goglio, P.; Vitali, A.; Williams, A.G. Livestock and climate change: Impact of livestock on climate and mitigation strategies. *Anim. Front.* **2019**, *9*, 69–76. [CrossRef] [PubMed]
9. Gerber, P.J.; Steinfeld, H.; Henderson, B.; Mottet, A.; Opio, C.; Dijkman, J.; Falcucci, A.; Tempio, G. *Tackling Climate Change through Livestock: A Global Assessment of Emissions and Mitigation Opportunities*; FAO: Rome, Italy, 2013.
10. Open Working Group on Sustainable Development Goals (OWG). *Sustainable Development Goals*; Technical report by the Bureau of the United Nations Statistical Commission (UNSC) on the process of the development of an indicator framework for the goals and targets of the post-2015 development agenda; United Nations Foundation: Washington, DC, USA, 2015.
11. Food and Agriculture Organization (FAO). *Sustainable Diets and Biodiversity—Directions and Solutions for Policy, Research and Action*; Burlingame, B., Dernini, S., Nutrition and Consumer Protection Division, Eds.; FAO: Rome, Italy, 2012.
12. Food and Agriculture Organization of the United Nations; World Health Organization. *Sustainable Healthy Diets: Guiding Principles*; FAO: Rome, Italy, 2019.
13. Trijsburg, L.; Talsma, E.F.; Crispim, S.P.; Garrett, J.; Kennedy, G.; de Vries, J.H.M.; Brouwer, I.D. Method for the Development of WISH, a Globally Applicable Index for Healthy Diets from Sustainable Food Systems. *Nutrients* **2021**, *13*, 93. [CrossRef]
14. Frederick Grassle, J. Marine Ecosystems. In *Encyclopedia of Biodiversity*, 2nd ed.; Elsevier: Amsterdam, The Netherlands, 2013; pp. 45–55. [CrossRef]
15. Hummel, M.; Hallahan, B.F.; Brychkova, G.; Ramirez-Villegas, J.; Guwela, V.; Chataika, B.; Curley, E.; McKeown, P.C.; Morrison, L.; Talsma, E.F.; et al. Reduction in nutritional quality and growing area suitability of common bean under climate change induced drought stress in Africa. *Sci. Rep.* **2018**, *8*, 16187. [CrossRef]
16. Smith, M.R.; Myers, S.S. Impact of anthropogenic CO_2 emissions on global human nutrition. *Nat. Clim. Chang.* **2018**, *8*, 834–839. [CrossRef]
17. Bista, D.R.; Heckathorn, S.A.; Jayawardena, D.M.; Mishra, S.; Boldt, J.K. Effects of Drought on Nutrient Uptake and the Levels of Nutrient-Uptake Proteins in Roots of Drought-Sensitive and -Tolerant Grasses. *Plants* **2018**, *7*, 28. [CrossRef]
18. Schmutz, J.; McClean, P.E.; Mamidi, S.; Wu, G.A.; Cannon, S.B.; Grimwood, J.; Jenkins, J.; Shu, S.; Song, Q.; Chavarro, C.; et al. A reference genome for common bean and genome-wide analysis of dual domestications. *Nat. Genet.* **2014**, *46*, 707–713. [CrossRef]
19. Lloyd, S.J.; Sari Kovats, R.; Chalabi, Z. Climate change, crop yields, and undernutrition: Development of a model to quantify the impact of climate scenarios on child undernutrition. *Environ. Health Perspect.* **2011**, *119*, 1817–1823. [CrossRef]
20. Challinor, A.; Wheeler, T.; Garforth, C.; Craufurd, P.; Kassam, A. Assessing the vulnerability of food crop systems in Africa to climate change. *Clim. Change* **2007**, *83*, 381–399. [CrossRef]

21. Beebe, S.; Ramirez, J.; Jarvis, A.; Rao, I.M.; Mosquera, G.; Bueno, J.M.; Blair, M.W. Genetic Improvement of Common Beans and the Challenges of Climate Change. In *Crop Adaptation to Climate Change*; Yadav, S.S., Redden, R.J., Hatfield, J.L., Lotze-Campen, H., Hall, A.E., Eds.; John Wiley & Sons, Ltd.: Hoboken, NJ, USA, 2011; pp. 356–369. ISBN 9780813820163.
22. Rouphael, Y.; Cardarelli, M.; Schwarz, D.; Franken, P.; Colla, G. Effects of drought on nutrient uptake and assimilation in vegetable crops. In *Plant Responses to Drought Stress: From Morphological to Molecular Features*; Aroca, R., Ed.; Springer: Berlin/Heidelberg, Germany, 2012; Volume 9783642326, pp. 171–195. ISBN 9783642326530.
23. Gong, M.; Chen, S.; Song, Y.; Li, Z. Effect of calcium and calmodulin on intrinsic heat tolerance in relation to antioxidant systems in maize seedlings. *Funct. Plant Biol.* 1997, *24*, 371. [CrossRef]
24. Wang, H.; Yang, Z.; Yu, Y.; Chen, S.; He, Z.; Wang, Y.; Jiang, L.; Wang, G.; Yang, C.; Liu, B.; et al. Drought Enhances Nitrogen Uptake and Assimilation in Maize Roots. *Agron. J.* 2017, *109*, 39–46. [CrossRef]
25. Nacry, P.; Bouguyon, E.; Gojon, A. Nitrogen acquisition by roots: Physiological and developmental mechanisms ensuring plant adaptation to a fluctuating resource. *Plant Soil* 2013, *370*, 1–29. [CrossRef]
26. Myers, S.S.; Zanobetti, A.; Kloog, I.; Huybers, P.; Leakey, A.D.B.; Bloom, A.J.; Carlisle, E.; Dietterich, L.H.; Fitzgerald, G.; Hasegawa, T.; et al. Increasing CO_2 threatens human nutrition. *Nature* 2014, *510*, 139–142. [CrossRef]
27. Kajala, K.; Covshoff, S.; Karki, S.; Woodfield, H.; Tolley, B.J.; Dionora, M.J.A.; Mogul, R.T.; Mabilangan, A.E.; Danila, F.R.; Hibberd, J.M.; et al. Strategies for engineering a two-celled C4 photosynthetic pathway into rice. *J. Exp. Bot.* 2011, *62*, 3001–3010. [CrossRef] [PubMed]
28. Masson-Delmotte, V.; Zhai, P.; Portner, H.-O.; Roberts, D.; Skea, J.; Shukla, P.R.; Rirani, A.; Moufouma-Okia, W.; Pean, C.; Pidcock, R.; et al. *Global Warming of 1.5 °C*; Intergovernmental Panel on Climate Change: Geneva, Switzerland, 2018.
29. Bennett, M.K. Wheat in National Diets. *Stanford Univ. Food Res. Inst.* 1941, *18*, 1–44.
30. The Core Writing Team; Pachauri, R.K.; Meyer, L. *Synthesis Report—Climate Change 2014 Contribution of Working Groups I, II and III to the Fifth Assessment Report*; Intergovernmental Panel on Climate Change: Geneva, Switzerland, 2015.
31. Smith, M.R.; Myers, S.S. Global Health Implications of Nutrient Changes in Rice Under High Atmospheric Carbon Dioxide. *GeoHealth* 2019, *3*, 190–200. [CrossRef] [PubMed]
32. Ewing, B.; Goldfinger, S.; Oursler, A.; Reed, A.; Moore, D.; Wackernagel, M. *Ecological Footprint Atlas 2009*; Global Footprint Network, Research Standards Department: Geneva, Switzerland, 2009.
33. Rose, D.; Heller, M.C.; Roberto, C.A. Position of the Society for Nutrition Education and Behavior: The Importance of Including Environmental Sustainability in Dietary Guidance. *J. Nutr. Educ. Behav.* 2019, *51*, 3–15.e1. [CrossRef] [PubMed]
34. Ranganathan, J.; Vennard, D.; Waite, R.; Dumas, P.; Lipinski, B.; Searchinger, T. GLOBAGRI-WRR model authors. In *Shifting Diets for a Sustainable Food Future*; World Resources Institute: Washington, DC, USA, 2016.
35. Alexandratos, N.; Bruinsma, J.; Global Perspective Studies Team; FAO Agricultural Development Economics Division. *World Agriculture towards 2030/2050: The 2012 Revision*. ESA Working Paper No. 12-03; FAO: Rome, Italy, 2012.
36. MacDiarmid, J.I.; Whybrow, S. Nutrition from a climate change perspective. *Proc. Nutr. Soc.* 2019, *78*, 380–387. [CrossRef]
37. Garnett, T.; Scarborough, P.; Finch, J. What is a healthy sustainable eating pattern? In *Foodsource: Chapters*; Food Climate Research Network, University of Oxford: Oxford, UK, 2016.
38. Hallström, E.; Carlsson-Kanyama, A.; Börjesson, P. Environmental impact of dietary change: A systematic review. *J. Clean. Prod.* 2015, *91*, 1–11. [CrossRef]
39. Oonincx, D.G.A.B.; de Boer, I.J.M. Environmental Impact of the Production of Mealworms as a Protein Source for Humans—A Life Cycle Assessment. *PLoS ONE* 2012, *7*, e51145. [CrossRef]
40. Lynch, J.; Pierrehumbert, R. Climate Impacts of Cultured Meat and Beef Cattle. *Front. Sustain. Food Syst.* 2019, *3*, 5. [CrossRef]
41. EAT Forum. EAT—The Science-Based Global Platform for Food System Transformation. Available online: https://eatforum.org/ (accessed on 3 August 2022).
42. Morrison, O. Industry Braces for EAT-Lancet: The Sequel. Available online: https://www.foodnavigator.com/Article/2022/06/06/industry-braces-for-eat-lancet-the-sequel (accessed on 4 August 2022).
43. Keys, A.; Mienotti, A.; Karvonen, M.J.; Aravanis, C.; Blackburn, H.; Buzina, R.; Djordjevic, B.S.; Dontas, A.S.; Fidanza, F.; Keys, M.H.; et al. The diet and 15-year death rate in the Seven countries study. *Am. J. Epidemiol.* 1986, *124*, 903–915. [CrossRef]
44. Grammatikopoulou, M.G.; Nigdelis, M.P.; Theodoridis, X.; Gkiouras, K.; Tranidou, A.; Papamitsou, T.; Bogdanos, D.P.; Goulis, D.G. How fragile are Mediterranean diet interventions? A research-on-research study of randomised controlled trials. *BMJ Nutr. Prev. Health* 2021, *4*, 115–131. [CrossRef]
45. Pett, K.D.; Willett, W.C.; Vartiainen, E.; Katz, D.L. The Seven Countries Study. *Eur. Heart J.* 2017, *38*, 3119–3121. [CrossRef]
46. Zagmutt, F.J.; Pouzou, J.G.; Costard, S. The EAT-Lancet Commission: A flawed approach? *Lancet* 2019, *394*, 1140–1141. [CrossRef]
47. Thorkildsen, T.; Reksnes, D.H. The Proof is Not in the EATing. *EuroChoices* 2020, *19*, 11–16. [CrossRef]
48. Zagmutt, F.J.; Pouzou, J.G.; Costard, S. The EAT-Lancet Commission's Dietary Composition May Not Prevent Noncommunicable Disease Mortality. *J. Nutr.* 2020, *150*, 985–988. [CrossRef] [PubMed]
49. Schoenfeld, J.D.; Ioannidis, J.P. Is everything we eat associated with cancer? A systematic cookbook review. *Am. J. Clin. Nutr.* 2013, *97*, 127–134. [CrossRef]
50. Ioannidis, J.P. Implausible results in human nutrition research. *BMJ* 2013, *347*, f6698. [CrossRef]

51. Zeraatkar, D.; Han, M.A.; Guyatt, G.H.; Vernooij, R.W.M.; El Dib, R.; Cheung, K.; Milio, K.; Zworth, M.; Bartoszko, J.J.; Valli, C.; et al. Red and Processed Meat Consumption and Risk for All-Cause Mortality and Cardiometabolic Outcomes: A Systematic Review and Meta-analysis of Cohort Studies. *Ann. Intern. Med.* **2019**, *171*, 703–710. [CrossRef]
52. Guyatt, G.; Oxman, A.D.; Akl, E.A.; Kunz, R.; Vist, G.; Brozek, J.; Norris, S.; Falck-Ytter, Y.; Glasziou, P.; de Beer, H.; et al. GRADE guidelines: 1. Introduction—GRADE evidence profiles and summary of findings tables. *J. Clin. Epidemiol.* **2011**, *64*, 383–394. [CrossRef]
53. Han, M.A.; Zeraatkar, D.; Guyatt, G.H.; Vernooij, R.W.M.; El Dib, R.; Zhang, Y.; Algarni, A.; Leung, G.; Storman, D.; Valli, C.; et al. Reduction of Red and Processed Meat Intake and Cancer Mortality and Incidence: A Systematic Review and Meta-analysis of Cohort Studies. *Ann. Intern. Med.* **2019**, *171*, 711–720. [CrossRef]
54. Vernooij, R.W.M.; Zeraatkar, D.; Han, M.A.; El Dib, R.; Zworth, M.; Milio, K.; Sit, D.; Lee, Y.; Gomaa, H.; Valli, C.; et al. Patterns of Red and Processed Meat Consumption and Risk for Cardiometabolic and Cancer Outcomes: A Systematic Review and Meta-analysis of Cohort Studies. *Ann. Intern. Med.* **2019**, *171*, 732–741. [CrossRef] [PubMed]
55. Platz, T. Methods for the Development of Healthcare Practice Recommendations Using Systematic Reviews and Meta-Analyses. *Front. Neurol.* **2021**, *12*, 1016. [CrossRef]
56. Brouwers, M.C.; Kho, M.E.; Browman, G.P.; Burgers, J.S.; Cluzeau, F.; Feder, G.; Fervers, B.; Graham, I.D.; Grimshaw, J.; Hanna, S.E.; et al. AGREE II: Advancing guideline development, reporting and evaluation in health care. *J. Clin. Epidemiol.* **2010**, *63*, 1308–1311. [CrossRef] [PubMed]
57. Harcombe, Z. US dietary guidelines: Is saturated fat a nutrient of concern? *Br. J. Sports Med.* **2019**, *53*, 1393–1396. [CrossRef]
58. Harcombe, Z.; Baker, J.S.; DiNicolantonio, J.J.; Grace, F.; Davies, B. Original research article: Evidence from randomised controlled trials does not support current dietary fat guidelines: A systematic review and meta-analysis. *Open Heart* **2016**, *3*, 409. [CrossRef]
59. DiNicolantonio, J.J.; Harcombe, Z.; O'Keefe, J.H. Problems with the 2015 Dietary Guidelines for Americans: An Alternative. *Mo. Med.* **2016**, *113*, 93.
60. Harcombe, Z. Designed by the food industry for wealth, not health: The "Eatwell Guide". *Br. J. Sports Med.* **2017**, *51*, 1730–1731. [CrossRef]
61. Lunny, C.; Ramasubbu, C.; Puil, L.; Liu, T.; Gerrish, S.; Salzwedel, D.M.; Mintzes, B.; Wright, J.M. Over half of clinical practice guidelines use non-systematic methods to inform recommendations: A methods study. *PLoS ONE* **2021**, *16*, e0250356. [CrossRef]
62. Grammatikopoulou, M.G.; Vassilakou, T.; Goulis, D.G.; Theodoridis, X.; Nigdelis, M.P.; Petalidou, A.; Gkiouras, K.; Poulimeneas, D.; Alexatou, O.; Tsiroukidou, K.; et al. Standards of nutritional care for patients with cystic fibrosis: A methodological primer and agree ii analysis of guidelines. *Children* **2021**, *8*, 1180. [CrossRef]
63. Wayant, C.; Puljak, L.; Bibens, M.; Vassar, M. Risk of Bias and Quality of Reporting in Colon and Rectal Cancer Systematic Reviews Cited by National Comprehensive Cancer Network Guidelines. *J. Gen. Intern. Med.* **2020**, *35*, 2352–2356. [CrossRef]
64. Kaiser, M. 58. 'What is wrong with the EAT Lancet report?'. In *Justice and Food Security in a Changing Climate*; Schübel, H., Wallimann-Helmer, I., Eds.; Wageningen Academic Publishers: Wageningen, The Netherlands, 2021; pp. 374–380.
65. Burnett, D.; Carney, M.A.; Carruth, L.; Chard, S.; Dickinson, M.; Gálvez, A.; Garth, H.; Hardin, J.; Hite, A.; Howard, H.; et al. Anthropologists Respond to the Lancet EAT Commission. *Rev. Bionatura* **2020**, *5*, 1023–1024. [CrossRef]
66. Hill, H.D.; Rowhani-Rahbar, A. Income Support as a Health Intervention. *JAMA Netw. Open* **2022**, *5*, e2143363. [CrossRef]
67. Gkiouras, K.; Cheristanidis, S.; Papailia, T.D.; Grammatikopoulou, M.G.; Karamitsios, N.; Goulis, D.G.; Papamitsou, T. Malnutrition and Food Insecurity Might Pose a Double Burden for Older Adults. *Nutrients* **2020**, *12*, 2407. [CrossRef]
68. Hirvonen, K.; Bai, Y.; Headey, D.; Masters, W.A. Affordability of the EAT–Lancet reference diet: A global analysis. *Lancet Glob. Health* **2020**, *8*, e59–e66. [CrossRef]
69. Drewnowski, A. Analysing the affordability of the EAT–Lancet diet. *Lancet Glob. Health* **2020**, *8*, e6–e7. [CrossRef]
70. Kousta, S. The cost of a healthy diet. *Lancet Glob. Health* **2020**, *4*, 9. [CrossRef] [PubMed]
71. Gupta, S.; Vemireddy, V.; Singh, D.K.; Pingali, P. Ground truthing the cost of achieving the EAT lancet recommended diets: Evidence from rural India. *Glob. Food Sec.* **2021**, *28*, 100498. [CrossRef]
72. Bloch, S. World Health Organization Drops Its High-Profile Sponsorship of the EAT-Lancet Diet | The Counter. Available online: https://thecounter.org/world-health-organization-drops-its-high-profile-endorsement-of-the-eat-lancet-diet/ (accessed on 25 June 2022).
73. Nutritioninsight Who Withdraws Endorsement of EAT-Lancet Diet. Available online: https://www.nutritioninsight.com/news/who-withdraws-endorsement-of-eat-lancet-diet.html (accessed on 25 June 2022).
74. Rappresentanza Permanente d'Italia ONU—Ginevra Press Release on the Launch of the EAT-Lancet Commission Report on Healthy Diets from Sustainable Food Systems (Geneva, 28 March 2019). Available online: https://italiarappginevra.esteri.it/rappginevra/en/ambasciata/news/dall-ambasciata/2019/03/comunicato-stampa-sul-lancio-del.html (accessed on 25 June 2022).
75. Zagmutt, F.; Pouzou, J.; Costard, S. Continuing the Dialogue on EAT-Lancet. Available online: https://www.epixanalytics.com/eat-lancet-criticism-correspondence.html (accessed on 25 June 2022).
76. MacMillan, S. ILRI/Livestock Science Leader Named to EAT-Lancet 2.0 Commission. Available online: https://www.ilri.org/news/ilri-livestock-scientist-named-eat-lancet-20-commission (accessed on 25 June 2022).
77. Knuppel, A.; Papier, K.; Key, T.J.; Travis, R.C. EAT-Lancet score and major health outcomes: The EPIC-Oxford study. *Lancet* **2019**, *394*, 213–214. [CrossRef]

78. Cacau, L.T.; De Carli, E.; de Carvalho, A.M.; Lotufo, P.A.; Moreno, L.A.; Bensenor, I.M.; Marchioni, D.M. Development and Validation of an Index Based on EAT-Lancet Recommendations: The Planetary Health Diet Index. *Nutrients* **2021**, *13*, 1698. [CrossRef]
79. Tepper, S.; Geva, D.; Shahar, D.R.; Shepon, A.; Mendelsohn, O.; Golan, M.; Adler, D.; Golan, R. The SHED Index: A tool for assessing a Sustainable HEalthy Diet. *Eur. J. Nutr.* **2021**, *60*, 3897–3909. [CrossRef]
80. Shamah-Levy, T.; Gaona-Pineda, E.; Mundo-Rosas, V.; Méndez Gómez-Humarán, I.; Rodríguez-Ramírez, S. Association of a healthy and sustainable dietary index and overweight and obesity in Mexican adults. *Salud Publica Mex.* **2020**, *62*, 745–753. [CrossRef]
81. Harray, A.J.; Boushey, C.J.; Pollard, C.M.; Delp, E.J.; Ahmad, Z.; Dhaliwal, S.S.; Mukhtar, S.A.; Kerr, D.A. A Novel Dietary Assessment Method to Measure a Healthy and Sustainable Diet Using the Mobile Food Record: Protocol and Methodology. *Nutrients* **2015**, *7*, 5375–5395. [CrossRef]
82. Seconda, L.; Baudry, J.; Pointereau, P.; Lacour, C.; Langevin, B.; Hercberg, S.; Lairon, D.; Allès, B.; Kesse-Guyot, E. Development and validation of an individual sustainable diet index in the NutriNet-Santé study cohort. *Br. J. Nutr.* **2019**, *121*, 1166–1177. [CrossRef]
83. Trichopoulou, A.; Costacou, T.; Bamia, C.; Trichopoulos, D. Adherence to a Mediterranean Diet and Survival in a Greek Population. *N. Engl. J. Med.* **2003**, *348*, 2599–2608. [CrossRef]
84. Verger, E.O.; Mariotti, F.; Holmes, B.A.; Paineau, D.; Huneau, J.F. Evaluation of a diet quality index based on the probability of adequate nutrient intake (PANDiet) using national French and US dietary surveys. *PLoS ONE* **2012**, *7*, e42155. [CrossRef]
85. Looman, M.; Feskens, E.J.M.; De Rijk, M.; Meijboom, S.; Biesbroek, S.; Temme, E.H.M.; De Vries, J.; Geelen, A. Development and evaluation of the Dutch Healthy Diet index 2015. *Public Health Nutr.* **2017**, *20*, 2289–2299. [CrossRef]
86. Guenther, P.M.; Reedy, J.; Krebs-Smith, S.M.; Reeve, B.B. Evaluation of the Healthy Eating Index-2005. *J. Am. Diet. Assoc.* **2008**, *108*, 1854–1864. [CrossRef]
87. Previdelli, Á.N.; De Andrade, S.C.; Pires, M.M.; Ferreira, S.R.G.; Fisberg, R.M.; Marchioni, D.M. A revised version of the Healthy Eating Index for the Brazilian population. *Rev. Saude Publica* **2011**, *45*, 794–798. [CrossRef]
88. Garzillo, J.; Machado, P.; Louzada, M.; Levy, R. *Pegadas dos Alimentos e das Preparações Culinárias Consumidos No Brasil*; FSP/USP: São Paulo, Brazil, 2019.
89. Cacau, L.T.; Benseñor, I.M.; Goulart, A.C.; Cardoso, L.O.; Lotufo, P.A.; Moreno, L.A.; Marchioni, D.M. Adherence to the Planetary Health Diet Index and Obesity Indicators in the Brazilian Longitudinal Study of Adult Health (ELSA-Brasil). *Nutrients* **2021**, *13*, 3691. [CrossRef]
90. Marchioni, D.M.; Cacau, L.T.; De Carli, E.; de Carvalho, A.M.; Rulli, M.C. Low Adherence to the EAT-Lancet Sustainable Reference Diet in the Brazilian Population: Findings from the National Dietary Survey 2017–2018. *Nutrients* **2022**, *14*, 1187. [CrossRef] [PubMed]
91. Shahar, D.; Shai, I.; Vardi, H.; Brener-Azrad, A.; Fraser, D. Development of a semi-quantitative Food Frequency Questionnaire (FFQ) to assess dietary intake of multiethnic populations. *Eur. J. Epidemiol.* **2003**, *18*, 855–861. [CrossRef]
92. Kesse-Guyot, E.; Castetbon, K.; Touvier, M.; Hercberg, S.; Galan, P. Relative validity and reproducibility of a food frequency questionnaire designed for French adults. *Ann. Nutr. Metab.* **2010**, *57*, 153–162. [CrossRef]
93. Waijers, P.M.C.M.; Feskens, E.J.M.; Ocké, M.C. A critical review of predefined diet quality scores. *Br. J. Nutr.* **2007**, *97*, 219–231. [CrossRef] [PubMed]
94. Steenson, S.; Buttriss, J.L. Healthier and more sustainable diets: What changes are needed in high-income countries? *Nutr. Bull.* **2021**, *46*, 279–309. [CrossRef]
95. Springmann, M.; Spajic, L.; Clark, M.A.; Poore, J.; Herforth, A.; Webb, P.; Rayner, M.; Scarborough, P. The healthiness and sustainability of national and global food based dietary guidelines: Modelling study. *BMJ* **2020**, *370*, 2322. [CrossRef] [PubMed]
96. Kovacs, B.; Miller, L.; Heller, M.C.; Rose, D. The carbon footprint of dietary guidelines around the world: A seven country modeling study. *Nutr. J.* **2021**, *20*, 15. [CrossRef] [PubMed]
97. Delabre, I.; Rodriguez, L.O.; Smallwood, J.M.; Scharlemann, J.P.W.; Alcamo, J.; Antonarakis, A.S.; Rowhani, P.; Hazell, R.J.; Aksnes, D.L.; Balvanera, P.; et al. Actions on sustainable food production and consumption for the post-2020 global biodiversity framework. *Sci. Adv.* **2021**, *7*, 8259. [CrossRef] [PubMed]
98. Mazac, R.; Renwick, K.; Seed, B.; Black, J.L. An Approach for Integrating and Analyzing Sustainability in Food-Based Dietary Guidelines. *Front. Sustain. Food Syst.* **2021**, *5*, 84. [CrossRef]
99. Smith, P.; Bustamante, M.; Ahammad, H.; Clark, H.; Ding, H.; Elsiddig, E.A.; Halberg, H.; Harper, R.; House, J.; Jafari, M.; et al. Agriculture, Forestry and Other Land Use (AFOLU). In *Climate Mitigaton of Climate Change. Contribution of Working Group III to the Fifth Assessment Report of the Intergovernmental Panel on Climate Change*; Edenhofer, O., Pichs-Madruga, R., Sokona, Y., Farahani, E., Kadner, S., Seyboth, K., Adler, A., Baum, I., Brunner, S., Eickemeier, P., et al., Eds.; Cambridge University Pres: Cambridge, UK; New York, NY, USA, 2014; pp. 811–922.
100. Harrison, M.R.; Palma, G.; Buendia, T.; Bueno-Tarodo, M.; Quell, D.; Hachem, F. A Scoping Review of Indicators for Sustainable Healthy Diets. *Front. Sustain. Food Syst.* **2022**, *5*, 536. [CrossRef]
101. Perignon, M.; Vieux, F.; Soler, L.G.; Masset, G.; Darmon, N. Improving diet sustainability through evolution of food choices: Review of epidemiological studies on the environmental impact of diets. *Nutr. Rev.* **2017**, *75*, 2–17. [CrossRef]

102. Eme, P.E.; Douwes, J.; Kim, N.; Foliaki, S.; Burlingame, B. Review of Methodologies for Assessing Sustainable Diets and Potential for Development of Harmonised Indicators. *Int. J. Environ. Res. Public Health* **2019**, *16*, 1184. [CrossRef]
103. Tsekos, C.A.; Vassilakou, T. Food Choices, Morality, and the Role of Environmental Ethics. *Philos. Study* **2022**, *12*, 147–152. [CrossRef]

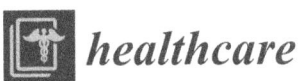

Review

The Experience and Enlightenment of the Community-Based Long-Term Care in Japan

Yun-Ru Zhou and Xiao Zhang *

School of Public Health, Southeast University, Nanjing 210009, China
* Correspondence: zhangxiao@seu.edu.cn

Abstract: (1) Background: China's population aging situation is severe, but the construction of the long-term care insurance system is still in its infancy. Through summarizing the long-term care experience in Japan, this paper explores the suggestions for the development of long-term care in China. (2) Methods: Based on literature research and policy review, we sorted out the relevant practices and safeguard measures of the long-term care insurance system in Japan, and summarized the characteristics of Japanese community care. (3) Results: In the development of long-term care services, Japan has gradually established a multi-level, systematic, and precise elderly care service model. Its community care has the characteristics of policy support, intensive intervention, complete elements, and strict evaluation. China's long-term care services should learn from Japan's experience, strengthen institutional guarantees, improve relevant supporting policies, encourage multiple subjects to participate in community care based on integrating community resources, and establish community care evaluation mechanism.

Keywords: long-term care; community care; preventive service; development experience

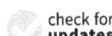

Citation: Zhou, Y.-R.; Zhang, X. The Experience and Enlightenment of the Community-Based Long-Term Care in Japan. *Healthcare* **2022**, *10*, 1599. https://doi.org/10.3390/healthcare10091599

Academic Editors: Sofia Koukouli and Areti Stavropoulou

Received: 7 July 2022
Accepted: 19 August 2022
Published: 23 August 2022

Publisher's Note: MDPI stays neutral with regard to jurisdictional claims in published maps and institutional affiliations.

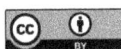

Copyright: © 2022 by the authors. Licensee MDPI, Basel, Switzerland. This article is an open access article distributed under the terms and conditions of the Creative Commons Attribution (CC BY) license (https://creativecommons.org/licenses/by/4.0/).

1. Introduction

In recent years, China's population aging situation is severe. According to the "China Statistical Yearbook 2021", as of 2020, the number of people aged 65 and over in China has reached 190.64 million [1]. A prediction study by Xiamen University on the scale of disability among the elderly in urban and rural areas in China shows that the total number of disabled elderly in China will rapidly increase from 43.75 million in 2020 to 91.4 million in 2050 [2]. The process of disability and dementia among the elderly in China is accelerating. With the progress of the economy, people have also put forward higher requirements for social security welfare. The demand for care services for disabled and dementia people has also given birth to China's long-term care insurance (LTCI). In 2016, China officially started the pilot work of LTCI and set up 15 pilot cities. In 2020, the number of pilot cities increased to 49. The National Medical Insurance Administration has also issued a series of guidance documents, policies, and regulations. However, China is still in the initial stage of promoting the construction and development of LTCI at the national level, and there are still many problems that need to be further solved and clarified.

"The 14th Five-Year Plan for National Economic and Social Development of the People's Republic of China and the Outline of the Vision for 2035" (2022) put forward the development goal of "building an elderly care service system coordinated by home and community institutions and combining medical care and health care" [3]. Before this, Sun Juanjuan (2021) had already proposed that it is necessary to build a multi-level care service system with families, communities, and institutions as the main body, expand the coverage of services, and make services penetrate into families and communities [4]. However, from the practices of the pilot cities, it can be seen that the long-term care services currently provided are home care and institutional care, and few cities independently carry out community care [5]. Xing Yuzhou (2021) believes that the current community elderly care service system in China not only needs to be improved in terms of the management system, but also faces problems such as a shortage of service personnel and insufficient specialization [6]. Therefore, China's current main task is to explore how to develop community care.

Long-term care (LTC) was derived from the report entitled "Establishing an International Consensus on Long-Term Care Policies for the Elderly" which was reported by the World Health Organization in 2000. It refers to a system of activities carried out by informal providers of caregivers (family, friends, and/or neighbors) and professionals (health, social, and others), which can ensure that people with limited self-care skills can maintain the highest possible quality of life based on individual preferences choice and enjoy the maximum possible independence, autonomy, participation, personal fulfillment, and human dignity [7]. Countries around the world usually provide basic living care or funds/service guarantees for medical care closely related to basic life for such people in the form of establishing LTCI [8].

LTCI was first developed in the United States around the 1980s and was introduced to Asia around 2000. Germany was the first country in the world to formally legislate public LTCI (1995) [9], while Japan was the first Asian country to establish public LTCI. LTCI in the United States is mainly composed of public security plans (Medicare, Medicaid) and commercial LTCI [10]. According to the research of Jing Tao and Yang Shu (2018), Medicare cannot provide real long-term care services or meet the long-term care needs of the disabled elderly. In addition, Medicaid plays a pivotal role in the long-term care system for the elderly in the United States, but it has strict restrictions, mainly for low-income individuals or families [11]. Germany decides whether to participate in public LTCI or commercial LTCI according to the income status of its citizens. Its LTC services include home care, partial institutional care, and full institutional care [10]. LTCI in Japan is compulsory for all citizens over the age of 40, and the insurance funds are jointly raised by social insurance and taxation [12]. It provides home care, institutional care, and community care.

Many Chinese scholars believe that China can learn from Japan's experience. Liu Xiaomei and other scholars (2019) believe that China has a rapidly increased demand for long-term care in an aging society which is similar to Japan, so we can draw inspiration from Japan's experience [13]. Zhao Jianguo and Shao Siqi (2019) both believe that Japan entered an aging society 30 years earlier than China, and Japan's experience in the construction of the elderly care system is very important for China to "completely build a home-based, community-based, institution-supported elderly care service system with complete functions, moderate scale, and coverage of urban and rural areas" [14]. Japan adopted a complete public LTCI model, the beneficiaries are only limited by age, not income level, and the development of community care is particularly prominent. The LTCI system currently being piloted in China is similar to that in Japan. In addition, because Japan and China both belong to East Asian countries, they are relatively similar in terms of physiological characteristics, living habits, cultural heritage, and social welfare concepts. Therefore, this paper takes Japan's LTCI system as the research object and mainly summarizes the development process of long-term care in Japan, especially community care, summarizes its characteristics, and puts forward suggestions for the development of community care in China.

2. Materials and Methods

The English literature was searched in PubMed with the phrases "long-term care" or "long-term care insurance" or "Community care" and "Japan" in the title or abstract. The articles that met the criteria were screened out by reading the title and abstract one by one, and the full text was obtained from literature databases and platforms such as PubMed, Medline, and Google Scholar. Chinese literature searched in literature databases such as China Journal Full-text Database (CNKI), Wanfang Data Knowledge Service Platform, etc. The abstract had to contain "long-term care insurance" or "community care" and "Japan". We selected articles that met the criteria by reading the title and abstract one by one, and read the full text selectively. The literature search period was from 2000 to 2021. At the same time, we browsed Japanese and Chinese government and agency websites related to LTCI to collect the required information. The data retrieval period ended in 2021. The data retrieval period ended at the end of 2021.

Inclusion criteria: We included relevant literature on LTCI policies or relevant laws and regulations.

Exclusion criteria: Literature without clear source; literature that mentions the name of the national (or regional) long-term care insurance policy, but lacks a description of the specific measures; literature that is published repeatedly.

The number of articles that were found in the initial search was 1378 (including 1258 English literature and 120 Chinese literature). The following types of documents were not included: Clinical trial, meta-analysis, randomized controlled trial, meeting abstract, editorial, proceedings paper, and other types such as opinions or comments (189 articles in total). According to the inclusion criteria and exclusion criteria, the final number of articles that were included in this paper was 28 (3 books not included).

Based on the literature research and policy review, this paper sorted out the safeguards of Japan's LTCI system, focused on the development of Japanese community care, and summarized the characteristics of Japanese community care. At the same time, based on the actual situation in China, it put forward relevant suggestions for the further development of community care in China.

3. Results

3.1. Long-Term Care Insurance in Japan

As one of the earliest Asian countries to establish the LTCI system, Japan has established a relatively complete care service system [15]. It is backed by law, has defined management departments, beneficiaries, finance sources, and care levels, and has rigorous care needs assessments, care market access, and supervision. The relevant information on its long-term care insurance system is shown in Table 1.

Table 1. The long-term care insurance system in Japan.

Country	Japan
Laws	Long-Term Care Insurance Act (2000)
Management department	Municipalities and Prefectures
The subject of the service being provided	For-profit corporations, non-profit organizations
Beneficiaries	Category I: the elderly aged 65 years and above Category II: people aged 40–64 years with disabilities
Finance	Half comes from taxes (25% from the Central Government, 12.5% from the prefectures, and 12.5% from the municipalities) and half comes from premium contributions.
Service/Payment Content	Institutional and domiciliary services
Care Levels	Seven care levels: two requiring support (levels 1 and 2) and five requiring long-term care (levels 1–5)

With the rapid change in the population structure and the disintegration of traditional family structures, in response to the expected shift from traditional home care to social care, the Japanese government took steps in the mid-1990s to promote the "socialization of care" for the elderly. In 2000, based on the "Long-Term Care Insurance Act", Japan launched the LTCI system to reduce the burden on family caregivers [16]. The purpose was to determine whether the elderly need to be cared for according to their physical conditions, and to provide corresponding care services according to the assessed care level.

The beneficiaries are divided into two categories: Category I beneficiaries are the elderly aged 65 years and above, and category II beneficiaries are people aged 40–64 years with disabilities. There are seven care levels, including two requiring support (levels 1 and 2) and five requiring long-term care (levels 1–5).

Municipalities, as insurance providers to the LTCI system, are responsible for implementing the LTC program and determining insurance premiums by measuring the balance between the needs of the population and the number of services available in the area. Half of the LTC service fees come from taxes (25% from the central government, 12.5% from the prefectures, and 12.5% from the municipalities) and half comes from premium contributions.

The Long-Term Care Insurance Act has been periodically revised every three years. The reforms in Japan's long-term care insurance are shown in Table 2. Due to an aging society, the LTCI has been facing escalating costs and recent reforms focus on cost containment, while keeping the quality and quantity of long-term care services.

Table 2. The reforms of Japan's long-term care insurance *.

Years	Contents
2003	Revision of the Category 1 premium, revision of long-term care fees
2005	(1) Enactment of the law to revise a part of the Long-term Care Insurance Law: amendments to LTC fees, premium rates, and portions of the Long-term Care Insurance Act (2) A review of facility benefit
2008	Strengthen government supervision: rectify nursing corruption and management system; strengthen the restraint mechanism of nursing institutions
2011	(1) Expand the content of nursing services (2) Improve the treatment of caregivers
2014	(1) Establishing the Community-based Integrated Care System: enriching services and making services more focused and efficient (2) Making Contribution Equitable: expanding reduction of premiums of people with low incomes, and reviewing co-payments
2017	(1) Promotion of initiatives for strengthening insurers' function, etc., toward independence support and prevention of serious conditions (2) Promotion of coordination between medical care and long-term care (3) Promotion of initiatives to realize a regional cohesive society (4) Increasing co-payment rate to 30% for those with particularly high income among persons bearing 20% co-payment (5) Introducing income-based payment system of long-term care levy (changing from capitation-based payment system)

* Compiled from relevant information on the official website of the Japanese Ministry of Health, Labour and Welfare.

Since the implementation of this system, the effect of LTC services has been obvious, and the system has been continuously improved. The mature LTCI system has laid the foundation for the formation of a community-based, small-scale, multi-functional elderly care service model in Japan [17].

3.2. Community Care in Japan

3.2.1. Development History

With the increase in the unmarried population, the acceleration of urbanization, and the increase in single-parent families or families with separated parents and children, the number of elderly people living alone in Japan is increasing [18]. In order to cope with the situation of rapid aging, after the implementation of LTCI, the construction of regional comprehensive services was strengthened, and it was proposed that community medical services should be effectively connected with LTC services, and the integrated community care system (ICCS) has been implemented since 2006. This system was designed to provide (1) medical care, (2) long-term care, (3) long-term preventive care, (4) living support, and (5) housing services collaboratively within a 30-min daily walk life circle (the ideal range for each community) [19]. This system is managed by municipal governments, using a fund from the LTCI system.

In 2012, the Japanese government launched the "Amendment to the Long-term Care Insurance Act to Strengthen Long-term Care Insurance Services", which clearly proposed to support the insured's sustainable life in the community environment where they are used to, and to integrate the originally independent living support and medical services. It is committed to building a community-based integrated care system that integrates medical care, long-term care, long-term prevention care, and living support and housing service [15], emphasizing the care concepts of self-help, mutual assistance, and public assistance.

In 2015, the "Long-term Care Insurance Act" was revised again, and some supplements were made: All care expenses (including home care) were handed over to the municipal community assistance centers for management; the community assistance services were enriched, home medical care was promoted, and a nursing prevention cooperation mechanism was implemented; community comprehensive care service seminars were to be regularly held; and it was stipulated that the occupancy level of special nursing care institutions should be above level 3, and further play the role of community elderly care functions and other related content [20].

In 2017, Japan incorporated disability services into community comprehensive care services to provide integrated, continuous/integrated services for the elderly and the disabled [21]. At present, the community has become the main carrier of social welfare such as pensions in Japan [22].

3.2.2. Characteristic

Comprehensive and Systematic Policy Support

In addition to the above-mentioned laws and regulations, Japan has also successively released the "Research Report on Nursing for the Elderly" (Ministry of Health, Labour and Welfare Elderly Nursing Research Association, 2003), and the "Report on the Community Comprehensive Care Service System Research Association" (Community Comprehensive Care Service System Seminar, 2013). "Law for Comprehensive Protection of Community Medical and Care Services" (2014) and other policy documents and research reports, to escort the implementation of community care.

Regarding the qualifications and incentives of caregivers, the Law on Social Welfare and Nursing Welfare Workers was promulgated in 1987, and a national qualification certificate was issued. When the Long-term Care Insurance Act was implemented in 2000, a care broker (nursing support specialist) was established. In 2018, the "Law on Improving the Treatment of Nursing Practitioners to Ensure the Reserve of Nursing Practitioners and Others" was promulgated to increase remuneration and activate the nursing talent market.

Regarding the construction of elderly care facilities and the environment, policy documents such as "Guidelines for Designing Housing for a Longevity Society" (1995), "Law on Promoting the Mobility of the Elderly and Disabled" (2000), and other policy documents have been promulgated successively. Relevant standards and requirements have been formulated for residential construction and community planning to provide a more comfortable and convenient retirement environment for the elderly [15].

In addition, Japan has also made policy regulations on the content of care services such as volunteer management, and has built a systematic and comprehensive policy system with the "Long-term Care Insurance Act" as the core.

Intensive Intervention and Early Prevention

After 2006, elderly with mild disabilities were included in the coverage of LTCI, and delayed the onset or worsening of disability further deterioration of this population by providing early intervention services to this population. Care prevention services (Services that prevent or reduce disability and improve life skills [23]) are provided in ICCS, focusing on care prevention management, developing care plans primarily for "requiring support" level 1 and 2 persons, and carrying out preventive work for those who can take care of themselves, etc. [24].

From the current point of view, the development of early prevention services can improve the health of the elderly, increase the healthy life expectancy of the elderly, and improve the quality of life of the elderly. In the long run, early intervention and prevention can help reduce the financial pressure on LTCI.

Integrate Resources and Complete Elements

Since 2006, Japan has positioned its long-term care policy as community-based integrated care, and is committed to building ICCS. Each community-integrated care service center is "small-scale and multi-functional". It provides services within a community, occupies a small area, and provides a variety of services. In addition to government-authorized care institutions and medical institutions, the subjects participating in the care service also include non-profit organizations, social workers, volunteers, and so on.

The ICCS includes five elements: "residence", "medical care", "long-term care", "care prevention", and "living support" [25]. "Residence" is the foundation; In addition to self-owned and rented houses, there are fully-equipped apartments for the elderly. "Medical care" refers to medical institutions, community hospitals, home medical care, visiting medical care, visiting rehabilitation, and other medical services. "Long-term care" includes institutional care and home care. "Care prevention" has been explained above. "Living support" includes the services provided by social workers and the support provided by volunteers from family and neighbors. The five elements are indispensable. They cooperate with each other to develop fragmented services into an integrated type and jointly maintain the normal operation of the ICCS [26].

Rigorous Evaluation and Continuous Improvement

The care work plan of ICCS in Japan is revised every three years and a strict evaluation will be carried out before revision. The PDCA (plan, do, check, action) cycle assessment is performed by using the "5W2H" (what, why, when, where, who, how, how much) assay.

The first step is to communicate with the client through the care meeting in the community to achieve information transparency and investigate the actual life and care needs of the elderly in the community, and then through quantitative analysis to find out the key points that the community needs to pay attention to and the society resource that needs to be explored. The second step is to share the situation, plans, and implementation results of each community through inter-community care conferences, which will help communities learn from each other to formulate more appropriate care plans. The third step is to discuss specific policies and formulate a final care plan and implement it strictly by the plan. Finally, the evaluation is carried out from multiple aspects during the implementation process, such as the service quality satisfaction evaluation of the service object, and the analysis and evaluation of the support status through the nursing support evaluation system.

At the same time, in order to ensure the quality of the care services, the government will also set up departments and agencies especially responsible for supervising care services, and promptly ban care service agencies with low service levels. Once the improper profit-making behavior of the care service institution is discovered, its qualification for care service will be canceled immediately.

Through the PDCA cycle evaluation mechanism, each community continuously improves service content and service quality, and then develops a community comprehensive care service center that conforms to the actual situation of each community.

3.3. The Enlightenment for China

3.3.1. Strengthen Institutional Guarantees and Improve Supporting Policies

At present, China has proposed to strengthen the functional connection between the construction of community elderly care service facilities and other community services in policy documents [27], but there is a lack of specific legal provisions and implementation rules. With the continuous exploration and development of China's LTCI system, we should seize the opportunity of the start-up of the LTCI system, combined with China's national conditions and the experience of pilot cities, further improve the relevant system guarantees through legislation. At the same time, according to the actual situation, stipulate the scope of each functional organization to realize the breadth and continuity of services [3], and to form a scientific and sound LTCI system.

In addition, it is also necessary to accelerate the introduction of supporting policies related to LTCI, and improve and standardize the behavior of the care industry constantly, including the qualification and incentives for caregivers, the standardization of elderly care facilities and environments, supervision, and demand assessment systems, volunteers management and other aspects of management and constraints to ensure that care services have laws to follow and violations must be investigated.

3.3.2. Optimize Community Care Service Resource Allocation

"Small-scale and multi-functional" community comprehensive care service centers can improve the utilization rate of care resources, provide convenient and fast services for care recipients, and effectively improve the satisfaction of care recipients. Therefore, various types of care service subjects should be encouraged and attracted to enter the community. We should integrate the elderly care service resources, and provide various types of services such as bed care, medical care, preventive education, and living assistance for care recipients in the community, to ensure that the care recipients can enjoy "residence", "medical care", "long-term care", "care prevention", and "living support" in the community.

At the same time, a community platform can be used to establish a coordination mechanism between care service agencies and care recipients, and help them formulate personalized care service plans according to their personal and family wishes. In addition, it is necessary to pay more attention to early mild symptoms. Through preventive education, regular screening, and early intervention, the development of severe diseases can be effectively avoided and the pressure on care funds can be reduced.

3.3.3. Encourage Diverse Subjects to Participate in Community Care Services

In Japan's community comprehensive care service centers, the main bodies involved in care services include government-authorized care institutions, medical institutions, and non-profit organizations, social workers, and volunteers. China should also form a pattern in which various subjects participate in community care services.

The most basic are professional care institutions and medical institutions. Professional care practitioners, doctors, and nurses provide corresponding care and medical services to care objects in the community. It is also possible to tap the social resources in the community and surrounding areas to provide assistance for the care services in the community, such as inviting social workers, non-governmental organizations, and non-profit organizations to regularly enter the community or even the homes of care recipients to provide health consultation, care needs surveys, life support, enrich entertainment life, and other services to alleviate the shortage of community care manpower. In addition, housewives, students, and elderly people in good health in the community can also be encouraged to participate, undertake part of the work of life support and psychological comfort, and formulate corresponding reward mechanisms, such as young people being included in individual volunteer hours, the elderly rely on payment in exchange for care services, etc.

3.3.4. Establish an Appropriate Community Care Assessment Mechanism

Drawing on the evaluation mechanism of Japan's ICCS, in addition to accepting supervision from the government, the community itself should also establish a service feedback and evaluation mechanism to ensure that the care recipients in the community can get better services. For example, regular assessments on the entities providing care services should be conducted, and institutions and care personnel with low service quality should be promptly dismissed. The evaluation should focus on the satisfaction of the care recipients in the community. The evaluation content may include service process, service quantity, service quality and satisfaction with care plan, etc. Then, a comprehensive overall service satisfaction evaluation should be conducted. Finally, according to the evaluation results combined with the needs investigation of the care recipients in the community, the care services in the community are adjusted accordingly. Dynamic adjustment or annual adjustment can be decided according to the actual situation of each region and community.

4. Discussion

In 2016, China started the pilot work of the LTCI system. However, China's LTC mainly relies on care service institutions at present, and the development of community nursing and institutional nursing is extremely unbalanced. Taking Nantong city as an example, by the end of 2021, the number of beds in care service institutions will exceed 96% of the city's designated beds, while there are only 3 hospitals and community health service centers providing care services, and the number of beds will account for less than 5% [28].

The traditional Chinese family culture makes people more willing to receive LTC services at home. Rather than living in LTC service institutions, the development of community care can not only satisfy people's desire to care for the elderly at home, but also effectively share the pressure of home care for family members. Therefore, this paper draws on the experience of establishing the ICCS in Japan, and puts forward relevant suggestions for the development of community care in China, expects that China's LTCI can also increase the emphasis on community care during the pilot process, enables home care, institutional care, and community care to develop together and share the responsibility for LTC. The most fundamental of which is to strengthen institutional guarantees, China can establish LTCI-specific laws or regulations to provide legal support for LTC services just like medical insurance. The supporting policies related to LTCI can also improve and standardize the behavior of the care industry; therefore, it is necessary to formulate LTCI-related management specifications as soon as possible such as the qualification and incentives for caregivers, the standardization of elderly care facilities, etc.

However, it should be noted that the LTCI system in Japan is not without its limitations, and faces many challenges. Two of the biggest issues are the sustainability of LTC funding and the shortage of nursing staff. The population is rapidly aging, and political turmoil and a natural disaster also burdened the country, and this has contributed to the potentially unsustainable problem of LTC funding. China's aging development is rapid, so the issue of LTC funding also needs to be paid great attention to, and it may be necessary to seek better financing methods to ensure the sustainability of funds. In addition, the low income of nursing staff has also led to a shortage of nursing staff, which is why we suggest encouraging diverse subjects to participate in community care services. In addition, we believe that how to improve the social recognition and treatment of nursing staff needs further research.

Author Contributions: Conceptualization, Y.-R.Z.; methodology, Y.-R.Z.; resources, Y.-R.Z. and X.Z.; writing—original draft preparation, Y.-R.Z.; writing—review and editing, X.Z.; supervision, X.Z. All authors have read and agreed to the published version of the manuscript.

Funding: This research received no external funding.

Institutional Review Board Statement: Not applicable.

Informed Consent Statement: Not applicable.

Data Availability Statement: The study did not report any data.

Conflicts of Interest: The authors declare no conflict of interest.

References

1. China Statistical Yearbook 2021. Available online: http://www.stats.gov.cn/tjsj/ndsj/2021/indexch.htm (accessed on 23 January 2022).
2. Zhang, L.; Fang, Y. Predictive research on the scale of disability and the cost of care for the elderly in urban and rural China from 2020 to 2050. *Chin. J. Health Stat.* **2021**, *38*, 39–42.
3. The 14th Five-Year Plan for National Economic and Social Development of the People's Republic of China and the Outline of the Vision for 2035. Available online: http://www.gov.cn/xinwen/2021-03/13/content_5592681.htm (accessed on 31 January 2022).
4. Sun, J. Elderly Care Service System in the Perspective of Healthy Ageing: Theory Analysis and Institution Conception. *J. Huazhong Univ. Sci. Technol. (Soc. Sci. Ed.)* **2021**, *35*, 1–8+72.
5. Wang, Q.; Yu, B. Pilot Analysis of China's Long-term Care Insurance System and Policy Suggestions for Future Development. *Health Econ. Res.* **2021**, *38*, 3–7.
6. Xing, Y.; Li, L. Accelerate the Construction of Urban Community Elderly Care Service System. *China Natl. Cond. Strength* **2021**, *10*, 17–21.
7. Jie, M. Comparison of international experience of the long-term care insurance system and its enlightenment to China. *Mod. Econ. Inf.* **2019**, *21*, 50–51.
8. Dai, W.D. *The OECD National Long-Term Care Insurance System Research*; China Social Sciences Press: Beijing, China, 2015; p. 5.
9. Chen, L.; Zhang, L.; Xu, X. Review of evolution of the public long-term care insurance (LTCI) system in different countries: Influence and challenge. *BMC Health Serv. Res.* **2020**, *20*, 1057. [CrossRef] [PubMed]
10. Li, X. The Long-Term Care Service System of the United States, Japan and Germany and Its Inspiration and Countermeasure to China. Master's Thesis, Dongbei University of Finance and Economics, Dalian, China, November 2017.
11. Jing, T.; Yang, S. Experience and reference of long-term care insurance system from the United States. *Chin. J. Health Policy* **2018**, *11*, 15–21.
12. He, P. The practice reflection and system trend of long-term care insurance fund-raising model in China. *Soft Sci. Health* **2021**, *35*, 8–14.
13. Liu, X.; Cheng, H.; Liu, H.; Liu, B. Vulnerability Analysis of Long-term Care Insurance System—The Enlightenment of Japan and Reflections on China. *Soc. Secur. Stud.* **2019**, *2*, 93–104.
14. Zhao, J.; Shao, S. Dimensional analysis and enlightenment of Japan's regional comprehensive care service system. *Soc. Sci. Front.* **2019**, *11*, 270–274.
15. Zhang, S. The Enlightenment of Japan's Community Comprehensive Care Service System to China. *Liaoning Econ.* **2020**, *3*, 32–33.
16. Annual Health, Labour and Welfare Report 2011–2012. Available online: http://www.mhlw.go.jp/english/wp/wp-hw6/index.html (accessed on 2 March 2022).
17. Li, X.H.; Zu, Z.L.; Yang, S.K. Analysis on the mode of elderly care and health industry in China and abroad. *Insur. Theory Pract.* **2019**, *3*, 141–150.
18. Comprehensive Survey of Living Conditions. Available online: http://www.mhlw.go.jp/toukei/list/20--21.html (accessed on 26 March 2022). (In Japanese).
19. Kojima, K.; Wan, J.L. Japan's Regional Differences of Ageing and Community Comprehensive Nursing System. *Soc. Policy Res.* **2017**, *6*, 3–14.
20. Takano, T. *In This Case, It Will Be Clear Long-Term Care Insurance*, 2nd ed.; Shoeisha Co., Ltd.: Tokyo, Japan, 2015; pp. 66–70.
21. Li, L.H. *Health Care in Japan*; China Labor and Social Security Press: Beijing, China, 2021; p. 137.
22. Zhang, J. Core Concepts and Development Paths of Community Welfare: A Comparative Study of China and Japan. *Chin. Soc. Secur. Rev.* **2018**, *3*, 133–147.
23. Zhang, J. Integrated Community Medical and Care Services: Exploration and Inspiration from Japan. *J. Anhui Norm. Univ. (Hum. Soc. Sci.)* **2021**, *49*, 74–82.
24. Tian, Y. Implication of the Long-term Care Policies for Older Adults in Japan and South Korea. *Soc. Constr.* **2017**, *4*, 10–19.
25. Ministry of Health, Labor and Welfare. Community Comprehensive Care in 2013. Available online: http://www.kantei.go.jp/jp/singi/kokuminkaigi/dai15/siryou1.pdf (accessed on 21 March 2022).
26. Shao, S. On Construction and reference of Japanese community comprehensive care service system. *J. Dongbei Univ. Financ. Econ.* **2018**, *6*, 69–76.
27. Several Opinions of the State Council on Accelerating the Development of the Elderly Service Industry. Available online: http://www.gov.cn/zwgk/2013-09/13/content_2487704.htm (accessed on 30 March 2022).
28. Zhou, Y. Research on the Practice of Long-term Care Insurance System—Take Nantong City as an Example. Master's Thesis, Southeast University, Nanjing, China, June 2022.

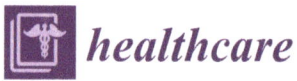

Article

Exploring Nurses' Working Experiences during the First Wave of COVID-19 Outbreak

Areti Stavropoulou [1,*], Michael Rovithis [2], Evangelia Sigala [1], Maria Moudatsou [3], Georgia Fasoi [1], Dimitris Papageorgiou [1] and Sofia Koukouli [3]

[1] Department of Nursing, School of Health and Care Sciences, University of West Attica, 12243 Athens, Greece; esigala@uniwa.gr (E.S.); gfasoi@uniwa.gr (G.F.); dpapa@uniwa.gr (D.P.)
[2] Department of Nursing, School of Health Sciences, Hellenic Mediterranean University, 71410 Heraklion, Greece; rovithis@hmu.gr
[3] Department of Social Work, School of Health Sciences, Hellenic Mediterranean University, 71410 Heraklion, Greece; moudatsoum@hmu.gr (M.M.); koukouli@hmu.gr (S.K.)
* Correspondence: astavropoulou@uniwa.gr

Abstract: During the COVID-19 outbreak, nurses employed in the clinical sector faced a number of difficulties associated with excessive workload, increased stress, and role ambiguity, which impacted nurses themselves and patient care. The aim of the present study was to investigate how Greek hospital nurses working in non-COVID units experienced the virus outbreak during the first wave of the pandemic. A descriptive qualitative research design was applied using a content analysis approach. To recruit the study participants a purposive sampling strategy was used. Ten nurses participated in the study. Data collection was conducted through semi-structured interviews. Content analysis revealed three themes namely, (a) emotional burden, (b) professional commitment, and (c) abrupt changes. Six subthemes were formulated and assimilated under each main theme respectively. Organizational changes, emotional burdens and feelings of fear and uncertainty, appeared to have a crucial effect on nurses and patient care. However, the professional commitment and the nurses' effort to provide excellent nursing care remained high. Nurses demonstrated that despite the burdens caused by the COVID-19 outbreak, the pandemic era created opportunities for thoroughness and accuracy in nursing care.

Keywords: COVID-19; nursing care; nurses' experiences; qualitative study

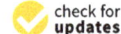

Citation: Stavropoulou, A.; Rovithis, M.; Sigala, E.; Moudatsou, M.; Fasoi, G.; Papageorgiou, D.; Koukouli, S. Exploring Nurses' Working Experiences during the First Wave of COVID-19 Outbreak. *Healthcare* 2022, 10, 1406. https://doi.org/10.3390/healthcare10081406

Academic Editor: Pedram Sendi

Received: 5 June 2022
Accepted: 25 July 2022
Published: 27 July 2022

Publisher's Note: MDPI stays neutral with regard to jurisdictional claims in published maps and institutional affiliations.

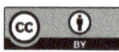

Copyright: © 2022 by the authors. Licensee MDPI, Basel, Switzerland. This article is an open access article distributed under the terms and conditions of the Creative Commons Attribution (CC BY) license (https://creativecommons.org/licenses/by/4.0/).

1. Introduction

In late 2019, the novel COVID-19 virus was identified as a rapidly spreading respiratory disease in Wuhan, China. Since then, the virus has spread worldwide, gaining a pandemic extent, with serious health, economic and social consequences. The latest evidence indicates that by April 2022, approximately 489 million people have been infected and over 6 million deaths have been reported globally [1].

Nurses have been at the forefront of caring for COVID-19 patients since the onset of the pandemic. Various studies highlighted the psychological impact on nurses working in COVID clinics, such as anxiety, stress, depression, and mental exhaustion [2,3]. The risk of infection, the fear of contamination, social isolation, and uncertainty were associated with work-related stress and anxiety among frontline health professionals [2]. In addition, lack of information about the novel virus, unpreparedness about the use of personal protection equipment (PPE), and changing policies have increased the levels of stress and uncertainty for all nurses, even for those who did not care for COVID patients [4]. Nurses globally appeared to share similar feelings of fear, moral conflict, need for preparedness and safety, sense of duty, and exhaustion [5]. Issues of vulnerability, family protection from possible infection, and yet professional commitment and collegiality appeared to be issues of significant importance for nurses all over the world [6]. Moreover, the COVID-19 pandemic led to unpredictable changes in health care organizations and nursing practice. Nurses faced many challenges such as high and abrupt demands in pandemic-related care, barriers in communicating with patients and families, and strict boundaries in physical contact with their patients [7]. Excessive workload, role ambiguity, and interpersonal conflicts at work, seemed to further impact nursing practice and patient care and expand stress, anxiety, and depression among nurses [8].

In addition, health care systems were not prepared to tackle pandemic and this lack of readiness was manifested through constantly evolving guidelines that caused confusion and discomfort among nurses [9–13]. This led to non-compliance and care inconsistencies, while nurses' performance in highly dependent clinical environments was hindered due to a lack of evidence-based treatment, insufficient knowledge about caring for COVID patients, poor patient prognosis, and lack of family presence [13–17].

Plenty of studies have been conducted worldwide to assess the psychological impact and the burnout frequency among frontline nurses during the pandemic [4,5,14,18–20]. Fewer focused on investigating the experiences of nurses working in general wards and the impact of the pandemic outbreak on the provision of nursing care [21–23].

In Greece, research evidence about the COVID-19 outbreak, has been mainly focused on investigating the mental health and the psychological impact of healthcare professionals and the general population, as well as the socio-economic effects and the health system responses to the pandemic crisis [24–30]. Data regarding nurses' experience from the first wave of the pandemic is lacking as research in this specific area seems to be rather limited in Greece.

In this respect, the aim of the present study was to describe how Greek nurses working in non-COVID units experienced the virus outbreak during the first wave of the pandemic. Furthermore, the impact of the pandemic on the provision of nursing care was explored.

Studying the nurses' experiences from the first wave of the pandemic is considered important, as the COVID-19 outbreak was an unprecedented, extraordinary public health challenge that brought up the need for new adjustments and innovative interventions in the health care field. This was an epoch-making and yet critical for the life and health era that nurses encountered for the first time. In this era when societies and health care systems were challenged by an unexpected and life-threatening event, nurses undertook the most crucial role of controlling the pandemic and caring for their patients. The nurses' experience at the very beginning of the pandemic, cannot be repeated or reoccur.

For this reason, the evidence raised from this study is unique, and it can be used as a reference point on how health professionals and health systems adapt and evolve when they face such challenges. Although, after the first wave of the pandemic, more waves have followed, the data derived from the very first days of the pandemic outbreak can be considered exclusive knowledge that may globally impact the further development of nursing science and practice.

2. Method

2.1. Design

A descriptive qualitative research design was applied using a content analysis approach. Qualitative description designs are particularly relevant when little is known about a phenomenon and the researchers seek information directly from those experiencing the phenomenon under investigation [31,32].

As Bradshaw [32] states, qualitative description research lies within the naturalistic paradigm, which supports the researcher to gain an understanding of a phenomenon through accessing the meanings conveyed by the study participants. The inherent inductive process, the subjectivity of the experience of the participant and the researcher, the active participation of the researcher in the research process, and the collection of the data in the natural setting of the participants who experience the phenomenon, are some of the main philosophical underpinnings of qualitative description approach [32]. To a further extent, evidence from qualitative description studies may offer methodologically sound and straightforward guidance on how to enhance healthcare practice, to foster more attentive work on the subject under investigation, and enforce organizational leadership and policies [31,32].

The researchers in the present study aimed to provide a rich description of the participants' experience and perspectives during the first days of the COVID-19 outbreak, a phenomenon for which little is known. Displaying an account of events and experiences as these were described from the participants' viewpoint was considered essential for gaining in-depth knowledge directly from those who encountered the phenomenon under study.

Learning from the participants' descriptions and using this knowledge to guide policy making and reframe practice are two of the inherently valuable attributes of descriptive qualitative designs [31,32].

For this purpose, this particular design was considered the most suitable for presenting how nurses experienced the COVID-19 outbreak during the first wave of the pandemic, within their clinical context.

2.2. Context and Participants

Registered nurses from the medical sector of a general hospital in Athens, Greece, participated in the study. A purposive sampling strategy was used to select study participants who provided nursing care in medical wards during the onset of the pandemic and had an adequate experience of the phenomenon under study. The inclusion criteria involved: (a) having a Bachelor's degree in Nursing, and (b) having at least two years of working experience in the clinical sector, as this time period was considered essential for the study participants to thoroughly present and discuss their experience regarding the research topic [33]. Nurse assistants and other healthcare professionals were excluded.

One member of the research team contacted the nurse managers of the proposed study sites and informed them about the nature and the aim of the research, so to gain their support and assistance in conducting the study. Informal meetings were held with potential participants within the hospital. Through these meetings, the study was advertised and appropriate information regarding the context of the research was provided to the participants. This process enhanced subjects' recruitment. Finally, ten female nurses from the medical sector participated and none of the participants withdrew from the study. The participants' working experience ranged from 7 to 25 years. They all had a Bachelor's degree in Nursing, while nine of them were MSc graduates.

2.3. Data Collection

The data collection phase was carried out from February to June 2020. In-depth, semi-structured interviews were used for gathering detailed information about the nurses' views and experiences. Interviews are considered the main tool of qualitative research, as it allows the researcher to gain a thorough understanding of the perceptions and beliefs of the people being asked [34]. The semi-structured interview consists of a flexible set of predefined questions and is used by the researcher as a guide to the issues which are considered important to cover within the interview [35]. It further provides the opportunity for the study participants to discuss and reveal their insights on complex or sensitive matters [36].

The interviews were conducted by a member of the authoring team who was experienced in applying qualitative interviewing techniques. The interviewer was a nurse, who was familiar with the context of the research without being actively involved in the work of the participants. This had a twofold effect, on the one hand, the participants felt comfortable expressing their opinions regarding the study topic, while, on the other hand, the appropriate neutrality regarding the role of the interviewer, was maintained [37]. Appropriate interviewing techniques were applied for encouraging the participants to provide detailed data [36]. The place and the time of interview were selected by the participants. Four interviews were conducted in a private area within the hospital and six interviews were arranged and completed via skype due to COVID-19 restrictions.

In the frame of the interviews, study participants provided evidence of their feelings and experience of the pandemic outbreak. Open-ended questions are displayed in Table 1.

Table 1. Interview scheme.

Interview Questions
I. How did you experience the COVID-19 outbreak at work?
a. How this event impacted care
b. How this event impacted you
II. How did you feel in terms of providing nursing care during that period?
a. Which were the bad and the good parts of it
III. How did you feel about the new conditions that evolved in your work?
IV. Other comments, thoughts, and feelings you would like to add

The interviews lasted from 20 to 30 min. They were all recorded and verbatim transcription took place immediately after the completion of each interview. All interviews were conducted in Greek and a backward translation technique was applied when the text was translated to English. This technique ensured the accuracy of translation and the correct rendering of the extracts' meaning [38]. Data saturation was achieved as no additional new information has been attained and further coding was not feasible after the ninth interview. Furthermore, saturation was also determined by the richness and thickness of the data which was obtained throughout the data collection phase. A wealth of the information gathered provided the best opportunity to answer the research question.

2.4. Data Analysis

Data were analyzed using a content analysis process. According to Sandelowski, this type of analysis fits better with the "straight description" of the data gathered in qualitative descriptive research designs [31]. Six steps of data analysis were used following Braun and Clarke framework [39], including familiarization with the data, coding the data, generating initial themes, reviewing and developing themes, refining, defining, and naming themes, and finally producing the report.

A member of the authoring team conducted the data analysis. In the first phase listening and reading the data repeatedly allows the analyst to be familiar with the data. Initial codes were formed (e.g., *emotional stress*) that identified basic elements of data (e.g., *uncertainty and fear*) having a meaning for the phenomenon under investigation. Following that, codes involving similar concepts were sorted out, leading to the generation of initial themes (e.g., *getting an emotional shock*). Reviewing and refining the initially formed themes led to the formulation of the final themes and subthemes accordingly, which reflected the essence of our data (Table 2).

Table 2. Coding and Generation of final themes.

Units of Analysis (Key Words and Phrases)	Basic Elements of Data	Initial Codes	Initially Generated Themes	Final Themes
"there was fear inside us" "it was fear and uncertainty"	Uncertainty and fear	Emotional stress	Getting an emotional shock	Emotional Burden
"the patients were there" "the work did not stop"	The patient and my work	Sense of duty	Being a responsible professional	Professional Commitment
"many changes happened at an organizational level" "nobody remained intact"	Shifts in personal and professional life	Reformed life	Experiencing a complete transformation	Abrupt Changes

2.5. Ethics

Before the commencement of the study ethical approval was requested and granted by the hospital's Scientific Board. (Ref. No. 15/9-7-2019). Furthermore, an informed consent form was given and signed by each participant before data collection. The participants were fully informed about anonymity and confidentiality issues. Voluntary participation and the subjects' right to withdraw from the study at any time without any penalty were also stressed. Permission was also given by the participants for tape recording the interview. To protect personal data code numbers were given to each one of the participants. Therefore, the interview excerpts used to illustrate the research findings, did not contain any identifying data.

2.6. Credibility of Research

Korstjens and Moser, suggest some techniques for enhancing trustworthiness in qualitative research [40]. Analyst triangulation and peer examination were two of the techniques applied in the present study. The former involved a second analyst who engaged to review the study findings and search for hidden concepts that might be overlooked. In this way, the integrity of the findings was reinforced. The latter involved rigorous feedback regarding the method the researchers' personal involvement and possible bias throughout the data collection and data analysis phase. Member check was also applied for confirming the findings' credibility [41,42]. The COREQ guidelines were used for reporting qualitative research as suggested by Tong et al. [43].

3. Findings

Ten female University graduate nurses participated in the present study. They were all employed as staff nurses in the medical sector with a minimum overall working experience of seven years. The demographic characteristics of study participants are presented in Table 3.

Table 3. Demographic characteristics of study participants.

Participants' Pseudonyms	Age	Marital Status	Years of Working Experience	Education
p1	47	married	24	BSc, MSc
p2	38	single	12	BSc, MSc
p3	47	married	25	BSc, MSc
p4	35	single	15	BSc, MSc
p5	31	single	8	BSc, MSc
p6	47	single	25	BSc, MSc
p7	37	married	13	BSc, MSc
p8	39	married	14	BSc, MSc
p9	42	single	17	BSc, MSc
p10	30	single	7	BSc

Data analysis revealed three themes namely, (a) emotional burden, (b) professional commitment, and (c) abrupt changes. Six subthemes were formulated and assimilated under each main theme respectively (Table 4).

Table 4. Themes and subthemes.

Themes	Subthemes
A. Emotional Burden	
	A1. The Fear of Contamination
	A2. The Uncertainty
B. Professional Commitment	
	B1. Caring for patients' well-being
	B2. The Work does not stop
C. Abrupt Changes	
	C1. The Organizational Shift
	C2. The Impact on Nurses and Care

3.1. Emotional Burden

Fear and uncertainty were the predominant feelings that participants experienced during the pandemic outbreak. Emotional distress was derived and enhanced by the unprecedented feelings and the ambiguous changes that an unknown situation brought up.

3.1.1. The Fear of Contamination

The nurses' anxiety about being contaminated was communicated throughout the interviews. The fear of being contaminated by the virus and transmitting it to their beloved ones was clearly reported. This feeling appeared to dominate the nurses' thoughts, despite the fact that in some cases remained hidden.

Mainly it was fear . . . . fear of not being contaminated . . . we were more afraid for our families not to be infected rather than for us. Generally, there was fear inside us but we tried to hide it, not to be shown to others (p1).

We were afraid of being contaminated, because potentially everyone could be positive (p2).

I was very worried . . . I wanted to stay safe and healthy, I was afraid of bringing the virus to my family (p9).

3.1.2. The Uncertainty

Feelings of uncertainty and vulnerability were also reported by the study participants. These feelings were reinforced by the COVID-19 restrictive measures, such as quarantine and lockdown.

It was a strange situation, there was a strange silence in the night shifts, it was uncertainty . . . and fear (p6).

There was fear and uncertainty . . . because at a time when everyone was telling people to stay at home we had to go out and come to the hospital . . . (p4).

This ambiguity seemed also to impact the nurses' perceived capability to provide the best patient care.

The situation is very ambiguous . . . The fear is still here, I think it will be with us for a long time. You want to do the best for the patient but on the other hand, you feel unprotected (p5).

3.2. Professional Commitment

The nurses' unique professional role was highlighted throughout the participants' statements, as the respondents were focused on their professional duty and the need to be next to the patients.

3.2.1. Caring for Patients' Well-Being

Many of the participants appeared to be frustrated or even reluctant to go to work in an era during which measures of social distance and lockdowns were applied worldwide. However, being next to the patients and provide care to them prevailed over hesitation and anxiety.

Our job is to be next to the patient, you have to take care for the sick person you wear your mask and gloves and you are there ... (p3).

I was frustrated ... I didn't want to go to work, I refused to go ... , on the other hand, I knew that the patients were there, waiting for me ... (p5).

We were anxious ... you are not sure if a patient has the virus or not ... then you start working and after a while, you forget the virus ... You cannot leave the patient ... you cannot ignore him ... (p6).

3.2.2. The Work Does Not Stop

The nurses continued to go to work as they used to do before the pandemic, since that was an imperative duty for them. PPE was referred to as an additional accessory, involved in patient care, necessary though for safely continuing their work.

We continue to work as we did before. Our work, our care did not stop ... we work as we used to do (laughing) having some additional accessories ... the mask ... the gloves (p1).

The work did not stop, we pay more attention to personal protection measures just to protect ourselves and our loved ones (p3).

Nurses also stressed their commitment to their work despite their psychological distress.

I am psychologically affected ... but I am still doing what I did before. When I have to go to the patients I'll go. When I have to give care, I'll do it. Nursing cannot stop (p8).

3.3. Abrupt Changes

During the first wave of the COVID-19 pandemic, unexpected and massive changes rapidly evolved worldwide. The health care systems were severely affected and major organizational alterations were implemented. This rapidly changing environment impacted both the healthcare professionals and the care provided within the healthcare organizations.

3.3.1. The Organizational Shift

Immediate and abrupt changes at an organizational level created frustration and anxiety for nurses. These new demands called for rapid adjustments that nurses tried to incorporate into their daily work.

Things were changed over a night ... the guidelines changed every day, many changes happened at an organizational level, reorganization of departments, staff deployment ... many changes were very annoying to us, to our work (p2).

At the end of the day, I do not know what bothered me the most, the fear of the virus or the changes that the top management imposed to us, the lack of information, the lack of equipment and material ... (p5).

There were big changes in the hospital, many new things that worried me, new rules, new equipment, new protection measures ... I tried to adjust and as time goes by I got used more or less to all these ... (p4).

3.3.2. The Impact on Nurses and Care

Within this rapidly changing environment, both organizational and personal strains appeared to affect nurses' performance in the delivery of care. Some of them reported that the use of PPE and the psychological burden caused certain limitations in dealing with the patient.

The pandemic affected me . . . the patient was alone and I could not go in and talk to him as I wanted to because of the protective measures . . . that was horrible (p10).

I have changed a lot, I am more distant with the patients, I am more distant at home, everything changed . . . the way you approach the patients, the things you do when you go back home, everything is new . . . and I am not relaxed the way I was before (p3).

Nobody remained intact in this situation . . . . although the work was reduced in our ward, which is a good thing, we were not happy . . . we were affected psychologically and this impacted on our work (p7).

Despite, the difficulties that COVID-19 caused, some nurses pointed out some positive aspects of the care delivered during the pandemic era. As previously reported, the better nurse/patient ratio due to reduced admissions and the strict compliance to safety measures, supported improved care. Feelings of anxiety and stress remained but this seemed not to hinder the provision of quality nursing care.

The work in our ward was better, we had fewer patients . . . we were not physically tired but we were more stressed . . . I suppose that now we have fewer patients and we can provide better care to them (p3).

We became more focused, more cautious, more diligent, when approaching patients, when we use the protection equipment, when we do hand hygiene (p9).

The pandemic added some more stress on me, but COVID did not stop me from providing excellent nursing care . . . (p8).

4. Discussion

The findings of the present study emphasized the nurses' experiences during the first wave COVID-19 pandemic. Emotional burden and feelings of fear, anxiety, and uncertainty, appeared to have a crucial effect on nurses' life and the care provided. However, the professional commitment and the nurses' effort to provide excellent nursing care remained high. In a rapidly changing environment involving a variety of stressors and burdens, nurses managed to show empathy for the patient, thoroughness, responsibility, and professional commitment. They faced abrupt changes including staff reallocation, rotation and understaffing, continuous use of PPE, and novel guidelines which should be strictly followed. These changes created a frustrating situation that impacted both nurses and patient care. Within this shifting and uncertain environment, some positive aspects were pointed out. These were mainly related to the reduced workload for non-COVID clinics, caused by the decreased number of patient admissions for routine treatment procedures. This enabled nurses to focus more intensively on patients' needs and safety and to provide thus a better quality of nursing care.

4.1. Emotional Burden: Fear and Uncertainty

Our findings revealed that fear and uncertainty were the most prevalent emotions among nurses throughout the pandemic's spread. The unexpected sentiments and the abrupt changes that COVID-19 brought up, resulted in emotional distress. The nurses' fear of becoming infected with the virus and infecting their loved ones was plainly expressed throughout the interviews.

Stress, anxiety, and fear were reported in the relevant literature as the most common emotions caused by the COVID-19 pandemic [4–6,9,13,44,45]. The fear of being contaminated was demonstrated specifically by the front-line nurses as they were in close contact with COVID-19 patients. Fear of death was also reported and several studies underscore that infection or death of colleagues and other health care professionals exacerbated nurses' fears and anxiety [12,16,17,45–48].

In line with our findings, the potential risk of transmitting the virus to their family and loved ones was also highlighted in the relevant literature as a factor that increased nurses' anxiety [11,49]. Emotional strain due to lack of understanding and feelings of guilt or self-blame for the infection of family members have been also reported by the frontline nurses [13,17,50].

Participants in the present study also expressed feelings of uncertainty and vulnerability that were reinforced by the COVID-19 restrictive measures and lockdown and influenced the nurses' ability to provide the best care to the patients.

In the same vein, findings from relevant studies have reported that nurses at the beginning of the pandemic have been left with a sense of uncertainty. As Galehdar et al., and Góes et al., point out the disease was unprecedented and therefore nurses worked under pressure due to a lack of available scientific information [11,45]. This ambiguous and unpredictable situation has inevitably brought about feelings of fear, uncertainty, and vulnerability in front-line nurses [47,51]. Uncertainty was also related to the variety and content of the information disseminated via media, which was referred to as one of the most stressful factors influencing nurses' emotions [4,10,11,15,44,45,49,52]. In addition, as the pandemic spread, nurses reported concerns about their future professional and personal lives [52], and this uncertainty and emotional stress led to physical and mental exhaustion, hindering thus their professional performance [11,16,47–50,53].

4.2. Professional Commitment: The Working Environment and the Patient

The importance of the nurses' distinct professional role was emphasized in the present study throughout the nurses' responses. The study participants were focused on their professional responsibilities and clearly demonstrated the necessity to care for their patients' well-being.

The significance of professional values and commitment were emphasized in various studies which explored frontline nurses' attitudes during the pandemic [9,11,12,45,49,50,54]. Specifically, a professional commitment was the foundation of nurses' motivation, while professional values and responsibility supported their commitment to work on the frontline without any hesitation and despite the fear and the risk of contamination [52]. Similarly, to the findings of the present study, Galehdar et al., Fan et al., and Góes et al., pointed out that nurses during the pandemic have made great efforts to preserve patients' well-being and to assist their family [11,45,50]. As such, opportunities to achieve their professional goals and values which enhanced their professional role and identity were raised [6,11,16,17,47,50].

Our study participants displayed their determination to keep working and caring for the patient as they did before the pandemic. PPE was regarded as an additional safety measure, which helped nurses to respond to their working responsibilities and to protect themselves and their families from the virus. This finding was in contrast with evidence raised from similar research in which nurses reported that PPE impeded vision and communication with the patient and prevented the provision of appropriate care [12,17,51–53]. Despite that, nurses maintained their professional commitment and expressed a sense of pride in achieving their professional goals [9,11,52].

4.3. Organizational Changes: The Impact on Nurses and Patient Care

The findings of the present study highlighted the unexpected changes that occurred during the first wave of the COVID-19 pandemic. Nurse participants referred to the rapidly changing environment that required immediate adjustments at an organizational, professional, and personal level. The nurses who tried to adapt to the new conditions felt frustration and anxiety by these sudden changes.

In the same vein, Fernadez et al. [15] illustrated the pressure on the nursing workforce during the COVID-19 outbreak which urged nurses to adapt to changes quickly, in a rather difficult and highly demanding environment. Bambi et al. [55] commented on the sudden organizational changes that were imposed by the hospital managers in order to effectively cope with the pandemic crisis, by pointing out that some of them (e.g., inappropriate staff skill mix due to staff shortage) hindered patients' safety and care. Furthermore, relevant research evidence confirmed the nurses' physical and psychological stress caused by the unexpected life and work changes. In this respect, nurses referred to supportive relationships, care, and understanding from colleagues and upper management as factors relieving negative feelings and facilitating a successful transition to new work patterns [5,12,15,17,52].

Our findings highlighted also the nurses' personal constraints, and the impediments to caring practices and communication caused by COVID-19. Thrysoee et al. [56] found that social distancing and fear of contamination affected nurses' life and caring practices.

In addition, the wide-ranging changes in health care organizations and the assignment of unfamiliar tasks to the staff increased nurses' burnout levels. This impacted negatively on nurses' personal and professional performance [57,58].

Despite the challenges faced, the nurses in our study identified a few positive aspects that supported the provision of care during the pandemic era. For example, improved nurse/patient ratio, lower number of admissions, and compliance with policies and safety procedures were referred to as factors that improved the standard of care provided in their wards.

In line with the findings of the present study, von Vogelsang et al. [59], who investigated the deficiencies in nursing care during the COVID-19 pandemic at inpatient wards, highlighted the crucial role of lower patients' admissions and the maintenance of nurse/patient ratio. However, during the first wave of the COVID-19 pandemic, the standards of care at non-COVID wards were regarded to be inadequate [60]. Even more, the pandemic crisis raised issues of inconsistencies in nursing care and low nursing performance due to nurses' mental health symptoms [61,62]. Stress, emotional exhaustion, and anxiety, impaired nurses' clinical performance and their ability to successfully attain the required nursing tasks [63,64].

Nurses in the present study stated that although levels of stress have increased due to the pandemic, this did not prevent them from providing excellent nursing care. This discrepancy between our findings and those of other studies might be explained by the nurses' strong sense of professional commitment and responsibility toward the patients. Furthermore, it might be stated that nurses in general wards experienced the pandemic outbreak less intensively [15,58,60,65]. Supporting health professionals who work both on the frontline and in the general wards is of critical importance and the role of nursing management in developing supporting strategies and maintaining quality practice has been widely recognized [5,66,67].

5. Limitations

This study involved ten nurses working in the medical sector during the first wave of the COVID-19 outbreak. Since this condition may limit the applicability of our findings, further research on this topic is recommended involving more participants from a variety of clinical sectors. Nurses' views of working in peripheral health care organizations located in non-metropolitan cities, may also contribute to further development of the knowledge gained so far in the relevant research field. Conducting interviews using alternative interview modes such as skype can also limit the researcher's access to body language and may inhibit the communication employed in face-to-face interviews. As such, the findings of this study should be viewed under these limitations.

6. Conclusions

Our findings stated that emotional disruption, fear, uncertainty, and frustration were amongst the dominant feelings that nurses working in general wards experienced. The abrupt changes caused by the pandemic drastically impacted nurses and care as the participants revealed that nobody remained intact. Professional values and commitment prevailed through over adversities and the virus did not stop nurses from providing excellent care despite the pandemic burdens. Within this changing environment, nurses identified some positive aspects and it appears that the pandemic created opportunities for practice improvement through increased caution, thoroughness, and accuracy in nursing care. This is an unexpected finding, as the prevailing perception at the period was that Greek nurses were under tremendous stress and overwhelmed due to the strain imposed on the health care system. This novel to us evidence may be utilized to enrich the current scientific knowledge on this topic and inform practice by providing an in-depth understanding of how nurses react and adapt in unexpected crisis situations. Further research on the experiences of health managers and leaders regarding organizational and governmental changes imposed by the pandemic, may also contribute to successful policy-making interventions during health crises.

Author Contributions: Conceptualization A.S., S.K. and M.R.; methodology A.S., M.R. and S.K.; data collection E.S.; data analysis, A.S. and M.M.; writing—original draft preparation, A.S., S.K., E.S., D.P.; writing—review and editing, M.R., M.M. and G.F.; supervision, A.S., G.F. and D.P. All authors have read and agreed to the published version of the manuscript.

Funding: This research received no external funding.

Institutional Review Board Statement: The study was conducted in accordance with the Declaration of Helsinki and approved by the Hospital's Scientific Board. (Ref. No. 15/9-7-2019).

Informed Consent Statement: Informed consent was obtained from all subjects involved in the study.

Data Availability Statement: Data generated during the present study is not possible to be shared due to issues of subjects' privacy and confidentiality.

Conflicts of Interest: The authors declare no conflict of interest.

References

1. World Health Organization. 2022 Weekly Epidemiological Update on COVID-19-5 April 2022. Available online: https://www.who.int/publications/m/item/weekly-epidemiological-update-on-covid-19-5-April-2022 (accessed on 11 April 2022).
2. Shreffler, J.; Huecker, M.; Petrey, J. The Impact of COVID-19 on Healthcare Worker Wellness: A Scoping Review. *West. J. Emerg. Med.* **2020**, *21*, 1059–1066. [CrossRef] [PubMed]
3. Batra, K.; Singh, T.P.; Sharma, M.; Batra, R.; Schvaneveldt, N. Investigating the Psychological Impact of COVID-19 among Healthcare Workers: A Meta-Analysis. *Int. J. Environ. Res. Public Health* **2020**, *17*, 9096. [CrossRef] [PubMed]
4. Nelson, H.; Hubbard Murdoch, N.; Norman, K. The Role of Uncertainty in the Experiences of Nurses During the COVID-19 Pandemic: A Phenomenological Study. *Can. J. Nurs. Res.* **2021**, *53*, 124–133. [CrossRef] [PubMed]
5. Zipf, A.L.; Polifroni, E.C.; Beck, C.T. The experience of the nurse during the COVID-19 pandemic: A global meta-synthesis in the year of the nurse. *J. Nurs. Scholarsh.* **2022**, *54*, 92–103. [CrossRef]
6. Fernandez, R.; Lord, H.; Halcomb, E.; Moxham, L.; Middleton, R.; Alananzeh, I.; Ellwood, L. Implications for COVID-19: A systematic review of nurses' experiences of working in acute care hospital settings during a respiratory pandemic. *Int. J. Nurs. Stud.* **2020**, *111*, 103637. [CrossRef]
7. Schroeder, K.; Norful, A.A.; Travers, J.; Aliyu, S. Nursing perspectives on care delivery during the early stages of the covid-19 pandemic: A qualitative study. *IJNS Adv.* **2020**, *2*, 100006. [CrossRef]
8. Rodríguez, B.O.; Sánchez, T.L. The psychosocial impact of COVID-19 on health care workers. *Int. Braz. J. Urol.* **2020**, *46*, 195–200. [CrossRef]
9. Bennett, P.; Noble, S.; Johnston, S.; Jones, D.; Hunter, R. COVID-19 confessions: A qualitative exploration of healthcare workers experiences of working with COVID-19. *BMJ Open* **2020**, *10*, e043949. [CrossRef]
10. Ohta, R.; Matsuzaki, Y.; Itamochi, S. Overcoming the challenge of COVID-19: A grounded theory approach to rural nurses' experiences. *J. Gen. Fam. Med.* **2021**, *22*, 134–140. [CrossRef]
11. Galehdar, N.; Kamran, A.; Toulabi, T.; Heydari, H. Exploring nurses' experiences of psychological distress during care of patients with COVID-19: A qualitative study. *BMC Psychiatry* **2020**, *20*, 489. [CrossRef]
12. Goh, Y.; Ow Yong, Q.Y.J.; Chen, T.H.; Ho, S.H.C.; Chee, Y.I.C.; Chee, T.T. The Impact of COVID-19 on nurses working in a University Health System in Singapore: A qualitative descriptive study. *Int. J. Ment. Health Nurs.* **2021**, *30*, 643–652. [CrossRef]
13. Kackin, O.; Ciydem, E.; Aci, O.S.; Kutlu, F.Y. Experiences and psychosocial problems of nurses caring for patients diagnosed with COVID-19 in Turkey: A qualitative study. *Int. J. Soc. Psychiatry* **2021**, *67*, 158–167. [CrossRef]
14. Guttormson, J.L.; Calkins, K.; McAndrew, N.; Fitzgerald, J.; Losurdo, H.; Loonsfoot, D. Critical Care Nurses' Experiences During the COVID-19 Pandemic: A US National Survey. *Am. J. Crit. Care* **2022**, *31*, 96–103. [CrossRef]
15. Fernández-Castillo, R.J.; González-Caro, M.D.; Fernández-García, E.; Porcel-Gálvez, A.M.; Garnacho-Montero, J. Intensive care nurses' experiences during the COVID-19 pandemic: A qualitative study. *Nurs. Crit. Care* **2021**, *26*, 397–406. [CrossRef]
16. Sheng, Q.; Zhang, X.; Wang, X.; Cai, C. The influence of experiences of involvement in the COVID-19 rescue task on the professional identity among Chinese nurses: A qualitative study. *J. Nurs. Manag.* **2020**, *28*, 1662–1669. [CrossRef]
17. Sun, N.; Wei, L.; Shi, S.; Jiao, D.; Song, R.; Ma, L.; Wang, H.; Wang, C.; Wang, Z.; You, Y.; et al. A qualitative study on the psychological experience of caregivers of COVID-19 patients. *Am. J. Infect. Control.* **2020**, *48*, 592–598. [CrossRef]

18. Nie, A.; Su, X.; Zhang, S.; Guan, W.; Li, J. Psychological impact of COVID-19 outbreak on frontline nurses: A cross-sectional survey study. *J. Clin. Nurs.* **2020**, *29*, 4217–4226. [CrossRef]
19. Cho, M.; Kim, O.; Pang, Y.; Kim, B.; Jeong, H.; Lee, J.; Dan, H. Factors affecting frontline Korean nurses' mental health during the COVID-19 pandemic. *Int. Nurs. Rev.* **2021**, *68*, 256–265. [CrossRef]
20. Hu, D.; Kong, Y.; Li, W.; Han, Q.; Zhang, X.; Zhu, L.X.; Zhu, J. Frontline nurses' burnout, anxiety, depression, and fear statuses and their associated factors during the COVID-19 outbreak in Wuhan, China: A large-scale cross-sectional study. *EClinicalMedicine* **2020**, *24*, 100424. [CrossRef]
21. Tiete, J.; Guatteri, M.; Lachaux, A.; Matossian, A.; Hougardy, J.M.; Loas, G.; Rotsaert, M. Mental health outcomes in healthcare workers in COVID-19 and non-COVID-19 care units: A cross-sectional survey in Belgium. *Front. Psychol.* **2021**, *11*, 612241. [CrossRef]
22. Fersia, O.; Bryant, S.; Nicholson, R.; McMeeken, K.; Brown, C.; Donaldson, B.; Mackay, A. The impact of the COVID-19 pandemic on cardiology services. *Open Heart* **2020**, *7*, e001359. [CrossRef]
23. Etesam, F.; Akhlaghi, M.; Vahabi, Z.; Akbarpour, S.; Sadeghian, M.H. Comparative study of occupational burnout and job stress of frontline and non-frontline healthcare workers in hospital wards during COVID-19 pandemic. *Iran. J. Public Health* **2021**, *50*, 1428. [CrossRef]
24. Kaparounaki, C.K.; Patsali, M.E.; Mousa, D.-P.V.; Papadopoulou, E.V.K.; Papadopoulou, K.K.K.; Fountoulakis, K.N. University students' mental health amidst the COVID-19 quarantine in Greece. *Psychiatry Res.* **2020**, *290*, 113111. [CrossRef]
25. Fouda, A.; Mahmoudi, N.; Moy, N.; Paolucci, F. The COVID-19 pandemic in Greece, Iceland, New Zealand, and Singapore: Health policies and lessons learned. *Health Policy Technol.* **2020**, *9*, 510–524. [CrossRef]
26. Kousi, T.; Mitsi, L.-C.; Simos, J. The Early Stage of COVID-19 Outbreak in Greece: A Review of the National Response and the Socioeconomic Impact. *Int. J. Environ. Res. Public Health* **2021**, *18*, 322. [CrossRef]
27. Siettos, C.; Anastassopoulou, C.; Tsiamis, C.; Vrioni, G.; Tsakris, A. A bulletin from Greece: A health system under the pressure of the second COVID-19 wave. *Pathog. Glob. Health* **2021**, *115*, 133–134. [CrossRef]
28. Parlapani, E.; Holeva, V.; Voitsidis, P.; Blekas, A.; Gliatas, I.; Porfyri, G.N.; Golemis, A.; Papadopoulou, K.; Dimitriadou, A.; Chatzigeorgiou, A.F.; et al. Psychological and Behavioral Responses to the COVID-19 Pandemic in Greece. *Front. Psychiatry* **2020**, *11*, 821. [CrossRef]
29. Kalaitzaki, A.; Rovithis, M. Secondary traumatic stress and vicarious posttraumatic growth in healthcare workers during the first COVID-19 lockdown in Greece: The role of resilience and coping strategies. *Psychiatriki* **2021**, *32*, 19–25. [CrossRef]
30. Kalaitzaki, A.; Tamiolaki, A.; Tsouvelas, G. From secondary traumatic stress to vicarious posttraumatic growth amid COVID-19 lockdown in Greece: The role of health care workers' coping strategies. *Psychol. Trauma Theory Res. Pract. Policy* **2022**, *14*, 273–280. [CrossRef]
31. Sandelowski, M. Focus on research methods: Whatever happened to qualitative description? *Res. Nurs. Health* **2000**, *23*, 334–340. [CrossRef]
32. Bradshaw, C.; Atkinson, S.; Doody, O. Employing a Qualitative Description Approach in Health Care Research. *Glob. Qual. Nurs. Res.* **2017**, *4*, 2333393617742282. [CrossRef] [PubMed]
33. Merkouris, A. *Methods in Nursing Res*; Ellin Editions: Athens, Greece, 2008.
34. Paraskevopoulou-Kollia, E.A. Methodology of qualitative research in social sciences and interviews. *Open Educ.-J. Open Distance Educ. Educ. Technol.* **2008**, *4*, 72–81.
35. Robson, C. *Real World Research: A Resource for Social-Scientists and Practitioner-Researchers*, 3rd ed.; Blackwell Publishing: Oxford, UK, 2011.
36. Boyce, C.; Neale, P. *Conducting in-Depth Interviews: A Guide for Designing and Conducting in-Depth Interviews for Evaluation Input*; Pathfinder International: Watertown, MA, USA, 2006; Volume 2.
37. Råheim, M.; Magnussen, L.H.; Sekse, R.J.T.; Lunde, Å.; Jacobsen, T.; Blystad, A. Researcher–researched relationship in qualitative research: Shifts in positions and researcher vulnerability. *Int. J. Qual. Stud. Health Well-Being* **2016**, *11*, 30996. [CrossRef]
38. Guillemin, F.; Bombardier, C.; Beaton, D. Cross-cultural adaptation of health related quality of life measures: Literature review and proposed guidelines. *J.Clin. Epidemiol.* **1993**, *46*, 1417–1432. [CrossRef]
39. Braun, V.; Clarke, V. Using thematic analysis in psychology. *Qual. Res. Psychol.* **2006**, *3*, 77–101. [CrossRef]
40. Korstjens, I.; Moser, A. Series: Practical guidance to qualitative research. Part 4: Trustworthiness and publishing. *Eur. J. Gen. Pract.* **2018**, *24*, 120–124. [CrossRef]
41. Anney, V.N. Ensuring the quality of the findings of qualitative research: Looking at trustworthiness criteria. *J. Emerg. Trends Educ. Res. Policy Stud.* **2014**, *5*, 272–281.
42. Noble, H.; Smith, J. Issues of validity and reliability in qualitative research. *Evid. Based Nurs.* **2015**, *18*, 34–35. [CrossRef]
43. Tong, A.; Sainsbury, P.; Craig, J. Consolidated criteria for reporting qualitative research (COREQ): A 32-item checklist for interviews and focus groups. *Int. J. Qual. Health Care* **2007**, *19*, 349–357. [CrossRef]
44. Arnetz, J.E.; Goetz, C.M.; Arnetz, B.B.; Arble, E. Nurse Reports of Stressful Situations during the COVID-19 Pandemic: Qualitative Analysis of Survey Responses. *Int. J. Environ. Res* **2020**, *17*, 8126. [CrossRef]
45. Góes, F.G.; Silva, A.C.; Santos, A.S.; Pereira-Ávila, F.M.; Silva, L.J.; Silva, L.F. Challenges faced by pediatric nursing workers in the face of the COVID-19 pandemic. *Rev. Lat.-Am. Enferm.* **2020**, *28*. [CrossRef]

46. Kalateh Sadati, A.; Zarei, L.; Shahabi, S.; Heydari, S.T.; Taheri, V.; Jiriaei, R.; Ebrahimzade, N.; Lankarani, K.B. Nursing experiences of COVID-19 outbreak in Iran: A qualitative study. *Nurs. Open.* **2021**, *8*, 72–79. [CrossRef] [PubMed]
47. Tan, B.Y.Q.; Chew, N.W.S.; Lee, G.K.H.; Jing, M.; Goh, Y.; Yeo, L.L.L.; Zhang, K.; Chin, H.-K.; Ahmad, A.; Khan, F.A.; et al. Psychological Impact of the COVID-19 Pandemic on Health Care Workers in Singapore. *Ann. Intern. Med.* **2020**, *173*, 317–320. [CrossRef] [PubMed]
48. Gao, X.; Jiang, L.; Hu, Y.; Li, L.; Hou, L. Nurses' experiences regarding shift patterns in isolation wards during the COVID-19 pandemic in China: A qualitative study. *J. Clin. Nurs.* **2020**, *29*, 4270–4280. [CrossRef]
49. Eftekhar Ardebili, M.; Naserbakht, M.; Bernstein, C.; Alazmani-Noodeh, F.; Hakimi, H.; Ranjbar, H. Healthcare providers experience of working during the COVID-19 pandemic: A qualitative study. *Am. J. Infect. Control.* **2021**, *49*, 547–554. [CrossRef]
50. Fan, J.; Hu, K.; Li, X.; Jiang, Y.; Zhou, X.; Gou, X.; Li, X. A qualitative study of the vocational and psychological perceptions and issues of transdisciplinary nurses during the COVID-19 outbreak. *Aging* **2020**, *12*, 12479–12492. [CrossRef]
51. Liu, Y.E.; Zhai, Z.C.; Han, Y.H.; Liu, Y.L.; Liu, F.P.; Hu, D.Y. Experiences of front-line nurses combating coronavirus disease-2019 in China: A qualitative analysis. *Public Health Nurs.* **2020**, *37*, 757–763. [CrossRef]
52. Lee, N.; Lee, H.-J. South Korean Nurses' Experiences with Patient Care at a COVID-19-Designated Hospital: Growth after the Frontline Battle against an Infectious Disease Pandemic. *Int. J. Environ. Res.* **2020**, *17*, 9015. [CrossRef]
53. Liu, Q.; Luo, D.; Haase, J.E.; Guo, Q.; Wang, X.Q.; Liu, S.; Xia, L.; Liu, Z.; Yang, J.; Yang, B.X. The experiences of health-care providers during the COVID-19 crisis in China: A qualitative study. *Lancet Glob. Health.* **2020**, *8*, e790–e798. [CrossRef]
54. Deliktas Demirci, A.; Oruc, M.; Kabukcuoglu, K. 'It was difficult, but our struggle to touch lives gave us strength': The experience of nurses working on COVID-19 wards. *J. Clin. Nurs.* **2021**, *30*, 732–741. [CrossRef]
55. Bambi, S.; Iozzo, P.; Lucchini, A. New Issues in Nursing Management During the COVID-19 Pandemic in Italy. *Am. J. Crit. Care* **2020**, *29*, e92–e93. [CrossRef] [PubMed]
56. Thrysoee, L.; Dyrehave, C.; Christensen, H.M.; Jensen, N.B.; Nielsen, D.S. Hospital nurses' experiences of and perspectives on the impact COVID-19 had on their professional and everyday life—A qualitative interview study. *Nurs. Open* **2022**, *9*, 189–198. [CrossRef] [PubMed]
57. Liberati, E.; Richards, N.; Willars, J.; Scott, D.; Boydell, N.; Parker, J.; Pinfold, V.; Martin, G.; Dixon-Woods, M.; Jones, P.B. A qualitative study of experiences of NHS mental healthcare workers during the COVID-19 pandemic. *BMC Psychiatry* **2021**, *21*, 250. [CrossRef] [PubMed]
58. Wu, Y.; Wang, J.; Luo, C.; Hu, S.; Lin, X.; Anderson, A.E.; Bruera, E.; Yang, X.; Wei, S.; Qian, Y. A Comparison of Burnout Frequency Among Oncology Physicians and Nurses Working on the Frontline and Usual Wards During the COVID-19 Epidemic in Wuhan, China. *J. Pain Symptom Manag.* **2020**, *60*, e60–e65. [CrossRef]
59. von Vogelsang, A.-C.; Göransson, K.E.; Falk, A.-C.; Nymark, C. Missed nursing care during the COVID-19 pandemic: A comparative observational study. *J. Nurs. Manag.* **2021**, *29*, 2343–2352. [CrossRef]
60. Nymark, C.; von Vogelsang, A.C.; Falk, A.C.; Göransson, K.E. Patient safety, quality of care and missed nursing care at a cardiology department during the COVID-19 outbreak. *Nurs. Open* **2022**, *9*, 385–393. [CrossRef]
61. Labrague, L.J.; de los Santos, J.A.A.; Fronda, D.C. Factors associated with missed nursing care and nurse-assessed quality of care during the COVID-19 pandemic. *J. Nurs. Manag.* **2022**, *30*, 62–70. [CrossRef]
62. Havaei, F.; Tang, X.; Smith, P.; Boamah, S.A.; Frankfurter, C. The Association between Mental Health Symptoms and Quality and Safety of Patient Care before and during COVID-19 among Canadian Nurses. *Healthcare* **2022**, *10*, 314. [CrossRef]
63. Labrague, L.J.; de los Santos, J. Fear of COVID-19, psychological distress, work satisfaction and turnover intention among frontline nurses. *J. Nurs. Manag.* **2021**, *29*, 395–403. [CrossRef]
64. Labrague, L.J. Pandemic fatigue and clinical nurses' mental health, sleep quality and job contentment during the covid-19 pandemic: The mediating role of resilience. *J. Nurs. Manag.* **2021**, *29*, 1992–2001. [CrossRef]
65. Sarboozi Hoseinabadi, T.; Kakhki, S.; Teimori, G.; Nayyeri, S. Burnout and Its Influencing Factors between Frontline Nurses and Nurses from Other Wards During the Outbreak of Coronavirus Disease -COVID-19- in Iran. *Investig. Educ. Enferm.* **2020**, *38*, e3. [CrossRef]
66. Tang, C.J.; Lin, Y.P.; Chan, E.-Y. 'From Expert to Novice', perceptions of general ward nurses on deployment to outbreak intensive care units during the COVID-19 pandemic: A qualitative descriptive study. *J. Clin. Nurs.* **2021**, Early View. [CrossRef]
67. Hofmeyer, A.; Taylor, R. Strategies and resources for nurse leaders to use to lead with empathy and prudence so they understand and address sources of anxiety among nurses practising in the era of COVID-19. *J. Clin. Nurs.* **2021**, *30*, 298–305. [CrossRef]

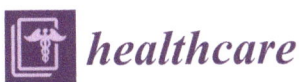

Article

Care and Safety of Schoolchildren with Type 1 Diabetes Mellitus: Parental Perceptions of the School Nurse Role

Marianna Drakopoulou [1,*], Panagiota Begni [2], Alexandra Mantoudi [1], Marianna Mantzorou [1], Georgia Gerogianni [1], Theodoula Adamakidou [1], Victoria Alikari [1], Ioannis Kalemikerakis [1], Anna Kavga [1], Sotirios Plakas [1], Georgia Fasoi [1] and Paraskevi Apostolara [1]

1. Department of Nursing, Faculty of Health Sciences, University of West Attica, 122 43 Athens, Greece; amantoudi@uniwa.gr (A.M.); mantzorou@uniwa.gr (M.M.); ggerogiani@uniwa.gr (G.G.); thadam@uniwa.gr (T.A.); vicalikari@uniwa.gr (V.A.); ikalemik@uniwa.gr (I.K.); akavga@uniwa.gr (A.K.); skplakas@uniwa.gr (S.P.); gfasoi@uniwa.gr (G.F.); vapostolara@uniwa.gr (P.A.)
2. 1st Health Center of Salamina, 189 00 Salamina, Greece; yiotabegni@gmail.com
* Correspondence: mdrakopoulou@uniwa.gr

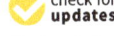

Citation: Drakopoulou, M.; Begni, P.; Mantoudi, A.; Mantzorou, M.; Gerogianni, G.; Adamakidou, T.; Alikari, V.; Kalemikerakis, I.; Kavga, A.; Plakas, S.; et al. Care and Safety of Schoolchildren with Type 1 Diabetes Mellitus: Parental Perceptions of the School Nurse Role. *Healthcare* 2022, *10*, 1228. https://doi.org/10.3390/healthcare10071228

Academic Editor: Pedram Sendi

Received: 17 June 2022
Accepted: 29 June 2022
Published: 30 June 2022

Publisher's Note: MDPI stays neutral with regard to jurisdictional claims in published maps and institutional affiliations.

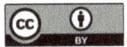

Copyright: © 2022 by the authors. Licensee MDPI, Basel, Switzerland. This article is an open access article distributed under the terms and conditions of the Creative Commons Attribution (CC BY) license (https://creativecommons.org/licenses/by/4.0/).

Abstract: Schoolchildren with type 1 diabetes mellitus (T1DM) need supervision in the management of their disorder by the school nurse, securing proper care and safety in the school environment. The aim of this study was to investigate the parents' perceptions regarding the care and safety of their children with T1DM at school. In this cross-sectional study, 356 parents of children with T1DM attending primary and secondary school (convenience sample) completed the "Parents' Opinions about School-based Care for Children with Diabetes" and the "Safety of children with T1DM at school". The majority (58.8%) noted that their children received some care from a school nurse, less than half (44.6%) declared feeling very safe concerning diabetes care, and 42.5% reported high levels of diabetes management satisfaction. Younger age of the child ($p < 0.001$), school nurses' advanced diabetic care skills ($p < 0.001$), existence of school nurse's office ($p < 0.05$) and higher educational level of the father were positively correlated with higher parental feelings of safety and satisfaction. The presence of a school nurse was associated with higher academic performance ($p < 0.001$), significantly fewer absences due to the disorder ($p < 0.001$) and better diabetes management ($p < 0.043$). The daily presence of a school nurse in school decreases absenteeism, greatly improves school performance and enhances diabetic management of schoolchildren with T1DM.

Keywords: type 1 diabetes mellitus; school nursing; school-based care; school-based safety; parental perceptions

1. Introduction

Type 1 diabetes mellitus (T1DM) is the commonest metabolic disorder in children [1]. It is a chronic autoimmune disease that leads to progressive destruction of the β pancreatic cells and culminates in non-secretion of insulin and persistent hyperglycemia [2]. Diabetes care requires lifestyle adjustments and a daily management routine [3], including the time spent in school [4], which may be up to seven hours daily [5,6]. Proper management of T1DM daily at school is associated with improved metabolic control, minimization of the risk of hypoglycemia and, in general, better quality of life, as it reduces the risk of microvascular complications or delays their development [7]. In addition, T1DM is associated with low academic achievement due to difficulties in glucose control, absenteeism and lack of concentration [8]. The school nurse's presence guarantees the proper management of metabolic control, as well as the safety and also the academic development of students who face special health problems such as T1DM [9].

A sense of security at school is important for adjustment and progress. Students' high self-esteem is associated with a strong sense of security at school [10–12]. In general, a safe school environment improves the educational experience and enhances the well-being and health of students [13]. The strategies that make school a safe environment focus on health education so that students may adopt behaviors that promote health and safety. Schools are, therefore, called upon to play an important role in promoting health and preventing illness and injury [14]. However, in a recent US study, it was found that the school staff was not well trained and did not have confidence in their diabetes management skills [15].

A 2017 qualitative study in Brazil revealed that successful management of diabetes requires the cooperation of school nurses, school staff and families of children with T1DM [16]. Although families largely determine the development of health-promoting behaviors, the school nurse can reinforce desirable behaviors and dampen down unwanted ones [17]. It thus emerges that there is a need for nursing care of the student with T1DM in the school environment, so that the school on the one hand is a safe environment and on the other offers the same level of access to educational opportunities to all children [18].

However, despite global research affirming the benefits of school nursing, there are developed countries where the majority of schools do not have school nurses [19], but even among countries that implement school nursing, there is variability in the practice of school nursing [20]. In addition to providing care to students in emergencies, the impact of providing integrated school nursing was investigated in a 2017 study in Turkey that concluded that integrated school nursing contributed positively to students' academic performance [21]. In schools where students report fewer problems, higher academic goals are set by them [10]. A similar study in public high schools in America found a possible link between students attending schools with a full-time school nurse and significantly higher graduation rates, lower student absenteeism and higher college enrollment scores. This, according to the researchers, was due to school nursing improving health indicators and at the same time contributing to the improvement of academic achievement [22]. During the turbulent period of adolescence, the management of T1DM becomes even more difficult. A 2017 survey in the US identified concerns that focused, among other things, on the lack of full-time nurses in schools, a lack of relevant T1DM teacher information, the lack of access among diabetic children to self-care supplies, and limited communication between parents and school staff about diabetes, resulting in diabetes having an impact on long-term well-being in adulthood [7]. The presence of a school nurse ensures the safety of all schoolchildren, both healthy and those facing health problems, such as T1DM, and, in this instance, guarantees proper management of metabolic control and academic development of children with diabetes [9].

In Greece, school nurses are usually employed in special education schools and private schools. According to the legislature, school nurses can also be employed in general public primary schools at the specific request of the parents of children with special healthcare needs. A medical diagnosis and report from a public hospital doctor is a necessary requirement, in which the need for the support of a school nurse has to be documented. So, a school nurse in general public education is annually employed in primary schools only if there are children with a special healthcare needs diagnosis [23].

Limited studies have been conducted in Greece to explore the views of parents of schoolchildren with T1DM regarding the care and safety provided by a school nurse to their children in the school environment. The present study sought to highlight the problems faced by diabetic children in school—and consequently by Greek families—throughout the country, as well as the role of school nurses in the management of T1DM in the school community, and to highlight their important contribution to the wider Greek society.

2. Materials and Methods

2.1. Instruments

In the present cross-sectional correlational descriptive study, a demographic and clinical characteristics questionnaire of the participants and the following two scales were used:

"Parents' Opinions about School-based Care for Children with Diabetes" by Driscoll et al. [24].

This is a 38-item questionnaire with sections on information about the child, the diabetes care training of the school personnel, parental opinions about the child's safety in school, staff handling of low or high blood glucose incidents at school, the medical staff in the child's school and school policies on managing diabetes.

"Survey for safety of children with T1DM at school" by Alaqeel [25]. This is a 30-item questionnaire examining diabetic management at school, negative peer comments, absenteeism and school performance for children with T1DM.

Participants were able to answer each question regarding their opinions on a 5-point Likert scale.

Cultural weighting of both the questionnaires for adaptation to the Greek language was performed following permission for use from the authors. A reverse translation of the questionnaire was performed, from English to Greek and vice versa by two independent translators following the standard guidelines for questionnaire translation to the Greek language.

Prior to the main study, a pilot study was conducted on nine parents of schoolchildren with T1DM in order to check for any difficulties in comprehension of the questionnaires' content. Based on the results of this pilot study, no modifications were made. The data obtained from these questionnaires were s not included in the study.

2.2. Participants and Data Collection

The sample consisted of 356 parents (288 mothers and 68 fathers) with a child with type 1 diabetes. As there are no school nurses in general public schools, only parents of children with special healthcare needs are familiar with the concept of school nursing. So, an online platform was created through Google forms for participation in the study and was made available to six (6) associations and two (2) online groups of parents of children with T1DM in primary and secondary education, from all parts of the country. Inclusion criteria were (a) being over 18 years of age, (b) being parents of children with T1DM in primary (6–12 years) or secondary (13–18 years) education, and (c) having an oral and written understanding of the Greek language.

For the realization of the study, permission was requested from the boards of the associations of parents of schoolchildren with T1DM, and their consent was secured. Permission was also sought from and granted by the website and group administrators, following which the questionnaire was disseminated. A convenience sample of parents of schoolchildren with T1DM was collected from March 2020 until May 2020. The study conformed to the rules of ethics that govern the research process.

3. Statistical Analysis

Quantitative variables were expressed as mean values (standard deviation) and as median (interquartile range), while qualitative variables were expressed as absolute and relative frequencies. Mann–Whitney test was used for the comparison of continuous variables between two groups. For the comparison of proportions, chi-square and Fisher's exact tests were used. Logistic regression analysis in a stepwise method (p for entry 0.05, p for removal 0.10) was used in order to find independent factors associated with parents feeling very/extremely safe with the care provided to their children during a normal school day and parents feeling very/extremely satisfied with the care provided to their children during a normal school day as dependent variables. Adjusted odds ratios (OR) with 95% confidence intervals (95% CI) were computed from the results of the logistic regression analyses. All reported p values are two-tailed. Statistical significance was set at $p < 0.05$, and analyses were conducted using SPSS statistical software (version 22.0).

4. Results

The demographic characteristics of the parents and children are presented in Table 1.

Table 1. Sample characteristics.

	n (%)
School	
Public	330 (93.2)
Private	24 (6.8)
School catchment area population density	
up to 1999 residents	22 (6.3)
2000–9999 residents	56 (15.9)
10,000–250,000 residents	178 (50.6)
more than 250,000 residents	96 (27.3)
Number of children in class, mean (SD)	20.7 (5.5)
Child's age, mean (SD)	11.0 (4.0)
Child's age at diagnosis, mean (SD)	5.9 (3.4)
Child's gender	
Male	156 (44.3)
Female	196 (55.7)
Father's age, mean (SD)	45.5 (6.8)
Mother's age, mean (SD)	42.5 (5.3)
Father's working status	
Full time	304 (88.4)
Part time	12 (3.5)
Unemployed	18 (5.2)
Retired	10 (2.9)
Father's educational level	
Primary school	6 (1.7)
Middle school	46 (13.2)
High school	94 (27)
College	70 (20.1)
University	90 (25.9)
Postgraduate studies	42 (12.1)
Mother's working status	
Full time	172 (48.6)
Part time	58 (16.4)
Unemployed	120 (33.9)
Retired	4 (1.1)
Mother's educational level	
Primary school	4 (1.1)
Middle school	12 (3.4)
High school	72 (20.3)
College	92 (26)
University	122 (34.5)
Postgraduate studies	52 (14.7)
Parental family status	
Living together	306 (86.9)
Living separately by choice (separated/divorced)	38 (10.8)
Living separately from need (e.g., parent working in another city)	4 (1.1)
Widowed	4 (1.1)
Siblings	264 (74.6)

The mean age of the children was 11 years (SD = 4.0 years), and 55.7% were girls. Mean age at diagnosis was 5.9 years (SD = 3.4 years), and 93.2% of the children attended public school. The average number of students in each class was 20.7 (SD = 5.5).

Information regarding the care of the child's diabetes is presented in Table 2.

About one out of ten (11.0%) children attended extended school, and in most cases, the children were responsible for their own diabetic management. In 34.4% of cases that did not attend extended school, it was due to diabetes. Additionally, 77.1% of children were allowed to check their glucose levels anywhere in the school, and 68.6% were allowed to inject insulin anywhere in the school. Further, 94.4% of children were allowed to use the toilet facilities whenever needed, and 94.9% had snacks that could be consumed during class. Most parents (85.9%) provided their children with medical supplies and snacks for diabetic management at school. In 58.8% of cases, there was a school nurse, and in 21.9%, there was a school nurse's office in school. Moreover, 89.9% of the participants knew how to get in touch with the person taking care of their child's diabetes at school, and 78.1% considered the role of the school nurse very important.

Table 2. Diabetic management in school.

	n (%)
Child attending extended school *	38 (11)
If yes, who manages his/her diabetes?	
Parent	8 (22.2)
Teacher	2 (5.6)
Principal	4 (11.1)
Child	12 (33.3)
School nurse	2 (5.6)
Other	8 (22.4)
If not, reason for not attending extended school has to do with the diabetes	90 (34.4)
Where is your child allowed to measure glucose levels?	
Anywhere in the school	270 (77.1)
In his/her classroom	52 (14.9)
In the nurse's office	42 (12)
Other	32 (9.1)
Where is your child allowed to inject insulin?	
Anywhere in the school	240 (68.6)
In his/her classroom	52 (14.9)
In the nurse's office	50 (14.3)
Other	38 (10.9)
Is your child allowed to use the restroom when needed?	336 (94.4)
Is your child allowed to have a snack during class?	332 (94.9)
Do you provide all medical supplies and snacks for your child's diabetes at school?	
No	16 (4.5)
Yes	304 (85.9)
Usually	34 (9.6)
School nurse in school	208 (58.8)
School nurse office in school	66 (21.9)
The school nurse is in school	
Full-time	164 (79.6)
Part-time	42 (20.4)
Knowledge of designated diabetes caregiver during school hours	248 (89.9)
How important is the presence of a school nurse?	
Not at all	2 (0.6)
A little	4 (1.2)
Moderately	18 (5.3)
A lot	50 (14.8)
Very	264 (78.1)

* Extended school: extracurricular activities and homework after normal school hours.

Furthermore, 44.6% of participants felt that their child was very/extremely safe during a normal school day (Table 3).

The parents' satisfaction with the handling of a low or high glucose incident was significantly higher in cases where their children's school had a nurse's office. Furthermore, the number of absences due to diabetes was significantly lower in cases where their children's school had a nurse's office. Additionally, the child's school performance and most recent HbA1c values were better in the instances where a school nurse was present.

Table 3. Participants' satisfaction with the management of low or high glucose incidents during school hours, the child's school performance in the previous year, the most recent levels of HbA1c and correlation of children's absences due to diabetes with the existence of a school nurse's office.

	School Nurse Office in School		p ‡‡
	No	Yes	
	Median (IQR)	Median (IQR)	
Level of satisfaction with management of incidents during school hours of your child having blood glucose of *less than* 70 mg/dL with symptoms?	3 (2–4)	3 (3–4)	0.011
Level of satisfaction with management of incidents during school hours of your child having glucose of *more than* 250 mg/dL with symptoms?	3 (1–4)	3 (2–4)	0.019
How was the child's school performance in the previous year characterized?	4 (3–5)	5 (4–5)	<0.001
Most recent levels of HbA1c	7 (6.5–7.6)	7 (6.2–7.2)	0.043
School absences during previous year due to diabetes	7 (3–20)	5 (2–7)	0.023

IQR: interquartile range; ‡‡ Mann–Whitney test.

Moreover, 42.4% of participants were very/extremely satisfied with the care provided for their children during a normal school day (Table 4).

Table 4. Association of participants' feeling safe for their child during school hours with information regarding management of their child's diabetes.

	How Safe Do You Think Your Child Is during School Hours?		
	Not at All/ A Little/Moderately	Very/Very Much Extremely	
	n (%)	n (%)	p
Is the school nurse providing most of the care for your child's diabetes during a normal school day?			
No	166 (74.1)	58 (25.9)	<0.001 +
Yes	30 (23.1)	100 (76.9)	
How do you evaluate the school staff's ability to manage your child's diabetes? (median (IQR))			
Teacher	0 (0–1)	1 (0–2.5)	0.009 ‡‡
School nurse	2 (1–4)	4 (4–4)	<0.001 ‡‡
Coach or trainer	0 (0–1)	0 (0–1)	0.985 ‡‡
Principal	0 (0–1)	0 (0–1)	0.878 ‡‡
Other	3 (2–4)	3 (3–4)	0.770 ‡‡
Does your child know how to measure his/her blood glucose without any supervision or help?			
No	24 (44.4)	30 (55.6)	0.087 +
Yes	170 (57)	128 (43)	
Is your child's glucose measured at school?			
No	16 (72.7)	6 (27.3)	0.098 +
Yes	178 (54.6)	148 (45.4)	
Does your child know how to inject insulin without any supervision or help?			
No	40 (40)	60 (60)	<0.001 +
Yes	156 (61.4)	98 (38.6)	
Is the school nurse trained to take care of your child's diabetes?			
No	44 (57.9)	32 (42.1)	
Yes	150 (55.1)	122 (44.9)	0.670 +
Would you allow the school nurse to take care of or help your child with their diabetes, assuming he/she was adequately trained?			
No	40 (66.7)	20 (33.3)	
Yes	154 (53.5)	134 (46.5)	0.061 +

+ Pearson's chi-square test; ‡‡ Mann–Whitney test.

The percentage of parents who felt very/extremely safe with the care provided to their child during a normal school day was significantly lower when their child or the parents themselves provided most of the care, while it was significantly higher when most of the care was provided by a school nurse. In addition, parents who felt very/extremely safe with the care provided to their child during a normal school day rated their teachers' and school nurse's diabetic care skills higher than those who felt not at all/a little/moderately safe. The percentage of parents who felt very/extremely safe with the care provided to their child during a normal school day was significantly lower among those who felt that the principal should be trained in the care and needs of children with diabetes and significantly higher among those who believed that some "other" school employee should be trained. In addition, the percentage of parents who felt very/extremely safe with the care provided to their child during a normal school day was significantly lower among those who preferred that the principal provide care and significantly higher among those who preferred that it be provided by the teacher or some "other" school employee. The percentage of parents who felt very/extremely safe with the care provided to their child during a normal school day was significantly lower when their child knew how to administer insulin without any supervision or assistance.

The age of the child, the parents' perception of the school nurse's level of ability in providing care for the child with diabetes during a normal school day, the existence of a school nurse's office and the father's level of education were found to be independently associated with parents feeling very/extremely safe and very/extremely satisfied with the care provided to their child (Table 5).

Table 5. Multivariate logistic regression results, with feeling very/extremely safe and satisfied with the care provided to their child as dependent variables.

Dependent Variable		OR (95% CI) +	p
Feeling very/extremely safe with the care provided to their child during a normal school day			
Child's age		0.82 (0.73–0.92)	<0.001
School nurse's ability to take care of your child's diabetes during a normal school day		6.36 (3.77–10.73)	<0.001
School nurse office in school	No (reference)		
	Yes	3.64 (1.53–8.67)	0.004
Being very/extremely satisfied with the care provided to your child during a normal school day			
Child's age		0.77 (0.68–0.86)	<0.001
School nurse's ability to take care of your child's diabetes during a normal school day		5.7 (3.39–9.59)	<0.001
School nurse office in school	No (reference)		
	Yes	2.4 (1.03–5.6)	0.044
	Primary/Middle school (reference)		
Father's educational level	High school/College	3.71 (1.01–13.63)	0.048
	University/Postgraduate studies	2.08 (0.57–7.63)	0.271

+ Odds Ratio (95% Confidence Interval).

Specifically, the older the children were, the less likely it was that the parents would feel very/extremely safe and be very/extremely satisfied with the care provided to their child during a normal school day. In the cases where the school had a school nurse's office, the probability that parents would feel very/extremely safe and very/extremely satisfied with the care provided to their child during a normal school day was 3.64 and 2.40 times higher, respectively. The more able they considered the school nurse to care for their child's diabetes during a normal school day, the more likely it was that the parents would feel very/extremely safe and very/extremely satisfied. When the father was a high school or college graduate, the probability that the parents would feel very/extremely satisfied with the care provided to their child during a normal school day was 3.71 times higher compared to when his educational level was primary/middle school.

5. Discussion

The prevalence of T1DM is increasing annually in Europe and in Greece [26,27], creating thousands of new cases each year. Therefore, the proper management of the diabetic child in school poses a challenge for school nurses.

An interesting finding of our study concerns the levels of parental perception of their children's safety and care during the school day. Parents felt safer when the nurse provided most of the care during the school day, compared to the proportion of parents who felt safer when the majority of care was provided by themselves or the child. This is supported by Wilt, who linked the security and satisfaction that parents feel with the school nurse/student ratio. The study showed that parents felt less secure and less satisfied when their children attended schools with higher nurse/student ratios [9].

The literature confirms that the presence of a full-time school nurse is vital for parents [7,28,29], as the school body is considered responsible for the health of each student, especially in primary school [30,31]. Furthermore, teachers also feel safer with the presence of a school nurse according to a study conducted in Greece. Teachers and other health professionals consider the school nurse an important member of the team [32]. School nurses do not only focus on children with diabetes, but on promoting student health in general [33]. The health and well-being of children at school is provided by the school nurse as a member of the healthcare team [34,35]. In the present study, in 58% of cases there was a school nurse to care for the child with diabetes. The results are similar in almost all studies worldwide. In Israel, a school nurse is only available a few days a month [18], or is hired only in a special school group, as is the case in private schools in Ireland [36], while in Brazil, the presence of school nurses is vital because teachers are not required to administer insulin [16]. Similarly in the US, depending on the state, a school nurse is hired, or else non-medical staff are allowed to provide care to the diabetic child [25]. In the state of Alabama, the school nurse is the only staff member authorized by law to administer medication. In general, parents expressed concern about the quality of care in the absence of a school nurse, while many believed that the constant presence of a school nurse would improve student care and reduce their concerns [37]. Contrarily, in another US state, if a school nurse was unavailable, they alternatively suggested the training of non-medical staff, stating that the parents feel just as safe [24]. Recent research, however, has shown that non-medical staff assigned to care for children with diabetes at school are not well trained and also do not feel confident in their ability to manage children with T1DM at school [15].

At the same time, almost half of our study participants were very satisfied with the care their children received during the school day. In two separate studies in the US, the results varied significantly; the highest rate of satisfaction (83.1%) was reported by parents in Skelley et al. [37], while in the Jacquez et al. study, parents found a lack of support from school and expressed concerns about the care their children received for their diabetes [28]. Conversely, an important finding was that in cases where children with diabetes were cared for by a school nurse, the levels of glycosylated hemoglobin were significantly lower. Extensive research has shown that optimal regulation of T1DM can prevent or delay the onset of chronic complications [7]. Researchers have also identified deficits in communication between schools, parents and health care providers and highlighted the necessity of adequate support, especially for adolescents with T1DM [38,39]. It is encouraging that 91% of the children in the study used insulin at school, and the school nurse was described by the majority of parents as "very capable" of delivering insulin to their children. The presence of a school nurse and the implied care enhances the sense of security of children in the school environment and improves their school performance as well as their metabolic regulation [40]. In contrast, in another study, only 34% of parents believed that a mild hypoglycemic episode could be recognized by teachers [38].

Other important findings were that children were allowed to control their blood glucose throughout the school (77.1%) and inject insulin anywhere in school (68.6%), and the majority were allowed to use the toilet facilities whenever needed. It has been shown that school rules usually do not facilitate the self-management of T1DM in school [41], as children are not allowed to control their blood glucose levels or inject insulin in the classroom [28]. Schwartz et al., in their study, report that almost half of children with diabetes experienced at least one incident of interference with diabetes self-care or restricted toilet use at school [29].

Our results also showed that parental satisfaction was higher when the father was a high school or college graduate, compared to when he was a primary/middle school graduate. This may mean that parents with higher academic achievements had better levels of communication with the school nurse and had knowledge of and appreciation for their role. In Wilt's study (2020), parental feelings of safety and satisfaction were higher than in previous studies and were associated with higher parental educational levels, similarly to our study [9].

The importance of the school nurse's role is paramount, as learning and health are interrelated. The average number of absences due to diabetes in this study was 6 days per year; however, the number of absences differs significantly between educational levels. Specifically, in high schools in Greece, where the majority do not have a school nurse, there were more absences. Half of the schoolchildren with chronic health problems were absent from school on a regular basis, and an additional 10% missed more than 25% of the school year [7]. T1DM is associated with low academic achievement due to glucose control difficulties, absenteeism, and lack of concentration [8].

A school nurse's presence is important for monitoring diabetic self-management in older schoolchildren, which ultimately promotes safety in the school environment [42]. Our study also revealed the fact that the older the children were, the less likely the parents were to feel safe and satisfied with the care of their children at school, since in the majority of high schools in Greece, the institution of the school nurse does not exist. In addition, another study found that the older the adolescent, the less compliant they were with diet and glucose control, and the longer the diabetes was established, the worse the metabolic control was [43].

Limitations

A limitation of cross-sectional studies is the inability to make a causal inference; thus, identified associations may be difficult to interpret. Moreover, the parents who participated in the present study were members of associations for T1DM, so they were informed about the role of the school nurse. Parents had to have email accounts or be members of social networking groups related to juvenile diabetes and be active on social media. HbA1c levels were reported by parents and not measured in one laboratory and may have varied.

It would be interesting to explore the perceptions of parents who are not members of associations and whose awareness is not as high. An example of such a population could be parents whose children attend outpatient diabetic clinics in public pediatric hospitals.

6. Conclusions

The sense of safety and satisfaction that parents of schoolchildren with T1DM have regarding the care their children receive in the school environment has been studied internationally in recent years, demonstrating the concern of parents about the diabetic profile of children at school. The presence of school nurses as permanent staff members in every school is considered necessary, as their daily presence helps to significantly reduce the absenteeism of diabetic schoolchildren, significantly increases their school performance and, at the same time, contributes to better regulation of T1DM.

A determining factor for better integration of the child with diabetes into the school environment is to increase the number of school nurses. According to Greek legislation, the recruitment of a school nurse is realized at the request of the parent and only following a medical diagnosis from a public hospital doctor. The school nurse's presence is necessary in all levels of education, since adolescents have significant diabetes management needs that increase due to the psychological burden they experience. National policies need to be reinforced so that schools in Greece will permanently employ school nurses in order to ensure that school is a safe environment for schoolchildren with diabetes, promoting learning and health. In the words of Lina Rogers Struthers 120 years ago: "It is true this must mean an increased expenditure, because only the best trained men and women can do this work properly. But the child's health is the most important resource in the earning capacity of the man."

Further studies in this field of research are recommended in order to generalize and reinforce our results

Author Contributions: Conceptualization, M.D. and P.B.; Methodology, A.M., S.P. and I.K.; Software, T.A., S.P. and I.K.; Validation, P.A. and A.M.; Formal Analysis, S.P. and I.K.; Investigation, M.D. and P.B.; Resources, G.G.; Data Curation, G.F.; Writing—Original Draft Preparation, M.D., T.A., V.A. and P.B; Writing—Review and Editing, A.M., M.M., G.G., A.K. and P.A.; Visualization, A.K.; Supervision, M.D. and G.F.; Project Administration, M.M. and V.A. All authors have read and agreed to the published version of the manuscript.

Funding: This research received no external funding.

Institutional Review Board Statement: The present study was conducted according to the guidelines of the Declaration of Helsinki, and approved by the "Panhellenic Association Fight against Type 1 Diabetes Mellitus" and the University of West Attica.

Informed Consent Statement: Informed consent was obtained from all subjects involved in the study.

Data Availability Statement: The data presented in this study are available on request from the corresponding author. The data are not publicly available due to privacy reasons.

Conflicts of Interest: All authors declare no conflict of interest in this paper.

References

1. Tönnies, T.; Rathmann, W.; Hoyer, A.; Brinks, R.; Kuss, O. Quantifying the underestimation of projected global diabetes prevalence by the International Diabetes Federation (Idf) Diabetes Atlas. *BMJ Open Diab. Res. Care* **2021**, *9*, e002122. [CrossRef] [PubMed]
2. Esposito, S.; Toni, G.; Tascini, G.; Santi, E.; Berioli, M.G.; Principi, N. Environmental factors associated with type 1 diabetes. *Front. Endocrinol.* **2019**, *10*, 592. [CrossRef]
3. Faro, B.; Ingersoll, G.; Fiore, H.; Ippolito, K.S. Improving Students' Diabetes Management Through School-based Diabetes Care. *J. Pediatric Health Care* **2005**, *19*, 301–308. [CrossRef]
4. Lehmkuhl, H.; Nabors, L. Children with diabetes: Satisfaction with school support, illness perceptions and HbA1c levels. *J. Dev. Phys. Disabil.* **2008**, *20*, 101. [CrossRef]
5. Wagner, J.; Heapy, A.; James, A.; Abbott, G. Brief Report: Glycemic Control, Quality of Life, and School Experiences among Students with Diabetes. *J. Pediatric Psychol.* **2006**, *31*, 764–769. [CrossRef] [PubMed]
6. Marks, A.; Wilson, V.; Crisp, J. The Management of Type 1 Diabetes in Primary School: Review of the Literature. *Issues Compr. Pediatric Nurs.* **2013**, *36*, 98–119. [CrossRef] [PubMed]
7. Kise, S.S.; Hopkins, A.; Burke, S. Improving school experiences for adolescents with type 1 diabetes. *J. Sch. Health* **2017**, *87*, 363–375. [CrossRef]
8. Minkkinen, J.; Lindfors, P.; Kinnunen, J.; Finell, E.; Vainikainen, M.-P.; Karvonen, S.; Rimpelä, A. Health as a Predictor of Students' Academic Achievement: A 3-Level Longitudinal Study of Finnish Adolescents. *J. Sch. Health* **2017**, *87*, 902–910. [CrossRef]
9. Wilt, L. The Role of School Nurse Presence in Parent and Student Perceptions of Helpfulness, Safety, and Satisfaction with Type 1 Diabetes Care. *J. Sch. Nurs.* **2020**, *38*, 161–172. [CrossRef]
10. Brand, S.; Felner, R.; Shim, M.; Seitsinger, A.; Dumas, T. Middle school improvement and reform: Development and validation of a school-level assessment of climate, cultural pluralism, and school safety. *J. Educ. Psychol.* **2003**, *95*, 570. [CrossRef]
11. Libbey, H.P. Measuring Student Relationships to School: Attachment, Bonding, Connectedness, and Engagement. *J. Sch. Health* **2004**, *74*, 274–283. [CrossRef] [PubMed]
12. Birndorf, S.; Ryan, S.; Auinger, P.; Aten, M. High self-esteem among adolescents: Longitudinal trends, sex differences, and protective factors. *J. Adolesc. Health* **2005**, *37*, 194–201. [CrossRef] [PubMed]
13. Zhang, X.; Xuan, X.; Chen, F.; Luo, Y.; Wang, Y. The Relationship Among School Safety, School Liking, and Students' Self-Esteem: Based on a Multilevel Mediation Model. *J. School Health* **2016**, *86*, 164–172. [CrossRef] [PubMed]
14. Liberal, E.F.; Aires, R.T.; Aires, M.T.; Osório, A.C.D.A. Safe school. *J. Pediatrics* **2005**, *81*, 155–163. [CrossRef] [PubMed]

15. Wright, A.; Chopak-Foss, J. School Personnel Knowledge and Perceived Skills in Diabetic Emergencies in Georgia Public Schools. *J. Sch. Nurs.* **2018**, *36*, 304–312. [CrossRef] [PubMed]
16. Sparapani, V.D.C.; Liberatore, R.D.; Damião, E.B.; Dantas, I.R.D.O.; de Camargo, R.A.; Nascimento, L.C. Children With Type 1 Diabetes Mellitus: Self-Management Experiences in School. *J. Sch. Health* **2017**, *87*, 623–629. [CrossRef] [PubMed]
17. Wilt, L. The Relationships Among School Nurse to Student Ratios, Self-Efficacy, and Glycemic Control in Adolescents With Type 1 Diabetes. *J. Sch. Nurs.* **2019**, *37*, 230–240. [CrossRef]
18. Lange, K.; Jackson, C.; Deeb, L. Diabetes care in schools—The disturbing facts. *Pediatric Diabetes* **2009**, *10*, 28–36. [CrossRef]
19. Helal, H.; Al Hudaifi, D.; Bajoudah, M.; Almaggrby, G. Role of the school nurse as perceived by school children parents in Jeddah. *Int. J. Innov. Educ. Res.* **2015**, *3*, 101–109. [CrossRef]
20. Doi, L.; Wason, D.; Malden, S.; Jepson, R. Supporting the health and well-being of school-aged children through a school nurse programme: A realist evaluation. *BMC Health Serv. Res.* **2018**, *18*, 664. [CrossRef]
21. Kocoglu, D.; Emiroglu, O.N. The Impact of Comprehensive School Nursing Services on Students' Academic Performance. *J. Caring Sci.* **2017**, *6*, 5–17. [CrossRef] [PubMed]
22. Darnell, T.; Hager, K.; Loprinzi, P.D. The Impact of School Nurses in Kentucky Public High Schools. *J. Sch. Nurs.* **2019**, *35*, 434–441. [CrossRef] [PubMed]
23. Government Gazette B 2038/2018 (30-5-2018). Duties and Responsibilities of the ΠΕ25 Sectors School Nurses and the ΔΕ01 Sector Special Support Staff in the Primary and Secondary Schools in General and Vocational Education. Available online: https://www.newseae.gr/nomothesia/nomothesia-ea/ypourgikes-apofaseis-ea/746-y-a-fek-v-2038-2018-kathikontologio-ton-pe25-sxolikon-nosilefton-kai-evp-sta-sxoleia-genikis-epaggelmatikis-ekpaidefsis-newseae-gr (accessed on 15 April 2022).
24. Driscoll, K.A.; Volkening, L.K.; Haro, H.; Ocean, G.; Wang, Y.; Jackson, C.C.; Clougherty, M.; Hale, D.E.; Klingensmith, G.J.; Laffel, L.; et al. Are children with type 1 diabetes safe at school? Examining parent perceptions: Caregiver perceptions and school safety. *Pediatr Diabetes* **2015**, *16*, 613–620. [CrossRef] [PubMed]
25. Alaqeel, A.A. Are children and adolescents with type 1 diabetes in Saudi Arabia safe at school? *SMJ* **2019**, *40*, 1019–1026. [CrossRef]
26. Patterson, C.C.; Dahlquist, G.G.; Gyürüs, E.; Green, A.; Soltész, G.; the EURODIAB Study Group. Incidence trends for childhood type 1 diabetes in Europe during 1989–2003 and predicted new cases 2005–2020: A multicentre prospective registration study. *Lancet* **2009**, *373*, 2027–2033. [CrossRef]
27. Ferentinou, E. *Compliance with Diet in Children with Diabetes Mellitus. Dissertation*; National and Kapodistrian University of Athens Medical School in Collaboration with TEI of Athens Nursing Department: Zografou, Greece, 2017.
28. Jacquez, F.; Stout, S.; Alvarez-Salvat, R.; Fernandez, M.; Villa, M.; Sanchez, J.; Eidson, M.; Nemery, R.; Delamater, A. Parent Perspectives of Diabetes Management in Schools. *Diabetes Educ.* **2008**, *34*, 996–1003. [CrossRef]
29. Schwartz, F.L.; Denham, S.; Heh, V.; Wapner, A.; Shubrook, J. Experiences of Children and Adolescents with Type 1 Diabetes in School: Survey of Children, Parents, and Schools. *Diabetes Spectr.* **2010**, *23*, 47–55. [CrossRef]
30. Kirchofer, G.; Telljohann, S.K.; Price, J.H.; Dake, J.A.; Ritchie, M. Elementary School Parents'/Guardians' Perceptions of School Health Service Personnel and the Services They Provide. *J. Sch. Health* **2007**, *77*, 607–614. [CrossRef]
31. Mastrogiannis, D.; Deltsidou, A.; Noula, M.; Poulaka, M.A.; Gesouli-Voltyraki, E.; Fouka, G.; Plakas, S.; Mantzorou, M. Exploring educationalists' views on the need for school nurses in secondary schools in Greece. *Br. J. Sch. Nurs.* **2013**, *8*, 303–307. [CrossRef]
32. Boutsoli, P.; Palantza, I.; Adamakidou, T. The Perceptions of Teachers, of School Nurses and Others Professionals who Work in Schools about the Role of the School Nurse. *Interscientific Health Care* **2021**, *13*, 56–59.
33. Särnblad, S.; Åkesson, K.; Fernström, L.; Ilvered, R.; Forsander, G. Improved diabetes management in Swedish schools: Results from two national surveys: Särnblad et al. *Pediatr Diabetes* **2017**, *18*, 463–469. [CrossRef] [PubMed]
34. Mäenpää, T.; Åstedt-Kurki, P. Cooperation between parents and school nurses in primary schools: Parents' perceptions. *Scand. J. Caring Sci.* **2008**, *22*, 86–92. [CrossRef]
35. Mäenpää, T.; Åstedt-Kurki, P. Cooperation between Finnish primary school nurses and pupils' parents. *Int. Nurs. Rev.* **2008**, *55*, 219–226. [CrossRef] [PubMed]
36. McCollum, D.C.; Mason, O.; Codd, M.B.; O'Grady, M.J. Management of type 1 diabetes in primary schools in Ireland: A cross-sectional survey. *Ir. J. Med. Sci.* **2019**, *188*, 835–841. [CrossRef] [PubMed]
37. Skelley, J.P.; Luthin, D.R.; Skelley, J.W.; Kabagambe, E.K.; Ashraf, A.P.; Atchison, J.A. Parental Perspectives of Diabetes Management in Alabama Public Schools. *South. Med. J.* **2013**, *106*, 274–279. [CrossRef] [PubMed]
38. Amillategui, B.; Calle, J.R.; Alvarez, M.A.; Cardiel, M.A.; Barrio, R. Identifying the special needs of children with Type 1 diabetes in the school setting. An overview of parents' perceptions: Original article. *Diabet. Med.* **2007**, *24*, 1073–1079. [CrossRef]
39. Lewis, D.W.; Powers, P.A.; Goodenough, M.F.; Poth, M.A. Inadequacy of In-School Support for Diabetic Children. *Diabetes Technol. Ther.* **2003**, *5*, 45–56. [CrossRef]
40. Stefanowicz, A.; Stefanowicz, J. The role of a school nurse in the care of a child with diabetes mellitus type 1—The perspectives of patients and their parents: Literature review. *Slov. J. Public Health* **2018**, *57*, 166–174. [CrossRef]
41. Hayes-Bohn, R.; Neumark-Sztainer, D.; Mellin, A.; Patterson, J. Adolescent and Parent Assessments of Diabetes Mellitus Management at School. *J. Sch. Health* **2004**, *74*, 166–169. [CrossRef]

42. Pinelli, L.; Zaffani, S.; Cappa, M.; Carboniero, V.; Cerutti, F.; Cherubini, V.; Chiarelli, F.; Colombini, M.; La Loggia, A.; Pisanti, P.; et al. The ALBA Project: An evaluation of needs, management, fears of Italian young patients with type 1 diabetes in a school setting and an evaluation of parents' and teachers' perceptions. *Pediatric Diabetes* **2011**, *12*, 485–493. [CrossRef]
43. Liakopoulou, M.; Kanaka-Gantenbein, C. Type 1 Diabetes mellitus in childhood and adolescence: A "hand in hand" team approach between Paediatric Endocrinologists and Child Psychiatrists. *Ann. Clin. Paediatr.* **2010**, *57*, 424–429. Available online: https://www.iatrikionline.gr/Deltio_57d_2010/3.pdf (accessed on 28 April 2022).

MDPI
St. Alban-Anlage 66
4052 Basel
Switzerland
www.mdpi.com

Healthcare Editorial Office
E-mail: healthcare@mdpi.com
www.mdpi.com/journal/healthcare

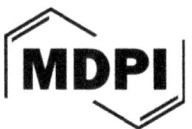

Disclaimer/Publisher's Note: The statements, opinions and data contained in all publications are solely those of the individual author(s) and contributor(s) and not of MDPI and/or the editor(s). MDPI and/or the editor(s) disclaim responsibility for any injury to people or property resulting from any ideas, methods, instructions or products referred to in the content.

www.ingramcontent.com/pod-product-compliance
Lightning Source LLC
LaVergne TN
LVHW070154100526
838202LV00015B/1945